WOMEN'S health WISDOM 2002

Real-Life Solutions from the Editors of *Health* Magazine

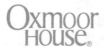
Oxmoor House

Hardcover ISBN: 0-8487-2509-3
Softcover ISBN: 0-8487-2580-8
ISSN: 1537-4394
Printed in the United States of America
Second Printing 2002

The articles in this book were printed in *Health* magazine and prepared in accordance with the highest standards of journalistic accuracy. Unless otherwise noted, these articles have not been updated since their original publication in 2001. Readers are cautioned not to use information from this book as a substitute for professional health care and advice.

To order additional publications,
call 800-633-4910

For more books to enrich your life,
visit oxmoorhouse.com

Cover photo by David Roth

Health
Editor/Vice President: Doug Crichton
Executive Editor: Lisa Delaney
Design Director: Paul Carstensen
Managing Editor: Candace H. Schlosser
Articles Editor: Elena Rover
Senior Editor: Warner McGowin
Beauty and Fashion Editor: Colleen Sullivan
Special Projects Editor: Emily Looney
Associate Editor: Abigail M. Walch
Editorial Coordinator: Christine O'Connell
Assistant Editors: Su Reid, Leah Wyar (Beauty)
Art Director: Amy Heise
Concept Director: Lori Bianchi Nichols
Graphic Designers: Christen Colvert, Soo Yeon Hong
Photo Coordinator: Angie Wilson Kelly
Assistant Photo Coordinator: Jeanne Dozier
Senior Copy Editor: Heather Gibson Cossar
Research Editors: Martha Yielding Scribner,
    Eric Steinmehl
Assistant Copy Editor: Julie R. Hall
Production Manager: Faustina S. Williams
Production Assistant: Julie Fricke
Office Manager: Stephanie Wolford
Editorial Assistants: Emily S. Delzell, Sara Jane Weeks

Health.com Editor: Jerry Gulley II
Health.com Managing Editor: Vanessa Rush

OXMOOR HOUSE, INC.
Editor-in-Chief: Nancy Fitzpatrick Wyatt
Executive Editor: Katherine M. Eakin
Senior Health Editor: Sandy McDowell
Art Director: Cynthia R. Cooper

Editor: Patricia Wilens
Editorial Consultant: Bill Gottlieb
Copy Editor: L. Amanda Owens
Editorial Assistant: Suzanne Powell
Designer: Melissa Jones Clark
Contributing Designer: Amy Bickell
Contributing Indexer: Katharine Wiencke
Publishing Systems Administrator: Rick Tucker
Director, Production and Distribution: Phillip Lee
Books Production Manager: Theresa L. Beste
Associate Production Manager: Larry Hunter
Production Assistant: Faye Porter Bonner

CONTENTS

VII. Stress Management: A Woman's Guide to Energy, Confidence, and Calm

VIII. Relationships and Sex: A Road Map Through the Maze of Love and Family

EDITOR'S NOTE

Reading this book clearly shows you're a woman who makes her health a top priority. Good thing, because this is one priority with powerful payoffs: feeling, looking, and being your absolute best. *Women's Health Wisdom 2002* makes it easy to be healthy.

• Ninety-three percent of readers surveyed said they've taken action because of *Health* magazine. And now, for the first time, we've compiled the best of the best from a year's worth of issues into one information-packed volume.

• This authoritative book is chock-full of real-life solutions and practical advice to inform and inspire you to make the coming year your best ever.

• Eight comprehensive chapters—Breakthroughs in Women's Health, Weight Loss, Fitness, Anti-Aging Secrets, Wellness, Food and Nutrition, Stress Management, and Relationships and Sex—make it easy to find what you're looking for. In addition to discovering Contributing Editor Petra Kolber's head-to-toe BodyWork sections (starting on page 114), you'll learn why—and when—women like you decided to make their health a priority (page 54). And our "The Face of Health" feature shows why beauty is a lot more than just skin-deep (page 144).

• If your days often feel like a high-wire act, you'll find in these pages easy-to-follow ways to bring more balance and grace to your everyday life.

I hope you enjoy this first annual in our *Women's Health Wisdom* series and that it becomes an indispensable companion on your journey to living well and healthfully.

Warm regards,

Doug Crichton
Editor-in-Chief, *Health*

chapter 1

breakthroughs
in women's
health

what you need to know

Want to know the secrets to a long and healthy life?

Start with these
10 MEDICAL BREAKTHROUGHS
that could change (or save!) your life

We asked ace reporters to poll the experts and comb the journals for the medical developments that are most likely to change our lives. Take a look at what they turned up.

A MAP OF ALL OUR GENES

Gregor Mendel would have smiled. Almost a century and a half after the Austrian monk invented the study of genetics with his painstaking experiments on smooth and wrinkled peas, researchers recently reaped a prize harvest: They determined the order of nearly all 3.1 billion units of DNA that make up the human genetic code.

The sequencing of the human genome is the biggest and boldest biological enterprise ever launched, costing about $2 billion and requiring millions of times the computing power used to land Neil Armstrong on the moon. "Without a doubt, this is the most important, most wondrous map ever produced by humankind," William Jefferson Clinton gushed.

In all of history? Well, maybe not, but the former president could be forgiven his exuberance. In an amazing feat of packaging, six feet of DNA is stuffed inside nearly all of the body's 100 trillion cells. That genetic payload carries all the biochemical instructions for making and growing a human being. Minor variations in sequence hugely influence who each of us is and how we will live, age, and die.

So, what's next? Scientists foresee genetic tests to identify those most at risk for cancer and other ailments so that people can gain time to take preventive measures. Medicine makers are already mining the data for clues to new designer drugs. And for those of us who crave a better sense of where we came from, the human genome promises to reveal with unprecedented accuracy our place in the evolutionary tree of life.

Of course, all that won't happen tomorrow. For one thing, the sequencing's not really done. The toughest 3 percent of the genome is still unread, and

Genetic tests may soon be able to identify those most at risk for cancer and other ailments—gaining valuable time for life-saving preventive measures.

a significant chunk needs some serious spell-checking. Even when those tasks are complete, what we'll have is just a long string of code—sort of like *War and Peace* in Greek, with no punctuation. Scientists can't yet tell how many genes are in there, much less how most of them function. And lots more legal work needs to be done to ensure that people won't be at risk of losing jobs or health insurance just because they harbor a molecular glitch. What was true for Mendel remains true today: The genetic future has the potential to be wrinkly or smooth. —*Rick Weiss*

A PROMISING FIX FOR DIABETES

The warning was all too familiar: Charlene Faltermeier had just rung up a bag of groceries at her supermarket when she began to see spots. She had barely enough time to call her supervisor and gulp a few sugar cubes before collapsing on the floor in a convulsion. When she awoke, she had an IV of glucose dripping into her arm and a stretcher waiting outside the store. "The paramedics asked me my name, and I didn't know it," she said. "I didn't know where I lived."

It wasn't Faltermeier's first coma. Like others with Type I diabetes, she lacked crucial clusters of insulin-producing cells, called islets, in her pancreas, which meant her blood sugar often took unpredictable, coma-inducing dives. By the time she received an experimental islet transplant last year, she was injecting insulin four times a day and was still unable to stay on an even keel—racking up $18,000 in ambulance bills alone. But now, eight months after receiving new islets, the active 31-year-old no longer needs insulin injections at all.

The idea behind the procedure is simple: Replace lost cells with healthy ones and then let them churn out insulin. But until 2000, the success rate for such transplants was dismal, hovering at around 8 percent. (In contrast, the survival rate of transplanted kidneys and livers at one year approaches 90 percent.) University of Alberta surgeon James Shapiro turned around the stats on islet cell transplants by creating

a new cocktail of anti-rejection drugs, doubling the number of cells in each transplant, and hurrying them straight from donor pancreas to waiting patient within minutes instead of the typical several hours.

"It worked better than I could have dreamed," he says. With only two or three simple injections, patients get what amounts to a full pancreas transplant—without the complications and expense of surgery.

The next step is a big one: Scientists must now figure out a way to grow islet cells in the lab—enough for about a million Type I diabetes patients waiting in the wings. —*Evelyn Spence*

> With only two or three simple injections, patients get what amounts to a full pancreas transplant—without the complications and expense of surgery.

A NEW REASON TO SKIP REFINED CARBS

If Americans eat less fat than 30 years ago, why are we plumper than ever and much more likely to have heart disease? In a little-noticed study, Harvard researchers turned up at least a partial explanation: Refined carbohydrates may be as bad for the heart as saturated fats—or perhaps even worse.

Boston internist Simin Liu and colleagues at the School of Public Health analyzed the eating habits of 75,000 women over 10 years to track the effects of foods with a high glycemic load, a fancy description for the starchy carbohydrates that send blood sugar soaring. Included are culprits you might expect, such as white bread and white rice, but also surprises, like potatoes and low-fiber cereals. Women whose diets were highest in those foods had an 85 percent greater risk of heart attack than those who ate the least. (No one was shunning carbs: Even the women at the low end were eating the equivalent of about three potatoes or four slices of white bread a day.)

The increased incidence of heart disease was most pronounced among women who were mildly to moderately overweight. "Those women were doing exactly what the dietary guidelines tell them to do," says Liu. "Consume less fat and alcohol and more complex carbohydrates. But they weren't paying attention to the

Research shows that women whose diets are high in starchy carbohydrates have an 85 percent greater risk of heart attack than those who eat less.
The culprits? Favorites like white bread, soda pop, mashed potatoes, and corn flakes.

type of carbohydrate." Their favorites: white bread, soda pop, mashed potatoes, corn flakes, and the like.

Why such starches (primarily those that are highly refined) make trouble for the heart is not yet fully understood. Evidence suggests that easily digested foods that dump torrents of sugar into the bloodstream may reduce levels of good cholesterol, raise triglyceride levels, and interfere with the body's ability to use insulin.

Liu stresses that he isn't indicting all carbohydrates. His research also shows that foods with a low glycemic load—such as whole grain breads and cereals, fruits, vegetables, and legumes—may, if anything, help to keep the heart healthy and the arteries clear. —*Susan Freinkel*

A NEW PRIORITY: PAIN RELIEF

Mary Vargas was waiting to turn left into a flower farm in Connecticut when a distracted driver smashed into her Oldsmobile. From that day forward, pain accompanied the 23-year-old law student day and night. The spasms sometimes racked her neck muscles, joints, and nerves so badly she had to vomit. "I was always someone who felt like I could do anything—and all of a sudden I had so many limits," she says. "There were times I couldn't pick myself up off the floor."

Vargas is finally able to function normally, with the help of a spinal cord stimulator and powerful drugs. Prescription narcotics helped her finish law school, pass the bar in two states, and land her dream job. But it took four years of struggle to get doctors to prescribe anything strong enough to ease her pain.

Vargas's experience is typical. In a 1999 survey, the American Pain Society found that only about one out of four people experiencing pain receives proper care.

Most doctors underprescribe narcotics, experts say, either because they aren't up to speed on what works or because they worry that potent drugs will lead to addiction, despite evidence that most patients don't get hooked. But thanks to new treatment standards enacted in 2000 by the national commission that accredits hospitals, health plans, and long-term care facilities, people like Vargas no longer need to suffer.

The new rules require health facilities to screen all patients for pain, determine its intensity and nature, and treat it effectively on an ongoing basis.

Patients must also be taught to expect relief. Sadly, many patients think that it's normal to suffer, says University of Wisconsin pharmacologist June Dahl. Such stoicism can lead to long-term damage, she says. People in pain not only grow depressed, but also suffer from weakened immune systems, heal more slowly, and have more complications after surgery.

Hospitals are now rushing to change their ways—any that don't could lose their Medicare funding. "The new standards have put pain management on every hospital's radar screen," Dahl says. "It really makes administrators sit up and take notice." —*Sally Lehrman*

In a 1999 survey, the American Pain Society found that only about one out of four people experiencing pain receives proper care. But new standards require health-care providers to offer more effective treatment.

A MYSTERY OF SLEEP UNRAVELED

Everyone thought Emmanuel Mignot was nuts when he gave up a prestigious research post in France in 1988 to move to California and study a weird colony of Doberman pinschers who collapsed into sleep dozens of times a day. Mignot was fascinated by their

Studies show that hypocretin modulates activity of neurotransmitters, which have either an alerting or a sedating effect.

Further research into how it works will bring better treatments—not just for the few who can't stay awake, but also for the many who can't get to sleep.

bizarre condition, known as narcolepsy, which afflicts not just the odd canine, but also 1 in 2,000 humans. He was determined to find its cause, though grants were initially so hard to come by that he all but had to pay for the dogs' food himself.

No one is questioning the value of his research now. Not since teams led by Mignot, who moved on to Stanford University, and Jerome Siegel, of the University of California at Los Angeles, managed to trace the ailment to a previously unknown chemical in the brain. Sleep experts think that the chemical (now known as hypocretin, or orexin), which is missing in narcoleptics, serves in healthy people as a sort of master switch that largely controls whether we're wide awake or lost in dreamland.

"It could be the most significant breakthrough in sleep research since the discovery of the link between dreaming and REM sleep in the 1950s," says Thomas Kilduff, a neurobiologist at SRI International in Menlo Park, California.

Hypocretin's role is still not fully understood, but animal studies show that it modulates the activity of some neurotransmitters (including serotonin and dopamine) that are known to have either an alerting or sedating effect. Further research into how it works is likely to bring better treatments—not just for the unfortunate few who can't stay awake, but also for the many who can't get to sleep. After all, says Mignot, "There are lots of people who'd love to be narcoleptic just for one night." —*Susan Freinkel*

ROBOTS IN THE OPERATING ROOM

Surgeons tend to have big hands, and that used to mean big incisions. Doctors have operated through tiny holes for some surgery for decades, but they're not able to perform the most delicate maneuvers of microsurgery—like cutting blood vessels the size of a pen tip and sewing them with thread as thin as a human hair—without significant trauma to patients. But robots have begun to go where the human hand can't, reducing recovery time in all sorts of surgeries.

"It's like having your hands in a patient's chest without opening it," says cardiac surgeon Randall Wolf of Ohio State University. Instead of cracking the breastbone to get to the heart, the doctor can sneak instruments into half-inch portals, allowing patients to walk away in as few as 10 days instead of six to eight weeks, with a fraction of the pain and the risk of infection.

In July 2000, the FDA approved the use of robotic devices for general abdominal surgery; meanwhile, experimental trials using the gadgets for heart bypass, mitral valve repairs, fallopian tube reconnections, prostate surgeries, and kidney removals are well under way. The philosophy behind each technique is the same: Sitting at a console in the operating room or outside it, the lead surgeon is nearly a medical one-man band. By voice, he directs a camera that displays three-dimensional images of the patient's insides, magnified 10 to 20 times, on a video monitor. He grasps handles, made to mimic conventional surgical instruments, that

Robots have begun to go where the human hand can't, reducing recovery time in all sorts of surgeries. Instead of cracking the breastbone to get to the heart, a doctor can sneak instruments into half-inch portals, allowing patients to walk away in 10 days instead of six to eight weeks, with a fraction of the pain and the risk of infection.

around the corner

Some advances, though not yet ready for prime time, are too exciting to ignore. Here's a sampling of what's ahead.

Now you see it

A new type of contact lens that's designed to be worn overnight improves vision in nearsighted people all the next day. The lens works by temporarily changing the shape of the eye with little or no irritation. It's in the final stage of testing and is expected to go up for Food and Drug Administration (FDA) approval soon.

Smart fillings

Dentists often must replace old fillings because the lumps of metal have wiggled loose, enabling bacteria to creep into crevices and dig even bigger pockets of decay. To the rescue: "smart fillings," compounds that sense when dental decay is under way and release calcium phosphate—a tooth-building mineral found in saliva. If further tests confirm early results, the new fillings could be in use within the next five years.

Easy cancer test

Colon cancer is curable when caught early, yet it remains the third leading cancer killer, largely because the best screening tests—colonoscopy and sigmoidoscopy—are so uninviting, and stool tests, though less invasive, aren't very reliable. An improved screening method is on the way: Unlike other stool tests, which check for blood, the one under study detects genetic markers that are shed by cancerous and precancerous lesions. In one study it detected 91 percent of colorectal cancers and 73 percent of polyps.

No more itch

For millions of Americans plagued by eczema, this year should bring the first good treatment in more than 40 years. The drug Tacrolimus gets into the skin better than existing ointments, to greatly ease eczema's miserable itching, redness, and pain. And unlike topical steroids, Tacrolimus has few side effects.

Blecchhh!

Within the year, smokers may be able to get help kicking the habit with a mouthwash that makes tobacco smoke taste like burnt rubber. Unlike traditional patches and gums, the rinse contains no nicotine, so it's safe for pregnant women and patients with heart disease.

are routed to a computer, which guides pencil-thin arms and flexible metal wrists with precision accuracy. Foot pedals freeze the arms in place. Unlike older, handheld devices—metal sticks that exaggerate the doctor's slightest tremor and pivot like teeter-totters—the latest robotic arms are rock-steady. —*Evelyn Spence*

A MORE DISCERNING CANCER DIAGNOSIS

Two patients, one cancer—a malignancy of the lymph nodes known as large B-cell non-Hodgkin's lymphoma. Bombarded with identical treatments, one patient beats back the cancer, while the other succumbs. Why such different fates?

A powerful new technology has enabled doctors to better differentiate between slow-moving and aggressive malignancies, pointing the way to better diagnoses and more effective treatments—not just for lymphoma, but potentially for all cancers. The tool—a postage-stamp-sized glass or silicon wafer dotted with thousands of snippets of DNA—allows scientists to look deeply into the genetic structure of cancer cells, gaining a far richer portrait than they could ever get by peering through a microscope. Using the so-called gene chip, scientists from six centers across the country recently discovered that large B-cell lymphoma is not one disease but at least two distinct cancers, one much more easily thwarted than the other.

To tease apart the crucial differences, researchers covered a microscope slide with 18,000 tiny droplets of salt water, each containing a different gene known to play a role in the lymph system. They then compared those genes with DNA fragments taken from the tumors of lymphoma patients and treated with a fluorescent dye so that they would light up when they encountered matching genes. Each match indicated a gene that might contribute to lymphoma.

The most exciting news came when the researchers correlated the patterns of genetic matches with the cancer patients' outcomes. Certain clusters of genes, it turned out, were active in cancers that yielded to treatment, while a different assortment lit up in those that stubbornly resisted therapy.

"Once this is confirmed in further research, it will change the way we do business," says Ronald Levy,

New gene technology enables doctors to better differentiate between slow-moving and aggressive malignancies, pointing the way to better diagnoses and more effective treatments.

chief oncologist at Stanford University, who collaborated in the discovery. A patient with the resistant version of lymphoma, for example, will immediately be given experimental treatments, Levy says, instead of wasting precious time on standard therapy.

Eventually, researchers hope to winnow the genes on such chips to just those that determine whether a cancer will be aggressive or mild, drug-resistant or treatable. For now, they're confident that the less refined chips could soon become a routine part of lymphoma diagnosis. And they're already at work on gene chips for melanoma and breast, lung, prostate, colon, brain, and other cancers.—*Susan Freinkel*

A NEW STRATEGY TO BUILD A STRONGER HEART

Move over, stair climbers, and heft a barbell or two. Findings published recently suggest that the most important muscle strengthened by weight lifting is your heart. The power of pumping iron to pull down high levels of bad cholesterol, blood fats, and hypertension was so impressive that the American Heart Association (AHA) has endorsed weight training as crucial to cardiovascular health.

"It's a major turnaround," says Barry Franklin, past president of the American College of Sports Medicine. For years, people associated weight training simply with bodybuilding. Even the more recently recognized health benefits—stronger arms, legs, and bones—have had little to do with cardiovascular spunk. But then a Northern Illinois University

researcher analyzed 11 studies conducted over three decades and found that weight training lowers resting blood pressure independent of any changes in body weight. (It also, of course, reduces body fat and increases lean muscle mass.) George Kelley, now an exercise scientist at the MGH Institute of Health Professions in Boston, found that systolic pressure fell by an average of 2 percent and diastolic by 4 percent after about four weeks. At the same time, participants increased their muscular strength by an average of 34 percent.

"Unfortunately," says Kelley, "only 16 percent of American adults lift weights." The good news: You needn't become a gym rat to get your ticker in shape. The AHA now urges that in addition to the usual aerobic sessions, you simply add several weight-training exercises to your routine. One set of 10 exercises (8 to 15 repetitions each) performed two or three times a week will do wonders for your heart. —*Evelyn Spence*

A COMFORTING WAY TO LOSE WEIGHT

The dismal truth about diets is that they too often fail. For every Duchess of York (Weight Watchers' pitch princess), there are eight or nine commoners who see the pounds creep back as soon as they quit dieting, regardless of the approach they've tried. That consistently sorry record—coupled with rising rates of obesity in America—has led some experts to wonder whether the phrase "permanent weight loss" is as much a marketing oxymoron as "jumbo shrimp."

But this year brought fresh hope for those yearning for an answer. Using a program developed at the University of California in San Francisco, a group of 23 obese men and women were able to keep off an

The most important muscle strengthened by weight lifting is your heart. The power of pumping iron to pull down high levels of bad cholesterol, blood fats, and hypertension is so impressive that the American Heart Association endorses weight training as crucial to cardiovascular health.

average of 17 pounds for a full six years. Equally important, the weight loss continued after the 18-week program ended. That, says Laurel Mellin,

The research supports the idea that some people seek love or comfort in food. The program helps overweight patients recognize those behaviors and offers exercises that teach self-nurturing and limit-setting.

who created the therapy, is a first for a nonsurgical obesity treatment.

The Solution, as Mellin calls her program, is based on the notion that some overweight people seek love or comfort in a bag of chips—just as others look for help in a bottle of booze, a shopping binge, or other excessive behaviors. For example, Hawley Riffenburg, a California software engineer who dropped 45 pounds through Mellin's program, says that in the past when she had trouble dealing with colleagues at work, she might soothe herself with a cookie. The program helped her recognize how those frustrating interactions upset her and offered exercises that teach self-nurturing and limit-setting. Now when communication snafus come up, instead of heading for the kitchen, she says, "I'll find someone else to talk to."

Weight loss, says Mellin, isn't the only positive result. Study participants also began exercising much more, their blood pressure improved, and their depression substantially lifted.

Such results are still preliminary, and most experts agree that Mellin's program doesn't get at the root of every weight problem. Still, "the results are very significant," and not just for people severely overweight, says John Foreyt, an obesity specialist at Baylor College of Medicine. With recent research suggesting that most people's weight swings within a narrow, genetically fixed range, the skills Mellin teaches might help anyone stay at the low end of the range.

Unlike most weight programs, this solution comes cheap. For just $5 a week, people can pursue the program through its Web site, www.weightsolution.com.
—*Susan Freinkel*

FRESH HOPE FOR REWIRING INJURED BRAINS

A stroke at age 59 left James Faust wholly paralyzed on his right side. Rehabilitation helped, but he still needed a cane to walk. His arm hung like rope from his shoulder, so useless he considered having it amputated. After two years, the doctors, echoing the bleak conventional wisdom on stroke recovery, told him he'd never get any better.

Instead, Faust found a new type of intensive rehabilitation therapy that won him back use of both his arm and his leg. Now, says the retired salesman, "I can brush my teeth, comb my hair, shave, drive a car, dress myself—do almost anything I want to."

The simple treatment—which involves restraining the healthy arm or leg for a time to force the impaired one to work harder—defies the long-held belief that rehabilitation can only help in the first few months after a stroke. Developed by researchers at the University of Alabama at Birmingham (UAB), constraint-induced movement therapy won the attention of experts when a study showed that it helped 13 stroke patients who'd been disabled for an average of five years. In each case, the areas of the brain reactivated had long been out of commission.

Once the healthy limb is restrained, patients practice such basic but taxing tasks as sorting beans or picking up pennies. After just two weeks of daily eight-hour sessions, all 13 participants in UAB psychologist Edward Taub's most recent study regained substantial use of an arm. When the researchers used magnetic resonance to map activity in the patients' brains, they found a corresponding change: The brain area devoted to control of the affected arm expanded after the treatment to normal size.

The findings are a revelation, says Edgar Kenton, a neurologist who heads up the American Heart Association's advisory committee on stroke. "We no longer consider the area in the brain where the stroke occurred as totally dead."

Indeed, the study adds to a growing body of evidence that the brain is extraordinarily resilient and capable of growth throughout life. Faust, for one, is thrilled. "This program," he says, "got me back my life." ✳ —*Susan Freinkel*

NEW SURGERY MAY CURE MANY CASES OF BLINDNESS

Imagine seeing the world through a fun-house mirror. Then you'll get an idea of what it's like to have age-related macular degeneration and why a new surgery has experts abuzz.

Some 13 million Americans have AMD. Typically, they find their sight slipping into blurs and blotches. For 1 in 10, the ailment advances into wet AMD, where blood vessels grow like tentacles, then leak fluid—leaving most

victims legally blind within months. In the past, the only option available was to halt the damage.

Now, limited macular translocation can really restore eyesight. Essentially, doctors pinch the eyeball so that the light-sensitive retina can find a path of vision.

The success rate is stunning. After operating on 101 patients, Eugene DeJuan, an ophthalmologist at Johns Hopkins who devised the treatment,

found that half of the patients could read two extra lines on an eye chart after six months. Ten percent of patients tested went from legally blind to 20/40.

Hopkins is one of several eye centers offering the outpatient procedure. But move fast. If treated within three months of diagnosis, 90 percent of DeJuan's patients did well. After a year, however, the success rate fell to about 25 percent.

Chlamydia:
why every woman should be tested

Talk about overlooking the obvious: Chlamydia is the country's most common bacterial sexually transmitted disease, yet it's often not on the list of routine gynecological tests, especially for the young women it affects most. In fact, a recent study found that two out of three primary-care physicians did not screen sexually active teens for the sexually transmitted disease (STD). The often symptomless infection is easily cured with a simple course of antibiotics, but when left untreated, it can cause pelvic inflammatory disease and infertility and can heighten the risk of HIV infection.

Chlamydia infects an estimated 3 million people each year, and women—particularly teens and young adults—are at the most risk. "Chlamydia is an epidemic in this country right now," says Mary Leon, M.D., a gynecologist at New York's Nassau University Medical Center. "It's a very silent and insidious infection."

Yet aging does not guarantee immunity. "As women get older, they typically have one partner, and there might be a decrease in chlamydia. However, that is not necessarily true," says Leon. "Many women believe they are in a monogamous relationship and are absolutely shocked if they find out they are not. If a woman is concerned or even suspicious that she may not be in a monogamous relationship, then she should definitely ask her physician to test her." It's usually a fairly simple swab or urine test.

The U.S. Preventive Services Task Force recommends all women who are sexually active, have multiple sex partners, a history of STDs, or inconsistent use of condoms get tested annually. The best bet: Ask your doctor what you're getting tested for and make sure chlamydia is on the roster.

Why smoking is worse for women than men

Women seem to be particularly vulnerable to the ill effects of cigarette smoke, according to a Norwegian study. Researchers surveyed 65,000 people over the course of two years and found that female smokers reported more episodes of wheezing or breathlessness than did male smokers. The scientists speculate that women's smaller lungs play a vital role. Even if they smoke the same amount of cigarettes as men, women are exposed to higher concentrations of noxious gas.

are you fit to be a MOM?

Even if baby-making's not yet on your mind, staying in shape now—physically and mentally—can make the difference in future fertility.

BY MICHELE BENDER

Sure, most women take excellent care of themselves once they know they've got a baby on the way. But there's a lot you can do to keep your reproductive health in top shape and give yourself the best shot at conception in the months—in some cases, years—before you see that pink line on the pregnancy test.

Infertility—defined as the inability to get pregnant after a year of unprotected intercourse—affects 6.1 million American women and their partners. You don't have to be a statistic, though. "While some women have physical conditions that make it difficult to have a child, in many cases, simple lifestyle changes can have a profound effect on your ability to conceive," says Robert L. Barbieri, M.D., chairman of the department of obstetrics and gynecology at Brigham and Women's Hospital in Boston. With Alice D. Domar, Ph.D., and Kevin R. Loughlin, M.D., he co-authored *6 Steps to Increased Fertility* (Simon & Schuster, 2000) and offers these tips to optimize your chances of conceiving a healthy baby.

In most cases, simple lifestyle changes can have a profound effect on your ability to conceive.

Exercise, but don't overdo.

If there's any time to slack off on your exercise routine, it's when you're trying to get pregnant. Too much exercise can alter hormone levels and decrease (or stop) ovulation, causing infertility. How much is too much? Barbieri recommends that women who are trying to get pregnant work out aerobically no more than seven hours a week. But if you're still having problems after cutting back, stop exercising altogether. Domar, director of the Mind/Body Center for Women's Health at Beth Israel Deaconess Medical Center in Boston, recommends yoga and easy walking (less than two miles) for three months to determine if the physical stress of exercise is a factor in conception.

Relax.

That yoga class may also lower your levels of stress, which can play a part in fertility. Emotional stress produces high levels of prolactin, a hormone that interferes with menstruation. In a recent study conducted by Domar, more than half the women who had difficulty conceiving got pregnant within a year after participating in a stress-reduction program, compared with 20 percent in a control group who did not take part in the program.

Guard against STDs.

Left untreated, common sexually transmitted diseases (STDs), such as chlamydia and gonorrhea, can cause pelvic-inflammatory disease (PID), which can severely scar the Fallopian tubes within days of a woman contracting the disease. Twenty percent of women with PID become infertile. Most STDs are easily treated with antibiotics, but since women who are infected often have no symptoms and are unaware that they need to see a doctor, the best bet is prevention. Practice safe sex, get tested and treated ASAP in the event of a condom catastrophe, and include an STD screening in your annual gynecological checkup.

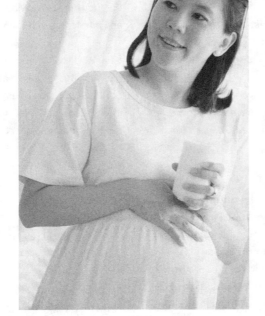

Stay away from cigarettes, even if you're not a smoker yourself.

Most pregnant women and prospective moms-to-be know that smoking is dangerous to the fetus. But recent research shows a clear relationship between cigarette smoke—including frequent exposure to secondhand smoke—and decreased fertility.

In a British study of 15,000 women, researchers demonstrated that those who smoked or were exposed to secondhand smoke took six months to a year longer to conceive than nonsmokers. "We suspect that smoking speeds up the rate at which a woman's supply of eggs is depleted," Barbieri says. Why this happens is unclear. Smoking may decrease the amount of oxygen and nutrients to the ovaries, affecting egg production. Smoking also decreases estrogen levels, another factor in ovulation.

Stay lean—but not too lean.

A low body mass index (BMI), a measure of body composition that strongly correlates to your body-fat percentage, could reduce your chances of conceiving. Women with low body fat may menstruate or ovulate infrequently or not at all. And even if they do ovulate, their hormone levels may not be sufficient to allow the fertilized egg to be implanted in the uterus.

According to the National Heart, Lung, and Blood Institute, a healthy BMI is between 18.5 and 24.9. (Find your BMI by multiplying your weight in pounds by 703, then dividing it by your height in inches squared.) There is a slight reduction in fertility associated with a BMI of below 20 and a significant reduction with a BMI of less than 17. The good news is that this can often be reversed by putting on a few pounds.

Too much body fat is not good for baby-making, either. Your odds of getting pregnant drop significantly with a BMI of more than 30 (the clinical definition of obesity), and there is a slight drop between 28 and 30. According to the American Society for Reproductive Medicine, being overweight can not only affect the hormonal signals to the ovaries but also release insulin levels in women that can cause them to overproduce testosterone and stop releasing eggs. This can usually be reversed by losing weight and getting down to a healthier BMI.

Cut down on alcohol—way down.

Although studies on alcohol consumption and fertility aren't as conclusive as they are for smoking, even a simple glass of wine with dinner may cause problems.

Research shows that women who smoke or are exposed to secondhand smoke take six months to a year longer to conceive than nonsmokers.

it takes two: his side of the infertility solution

The man—not the woman—is the problem in 40 percent of infertile couples. Like women, prospective daddies should ease up on Heinekens and skip the marathon this year. There are other strategies for fertility-boosting that apply to males only.

GO DRUG-FREE. Marijuana has been associated with a decrease in a man's ability to perform sexually and with the development of abnormally shaped sperm.

BUY A NEW BIKE SEAT. Studies have shown that bicycling more than 50 miles a week on a hard, narrow seat can affect blood flow to the penis and cause nerve damage.

Look for doughnut-shaped bike seats that take the pressure off the privates—Serfas and Terry are two popular brands.

LAY OFF THE STEROIDS. Men may think they're getting buff on the inside as well as the outside by using steroids, but they may actually be depressing hormone secretion and interfering with sperm production.

STAY OUT OF EXCESSIVE HEAT. It has been shown that soaking in hot water, such as a steaming hot tub, sauna, or shower, can slow sperm production. Sitting for too long in a hot car seat or wearing tight pants or tight underwear can have the same effect.

According to a 1998 Danish study, fertility decreased in women who had as few as one cocktail a day; the more the women drank, the more trouble they had getting pregnant. Women who had more than 10 drinks a week had about half the odds of conceiving as those women who had fewer than five drinks per week. The women who abstained from drinking altogether had the best chances of conceiving.

Adopt a two-cup maximum.

Caffeine's impact on conception does need more research, but early returns suggest that you may need to curtail your Starbucks habit during baby-making. A European study of more than 3,000 women found that drinking five cups of coffee had a negative effect on fertility. Whether you're trying to conceive or you're already pregnant, most doctors recommend limiting your intake to two cups a day. And if you are pregnant, this is even more important: About four cups or 500 milligrams of caffeine daily is associated with first-trimester miscarriages. Coffee's not the only culprit. Caffeine in tea, soda, and over-the-counter products, such as No-Doz (which has 200 milligrams per tablet), should also be carefully monitored by mothers-to-be. ✳

Michele Bender is a Health *contributing editor.*

GINGER:
the herbal cure for morning sickness?

A group of Thai researchers say they've discovered that 1 gram of baked ginger root, ground and taken in capsule form, reduced nausea and vomiting in pregnant women. The results, published in *Obstetrics and Gynecology*, compared 32 women who took the ginger supplement with 35 women who took a placebo. After four days, the nausea in the ginger group was significantly lower. At a one-week follow-up visit, 88 percent of those treated with the ginger reported ongoing improvement, compared with 29 percent of the control group.

Known as an herbal antidote for morning sickness, ginger's safety during pregnancy is questioned by some experts. Powdered ginger root may adversely affect fetal development. That doesn't mean you have to pass on the gingersnaps, but you should ask your doctor before adding any capsules to your diet.

OVERCOMING INFERTILITY:
don't count on the calendar

If you've ever tried to get pregnant, you've probably done most of your trying about midway between your menstrual periods. Gynecologists routinely advise women that their "fertile window" falls between 10 and 17 days after the start of their last period. But new research suggests that the timing of ovulation varies more than was previously suspected. That, of course, has implications for avoiding pregnancy too. Oops.

Epidemiologist Allen J. Wilcox of the National Institute of Environmental Health Sciences collected about 21,000 urine samples from 221 women during a total of nearly 700 menstrual cycles—a more thorough study than any done previously. Analyzing hormone markers in the samples, he discovered that as many as 70 percent of the women were in their fertile window before or after days 10 and 17.

For instance, nearly 20 percent of women tested were fertile by day 7, while another 5 percent were still in their fertile window at the end of their cycles. Even many women who had regular cycles ovulated outside of days 10 through 17. "If you're relying on the calendar to protect you," Wilcox says, "there's no safe time."

Most women in the study ranged from 25 to 35, but don't think you're off the hook if you're in your 40s. "As women approach menopause, their cycles typically become less regular, making ovulation even less predictable," Wilcox says. "This may explain some of those unexpected pregnancies among older women."

If you really want to get pregnant, fertility specialist Robert Stillman, a spokesperson for the American Society of Reproductive Medicine, suggests that you use a home testing kit that can predict ovulation within a couple of days. (You're most likely to conceive on the day of ovulation and the few days leading up to it.)

And if you really want *not* to get pregnant? No matter how well you think you know your cycle, use birth control—each and every time.

When It Comes to Infertility Testing, Let the Man Go First

Often the woman goes to a gynecology specialist first, but it's more productive and cost-effective to start with the man.

It may not be proper etiquette for a man to go through a door before a woman, but when it comes to fertility problems, that might prove to be the best strategy. About half of all infertility cases involve a problem associated with the male, according to Peter Kolettis, M.D., a urologist at the University of Alabama at Birmingham. "Often the woman goes to a gynecology specialist first, but it's more productive and cost-effective to start with the man," he says.

Many common problems associated with male infertility, such as varicocele (dilated veins that drain the testicle), are actually easily corrected, and the risks of surgical complications are lower. "Correction of the male factor can also spare the woman having to take medications that increase the risk of multiple births," says Kolettis.

Ovulation online—how to track your personal fertility *accurately*

We enlist computers to assist us with everything from anniversary reminders to personal finances. So why not use their mighty math skills and scheduling talents for the most intimate female moment: ovulation? Visit www.my.webmd.com for an interactive ovulation calendar (it's on the "Health-E-Tools" page) that figures your most fertile days and identifies them with budding flowers. On the day your fertility hits its peak, a fat bee nuzzles up to the blossom. That should help get things buzzing.

PILLS for PMS
hope or hype?

Can a pill tame the worst premenstrual symptoms? There's a lot to consider before asking your doctor for a prescription.

BY NANCY ROSS-FLANIGAN

The ads have the feel of a summer garden party on one of those days when sunshine streams down from a sky that's been gloomy too long. Dotted with sunflowers and brightened by beaming faces, they convey the hopeful message that relief from the dark cloud of premenstrual misery—mood swings, bloating, irritability—is as close as your doctor's prescription pad.

Don't dismiss your monthly distress as mere premenstral syndrome (PMS), the ads admonish. You could be suffering from a more serious condition called: premenstrual dysphoric disorder (PMDD). But there's no need to despair; there's a new medicine that can deflate your bloated belly as it boosts your spirits.

Never heard of PMDD? Neither had a lot of other women until those ads came along—making some wonder whether the syndrome was indeed a true diagnosable condition. But PMDD—the severe end of the PMS spectrum, characterized by incapacitating mood and physical symptoms—is all too real for the women who suffer from it. Research on these severe premenstrual problems goes back 15 years or more, and so does the possibility of treating the condition with pills—specifically mood-altering drugs. (More recently, research has focused on

calcium as an answer to premenstrual problems. See "Calcium for PMS?" on page 22.)

Despite the mixed results of early research, there's now strong evidence that newer antidepressants relieve both physical and emotional symptoms in many sufferers. Hence, the new ads: Sarafem, the drug they promote, is fluoxetine hydrochloride, also known as Prozac. In clinical trials, daily doses of fluoxetine have been shown to reduce bloating, breast tenderness, tension, irritability, depression, and mood swings in women with PMDD.

Still, there's a lot to consider before asking your doctor for a prescription. To meet the official criteria for PMDD, a woman must check off at least five or more symptoms from a list of 11 (see box at right), and at least one must involve mood. Symptoms must be most

PMDD, more severe than PMS, can toy with a woman's body and darken her sunny nature. Many see the new drug treatments as a marketing ploy, but some women, now symptom-free, have a different story.

severe during the week before menstruation, improve significantly or disappear within a few days after your period starts, and cause problems at work or school, during social activities, or in relationships with others. While most women in their reproductive years have premenstrual complaints ranging from tender breasts and swollen gums to anger and anxiety, only 3 to 5 percent have symptoms—mainly mood-related—serious enough to make life miserable.

Beverly Palmer (her name has been changed) is one of those women. Before the 38-year-old flight attendant recognized the premenstrual pattern and sought treatment, she suffered for years with extreme tension, irritability, and emotional sensitivity.

"I cried, I yelled, I felt like an overwound spring," says Palmer, who lives in Las Flores, California. Normally a peacemaker, she'd turn sarcastic and pick fights with her husband just before every period. "If he told me the sky was blue, and I saw a cloud, then we had an issue," Palmer recalls. She'd end up sobbing hard enough to hyperventilate, leaving her bewildered mate "looking like he had been sideswiped," she says. But the looks that pained her most were on the faces of her two little girls, sitting sad and silent in the backseat of the car after Palmer exploded at them for taking too long to lace up their shoes.

Psychologist Jean Edicott, Ph.D., director of the Premenstrual Evaluation Unit at Columbia Presbyterian Medical Center, says PMDD has a wide-reaching effect on sufferers. "For women with PMDD, it really impairs their lives. For a week to 10 days of the month, they're having really major problems," she says. The severity of PMDD was confirmed in a study by Eli Lilly and Company researchers on the impact of premenstrual problems;

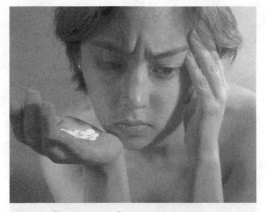

do you have PMDD?

The first step is paying attention to your body. Listed below are the criteria doctors use for diagnosing PMDD. Symptoms should occur during the last week of the luteal phase (the time between ovulation and the onset of your menstrual period) and be resolved within a few days after your period starts. Five or more of the following symptoms must be present and at least one must involve mood:

1. feelings of sadness or hopelessness, possible suicidal thoughts
2. feelings of tension or anxiety
3. mood swings marked by periods of teariness
4. persistent irritability or anger that affects other people
5. disinterest in daily activities and relationships
6. trouble concentrating
7. fatigue or low energy
8. food cravings or bingeing
9. sleep disturbances
10. feeling out of control
11. physical symptoms, such as bloating, breast tenderness, headaches, and joint or muscle pain

it was published in October 2000 in the *Journal of Women's Health & Gender-Based Medicine*. In the survey of 1,022 women between the ages of 18 and 49, a whopping 83 percent reporting PMDD symptoms said they had marital troubles, 78 percent said they had problems in relationships with their children, and 69 percent said their symptoms interfered with their social lives. It seems relationships often suffer more than work performance. While women often say they feel fuzzyheaded, forgetful, and slow just before their periods, researchers have found no evidence of impaired memory, attention, or learning.

PMS, the milder mannered sister of PMDD, is not as clearly delineated. Women with PMS may have any of 100 or more physical and emotional symptoms in the two weeks before their periods. Symptoms vary from woman to woman and even from month to month. With the syndrome so broadly and vaguely defined, it's very hard to say exactly how many women have it—estimates range from 30 to 80 percent. While PMS may interfere somewhat with everyday life, it's not as consistently devastating as PMDD, and it often can be managed through diet and lifestyle changes.

That said, not everyone who slams doors, snaps at her spouse, or suddenly turns tearful in the days leading up to her period has PMS or PMDD. Many women who think they have PMS or PMDD actually have chronic anxiety or depression that gets worse just before their periods, says Endicott. Since there are no medical tests for PMS or PMDD, the only way to know whether symptoms are confined to the premenstrual phase of a woman's cycle—the two weeks or so bounded by ovulation and the first day of menstrual bleeding—is to jot down the severity of symptoms daily for at least a couple of months, rating them on a scale from 1 (not present) to 6 (extreme). "When they do the daily ratings, a lot of women realize that something is going on all month. It gets worse premenstrually, but it's going on all the time," says Endicott.

So just what is at the root of this distress? Many researchers suspect the brain chemical serotonin, though its exact role in PMS and PMDD isn't clear. "If you look at what drives women to see a doctor for premenstrual problems, it's feeling irritable and out of control," says psychiatrist Diana Dell, M.D., of Duke University Medical Center, who has conducted clinical trials of various drug treatments for PMDD. "We have pretty good evidence from animal models that irritability may be a serotonin-deficit symptom."

Furthermore, a number of studies over the past 11 years have shown that antidepressants in the category known as selective serotonin reuptake inhibitors (SSRIs), which include Prozac and Zoloft, relieve a range of premenstrual symptoms—tension, irritability, mood swings, sadness, bloating, and breast tenderness—usually within a month or two after treatment begins. These PMDD-pacifying drugs act by keeping levels of serotonin elevated in the brain; antidepressants that don't affect serotonin levels generally have no effect on PMS or PMDD. And women who take the drugs for their symptoms don't have to take them all month—only in the two weeks before menstruation. They also can get the benefit from lower doses than are used for depression, so the side effects are minimized. SSRIs don't work for everyone—in studies, about 50 to 65 percent of PMDD patients get relief—and researchers aren't really sure why that is.

But for that 50 to 65 percent, symptom improvements translate into happier lives, Yale University School of Medicine psychiatrist Kimberly Yonkers,

calcium for PMS?

Can calcium ease symptoms of PMS and PMDD? Some researchers think so. Susan Thys-Jacobs, M.D., an assistant professor of medicine at Columbia University in New York, is convinced that calcium combats even severe premenstrual symptoms at least as effectively as antidepressants. In a multicenter study of women with moderate to severe premenstrual symptoms, she and her colleagues found that more than half of those who took 1,200 milligrams of calcium a day showed a greater than 50% improvement over a period of three months. Women in the study kept track of 17 symptoms, including mood swings, tension-irritability, anxiety-nervousness, abdominal bloating, cramps, low back pain, and food cravings. All improved.

Based on that study and others, some doctors tell their PMS and PMDD patients to try taking 600 to 1,200 milligrams of calcium daily for a few months before resorting to medication.

M.D., and colleagues have found. They studied 200 women with PMDD whose problems with relationships, family life, and social and leisure activities were similar to those of patients with severe depression. Women who took Zoloft said their productivity improved and they felt more sociable and interested in their hobbies. But the biggest change was in their relationships; 42 percent of women taking the drug reported improvement in that area, compared to 15 percent of those taking an inactive, dummy pill.

Not everyone believes in using SSRIs for PMS and PMDD. When Prozac was introduced by Eli Lilly and Company in 1988, many people raised concerns about overuse of the drug; there was a similar outcry when it came out under the name Sarafem last year. Since Eli Lilly's patent on fluoxetine for depression is being debated in the courts, the timing of Sarafem's appearance has made some people suspicious. Eli Lilly maintains, however, that the development of Sarafem began years before they knew one of Prozac's patents

"I cried, I yelled, I felt like an overwound spring," says one PMDD sufferer who was calm the rest of the month.

would be invalidated. And because the company has a seven-year method-of-use patent on fluoxetine for PMDD, don't expect generic versions of Sarafem to show up any time soon.

Critics also worry that women who take antidepressants for PMDD will be labeled as mentally ill, which they fear could lead to a host of consequences, from workplace discrimination to loss of parental rights. And just like Prozac before it, Sarafem raises serious questions about whether the drug is being used to treat an illness or simply to change normal—albeit unpleasant—personality traits.

If your tension and tearfulness have you making an appointment at your doctor's office, find out if he or she is comfortable treating premenstrual problems. Ask what approach the doctor uses, Yonkers advises. Be wary of a physician who advocates only one type of treatment or who wants to prescribe pills without having you keep a symptom diary. Track your symptoms for two or three months; then discuss them—and all the treatment options—with your doctor. Keep tracking them after starting treatment so you can see if you're getting results.

And buy yourself a bunch of sunflowers. They won't do a thing for your premenstrual problems, but they seem to have a way of making people smile. ☀

Nancy Ross-Flanigan is a contributing editor.

TAMPON SAFETY—IS ORGANIC BETTER?

"We want women to know they have a choice about what they put in their bodies," says LaRhea Pepper, president of Organic Essentials. Sounds like she's talking about vegetables—but no. She's referring to the latest step in the all-natural movement: feminine products.

Pepper claims that about half the women who buy the company's organic, all-cotton tampons say they're allergic to the rayon-cotton blend used in most tampons. "Our other customers are making a lifestyle choice," she says, by staying away from conventionally grown cotton treated with fertilizers and defoliants.

It's true that cotton is one of the most heavily treated crops in the nation, but does it pose a health threat to women? Not according to routine testing of tampons done by the Food and Drug Administration. But there may be another

good reason to go with all-cotton personal-care products, says Philip Tierno Jr., Ph.D., director of clinical microbiology and immunology at the New York University Medical Center, who studies toxicity in tampons. The wood pulp (or viscose rayon) used in major tampon brands may be harmful.

"There is no question that an all-cotton tampon is superior to conventional ones," Tierno says, because viscose rayon enhances the effect of the toxin that's associated with toxic shock syndrome (TSS). One reason major brands use viscose rayon, according to Tierno, is that it's cheap and widely available.

Procter & Gamble, which recently discontinued manufacturing its all-cotton Tampax Naturals, argues that studies have shown cotton and rayon to be equally safe and cautions that using an all-cotton tampon will not protect women

from TSS. Jessica R. Brown, M.D., a gynecologist in New York City, agrees. "Any tampon can cause problems if left in place too long," she says. "But vaginal irritation is more commonly caused by deodorant sprays, soaps, and fragrances."

Organic Essentials' all-cotton tampons don't come cheap. Sold in many health stores, a box of 20 costs $5.99—that's up to $2 more per box than a regular name-brand. Perhaps the high price is the main reason organic tampons account for less than 1 percent of the sales in the $800 million tampon industry in the United States.

Are these natural products worth the price? The jury's still out on that one. But if you're concerned about tampon safety and want to give all-cotton ones a try, you can find an Organic Essentials retailer by calling 800-765-6491.

Once-a-Month Birth Control?

At last, women in the United States have a reliable birth control option that doesn't require attention to daily doses or proper positioning of a device—or that offers convenience only in exchange for troublesome side effects. In October 2000, the Food and Drug Administration broke through a logjam and approved one of the first new birth control alternative in seven years: a once-a-month hormone injection called Lunelle.

Admittedly, we're not talking revolution here. Lunelle simply wraps estrogen and progestin—the same hormones found in oral contraceptives—into a new package. But it offers a welcome end to anxiety-provoking forgotten doses and lops off many annoying side effects of Depo-Provera, the longer acting injectable that's been around for years.

Depo-Provera, which requires a shot every three months, uses a concentrated dose of progestin to convince the body not to ovulate, causing many women to experience spotting. If a woman stays on the method a year or more, ovulation (and menstruation) can take as long as 13 months after the final injection to return. One last little Depo-Provera tip: Because it shuts down the ovaries, long-term use of the contraceptive may weaken a woman's bones. Fortunately, however, one study suggests that this effect is completely reversible once a woman stops using the method.

Lunelle's advantages? Its hormone combo is delivered in smaller doses, meaning fewer bleeding problems, no worry about bone loss, and a quicker return to fertility—usually within four months of the last injection. Women on Lunelle also avoided about a pound of the average five-pound weight gain that comes with the first year of Depo-Provera (hey, 20 percent is 20 percent).

True, a monthly trip to the doctor can be a pain in the neck (or the arm or the rear end), but in some cities it's possible to drop by the drugstore for a shot. And by 2003, Pharmacia expects to introduce a do-it-yourself version of Lunelle that can be injected at home.

on the horizon:
"patch"-work contraception

Women who may forget to take a birth-control pill every day may soon have a new contraceptive option: a medicated patch worn like a Band-Aid. Research shows the weekly Ortho Evra patch, which releases low levels of hormones through the skin and into the bloodstream, is just as effective as a daily oral contraceptive pill in preventing pregnancy. The device is pending Food and Drug Administration approval.

PUT HEAVY PERIODS ON ICE

For women with menorrhagia, a period is more than a nuisance; it's a life-altering force. "A woman who bleeds for more than seven days, or who routinely uses more than 10 pads a day during her period, is usually diagnosed with menorrhagia," says Seth J. Herbst, M.D., a board-certified member of the American College of Obstetrics and Gynecology. "It's a chronic condition that can severely compromise her health and quality of life."

Until recently, for many of the 10 million menorrhagic women, the ultimate treatment was hysterectomy (about 45 percent of U.S. hysterectomies are due to excessive menstrual bleeding). But a recent Food and Drug Administration approval now offers women a less invasive treatment.

Her Option Uterine Cryoblation Therapy System uses freezing temperatures to eliminate the uterine lining, so women experience either light or no periods at all. In this no-incision process, a probe is threaded through the cervix. "The tip of the probe is brought to a very low temperature to freeze and eliminate the uterine lining," Herbst says. The best candidates for the procedure are women whose excessive bleeding is due to benign causes and who don't plan to give birth again (the procedure destroys the endometrial lining necessary for a normal pregnancy). Check with your doctor to see if the procedure is right for you.

VIAGRA FOR WOMEN?

Men may not be the only ones who can pop a pill for improved sex lives.

A Stanford University School of Medicine study suggests that an over-the-counter dietary supplement could turn out to do for women what Viagra has done for men.

Stanford doctors studied 93 women, ranging in age from 22 to 73, who complained of a lack of sexual desire. For one month, half of the women took a placebo, while the other half took Argin-Max—a combination of ginkgo, ginseng, damiana, L-arginine, and 14 vitamins and minerals.

At the end of the month, two-thirds of the ArginMax group reported improved sexual desire and satisfaction, compared with about one-third in the placebo group. The supplement seemed to be especially effective in women nearing menopause, 91 percent of whom noted increased frequency of intercourse. And, happily, the ArginMax group reported no negative side effects.

Doctors don't know just exactly how this supplement works in a woman's body, but they believe that a key ingredient—the essential amino acid L-arginine—raises levels of nitric oxide, which may lead to an increased blood flow that can stimulate sexual arousal.

Before you start popping pills, though, you should know that some doctors still remain skeptical. "It's possible that this supplement may be effective in some women, but this study was too short in length and too small in number to know for sure," says Alan J. Wabrek, M.D., professor of obstetrics and gynecology at Upstate Medical University in Binghamton, New York. The Stanford doctors are planning a larger and longer study in the future.

Catering to women's sexual needs is no small feat. Close to half of all women asked say they experience some form of sexual dysfunction—either low desire, problems reaching orgasm, painful intercourse, or trouble getting aroused.

"Any woman who is experiencing sexual problems should consult her physician," Wabrek says. "Often the problem is physiological, and hormone replacement may help. Sometimes symptoms are really due to an underlying problem in the relationship, and counseling may be the answer. In other cases, a woman may be depressed or very stressed. Those issues need to be addressed first, and often the sexual problems resolve as well."

The final word: The secret to good sex doesn't come in a tablet, but this supplement might just give you the boost you need.

liposuction's secret side-effect: menstrual problems

If you're looking to liposuction as a quick fix for excess fat, here's a word to the wise: Apparently the procedure can make your period appear almost as swiftly as it makes your saddlebags disappear.

Dermatologists Min-Wei Christine Lee and Richard Glogau, then at the University of California at San Francisco, checked up on four women who'd had the surgery. They learned through interviews that prior to the procedure, all had had regular, 28-day menstrual cycles. After it, their periods were irregular. The researchers think that estrogen—or, rather, its absence—is to blame.

Makes sense, because the link between the hormone and fat has been well-documented. While the ovaries are the primary estrogen factory, fat cells also produce and store it. When fat is removed, estrogen goes with it. The good news is that a little dip in circulating estrogen isn't harmful—it's what triggers your period every 28 days. Or sooner than that: Lee thinks that the abrupt drop in estrogen caused by liposuction tricks the uterus into prematurely shedding its lining.

Of Lee's patients, only about 1 in 20 reports an unexpected period. The effect is temporary, since the ovaries boost estrogen production to fill the gap. Lee's patients all saw their cycles normalize within two months.

Because even a brief estrogen upset may render hormonal birth control methods like the Pill less effective, Lee advises using a backup method for two months after the procedure.

Cancer Alert:
If you took the Pill before 1975, *you must read this!*

Researchers at the Mayo Clinic have found that the risk of developing breast cancer is three times higher for women who took the Pill before 1975 and have a mother or sister with the disease than for women with the same family history who chose a different method of contraception.

Why? Because early formulations of the Pill packed triple the estrogen punch of today's version—and high doses of estrogen are what's thought to raise breast cancer risk. The study found that even short-term use of the pre-1975 Pill can raise your risk.

If you took the Pill in those days, get mammograms regularly and talk to your doctor about a new procedure called ductal lavage (for more information, see "Ductal Lavage: The New Test That Detects Breast Cancer Sooner," page 43).

As for today's Pill, it's too early to tell if it also raises your risk, but the going theory is that its estrogen level is low enough that it can be considered safe—at least for those people who aren't already at high risk of breast cancer.

why women have more stamina than men

Men may grow bigger muscles, but women's muscles have more stamina. A recent study compared the length of time men and women could hold a muscle contraction. The researchers found that the women lasted 75 percent longer. The explanation may be in the hormones: Estrogen seems to promote blood flow, and the more blood you can deliver to the muscles, the longer they work.

Genital herpes: new vaccine offers permanent relief

If you're sexually active and herpes-free, this statistic will scare you: One in five Americans has genital herpes. That's 50 million people with a contagious disease that you don't want to contract. But a recent meeting of the American Society of Microbiology brought encouraging news about a possible vaccine. Encouraging, at least, for those who have never had a cold sore.

At the meeting, Spotswood Spruance, an internist specializing in infectious diseases, presented the results of two studies of the vaccine conducted on 1,350 couples in which just one partner had genital herpes. The vaccine cut the risk of infection by 75 percent in women who had never had cold sores. Those are caused by the herpes simplex I virus (HSV-I); genital herpes is caused by the closely related herpes simplex 2.

That's not perfect protection by any means, but it's a whole lot better than nothing. However, the vaccine proved worthless for women who carried the cold sore virus. The researchers speculate that HSV-I may prime the immune system to recognize and combat the genital herpes virus and that the vaccine can't add much to this protection. The vaccine also failed to protect men, which makes it the first vaccine to work in one sex but not in the other.

Let's face it: Most women don't make it to maturity without herpes—either the dreaded genital sort or the irritating oral variety. So if the vaccine survives further testing, it may be of more use to your daughter than it is to you. Vaccinating young women at their first visit to a gynecologist could eventually cut the number of herpes cases by 30 percent, says Spruance, of the University of Utah. And that could indirectly protect men and women with cold sores too.

"Anything we can do to slow this epidemic is an advantage," says Hilary E. Baldwin, a dermatologic surgeon at the State University of New York in Brooklyn and an expert in sexually transmitted diseases. "And this is the best thing we've got so far."

RU-486: the facts, the lies, the surprises

American women have a new option for ending an unwanted pregnancy: the abortion drug mifepristone, better known as RU-486. When the Food and Drug Administration (FDA) approved the drug in 2000, pro-choice forces hailed the event as a "historic moment comparable to the arrival of the birth control pill." There's no doubt RU-486 will alter the landscape of abortion. But will it be as revolutionary—or as popular—as the Pill?

Part of its appeal is that it promises to take a profoundly personal decision out of the public spotlight. A woman who chooses an RU-486 abortion can pursue it in the privacy of her doctor's office and the quiet of her home. Pro-choice advocates also hope the drug's availability will increase the proportion of early abortions, which are safer, simpler, and less controversial than those done later. Mifepristone is approved for use in the first seven weeks, whereas most surgical abortions are performed between the eighth and twelfth weeks.

Still, using this seemingly simple "abortion pill" is more complicated than it sounds. The FDA-approved protocol requires three trips to the doctor: first to get the mifepristone, which blocks a hormone essential for pregnancy; then again three days later to take another pill, misoprostol, which causes the uterus to contract. The final checkup happens two weeks after that, to make sure the abortion is complete. (In practice, the regimen may be looser, but it's still no cakewalk.) The process is similar to a miscarriage, with many women reporting pain, cramping, nausea, and fatigue over the course of several days. And there are some risks: In American studies, 5 percent of the women experienced heavy bleeding, and a small proportion of this group had to have blood transfusions. About 5 percent needed a surgical procedure to complete the abortion.

It's also not clear how many doctors will be willing to dispense the drug. While abortion clinics will certainly offer it, many small-town physicians may be reluctant to become identified as abortion providers for fear of drawing pickets or worse. What's more, antiabortion activists have threatened federal legislation that would limit distribution of the drug to a certified cadre of physicians.

Still, in a recent survey, 44 percent of gynecologists and 31 percent of family physicians polled said they would be likely to offer the option, and mifepristone's backers are optimistic that many more will eventually sign on. In France, where RU-486 has been available for over 10 years, as many as one-fourth of abortions are now induced by the drug.

Coming soon: "smart" panty liners that will monitor your hormones

They've already got wings. What more could you ask from a panty liner? Plenty, according to Procter & Gamble. The maker of Always recently secured international patents for "smart" pads, which can alert you when your period is about to start (if you haven't figured that out yet) or if you're pregnant.

P&G's inventors have laced the pads with special sensors, including a wood resin that turns blue upon reacting with traces of blood in vaginal discharge. A second chemical turns red when acidity levels change. With both sensors tripped, the liner becomes purple, signaling impending menstruation. Hormone detectors can pick up changes that occur with pregnancy or just before ovulation. Other "biosensors" can spot a yeast infection or sexually transmitted diseases (STDs), including HIV—problems a panty shield might announce by glowing in the dark or emitting heat. Wow.

It's unclear when, or even if, these high-tech liners will hit the shelves, but they certainly have a weird logic: You can wear a pad that tells when you're going to menstruate, so that you'll, uh, be sure to be wearing a pad when the bleeding starts. Meanwhile, discovering you're pregnant or have an STD is, to be sure, crucial information. But who wants to get it from her skivvies? Some things you just shouldn't learn during a bathroom break.

cholesterol
why you need to be tested

Even if you're female and fit, heart disease could still be in your future. New research suggests you ought to be worried about your cholesterol. Here's why—and how—you should be tested.

BY DIANNE HALES

Lynne Naeve, a third-grade teacher in Glendale, California, was furious. For years she'd been jogging almost daily—she was a competitive runner, an aerobic dancer, a triathlete, for heaven's sake. Along with her husband, she'd been following the rigorously low-fat Pritikin diet, avoiding red meat and eating lots of fruits and vegetables. So when her doctor suggested baseline cholesterol testing 10 years ago, Naeve—then 39 and a size 2—scoffed. Until she saw the results. "I was shocked to find I had high cholesterol," says Naeve, whose peak level was an alarming 280 milligrams per deciliter of blood. "Even though my father had high cholesterol, I'd considered myself safe because I'm a woman. And I was mad because I'd been doing everything right."

Like Naeve, many women assume that being female and fit means they don't have to worry about heart disease; their biggest fear is cancer, particularly breast cancer. But heart attacks kill more women than breast cancer, stroke, and lung cancer combined. Given this grim reality, the best hope for the female heart lies in prevention. "In the last decade, we've had conclusive proof that when you lower cholesterol in women, the benefit is similar to that seen in men," says James Cleeman, director of the National Cholesterol Education Program of the National Heart, Lung, and Blood Institute (NHLBI). Yet at every age, women with high cholesterol are underdiagnosed, undertreated, and underinformed.

We've updated the facts in this article based on new guidelines from the National Cholesterol Education Program (NCEP), issued in May 2001. These guidelines are the ones that tell doctors when their patients ought to be getting tested and what numbers should set off alarm bells. Last updated in 1993, the old guidelines were due for a change. The new recommendations could provide a wake-up call to women who assume they're immune to heart problems.

Heart attacks kill more women than stroke, lung cancer, and breast cancer combined. There is conclusive proof that when you lower cholesterol levels in women, the benefit is similar to that seen in men. Yet women with high cholesterol are underdiagnosed and undertreated.

Much of the focus is on HDL, the good cholesterol. According to the new standard, a level below 40 mg/dL means trouble for both men and women. But, says Rose Marie Robertson, president of the American Heart Association (AHA), that may miss the mark. "We've learned that what's normal for a male may spell trouble for a female. We don't know why, but women seem to need more high-density lipoprotein, or HDL, than men do. Women with HDL under 45 mg/dL are at greater risk of heart disease, while men don't seem to be at risk unless their HDL dips below 35 mg/dL."

Some research also suggests that triglycerides, another type of blood fat, pose a particular hazard for a woman's heart. These are essentially little packets of fat that cells use for energy. They're crucial to health; in fact, if you don't get enough in your food, your liver will manufacture its own. But in excess, triglycerides can damage artery walls. When high triglycerides combine with low levels of protective HDL cholesterol, women's arteries seem to be especially vulnerable.

"Triglycerides are a greater risk factor in women than they are in men, even at lower levels," says Francine Welty, director of preventive cardiology and nutrition education at Harvard Medical School. The 2001 NCEP guidelines define a normal triglyceride level as 150 mg/dL or below. Both the American College of Cardiology and the AHA have also gone on record as saying that women have reason to worry if the blood fat goes above 150 mg/dL.

Rhonda Whitley, a 49-year-old Dallas nurse, is one woman who's begun paying attention to her triglycerides; last May, her levels jumped to 202 mg/dL, up from 150. The same tests showed that she had a very low HDL reading, just 18 mg/dL.

Whitley had reached menopause, a stage of life that often triggers ominous changes in blood fats: Good cholesterol starts to fall. Triglyceride levels rise. So do total cholesterol and bad (LDL) cholesterol—in fact, average levels in women actually pass those of men of the same age. The risk of a heart attack or other

major cardiovascular problem doubles. "Heart disease develops about a decade later in life in women than in men," says cardiologist Valentin Fuster, of Mount Sinai School of Medicine in New York City. "But once it begins, it gallops."

In the past, Whitley might simply have been put on hormone replacement therapy (HRT), long the treatment of choice for menopausal women with cholesterol trouble. After all, estrogen supplements are known to boost good cholesterol and quash levels of bad cholesterol.

Unfortunately, it now seems that one thing they may not do is protect against heart disease. In two landmark studies in the past few years, estrogen replacement failed to improve the cardiovascular health of women already diagnosed with heart disease. And in healthy women, HRT may harm more than help, at least initially. In the first two years of a massive research project called the Women's Health Initiative, women who started hormone replacement had a slightly raised risk of heart attack, stroke, or blood clots. "Everyone's gone back to the drawing board to try to understand why," says cardiologist Robert Rosenthal of HeartPlace in Dallas.

If not estrogen therapy, then what? Exercise, a healthy diet, and weight loss all move blood fats in the right direction, but they nudge rather than shove. "Lifestyle changes are great—they're a crucial part of treatment—but they generally don't lower cholesterol by more than 10 to 15 percent," says Nanette Wenger, a cardiologist at Emory University in Atlanta. "Most people with very high cholesterol or triglycerides will need medication."

As it happens, there couldn't have been a better time for estrogen to fall from favor, because there's an understudy in the wings just waiting to emerge as a star. The group of drugs called statins has revolutionized heart disease prevention by blocking cholesterol production in the liver, with few side effects. The drugs—Lipitor, Mevacor, Pravachol, and Zocor among them—cut bad cholesterol by 18 to 55 percent,

> Menopause often triggers ominous changes: Good cholesterol starts to fall, bad cholesterol and triglyceride levels rise. The risk of heart attack or other major cardiovascular problem doubles.

increased good cholesterol by 5 to 15 percent, and decreased triglycerides by 7 to 30 percent.

More important, they clearly save women's lives. In one study of postmenopausal women who'd already had a heart attack, those who took a statin for five years reduced their risk of heart attack and death by 43 percent. The drugs are effective at prevention, as well. The Air Force/Texas Coronary Atherosclerosis Prevention Study, which included 997 postmenopausal women—healthy, but with low good cholesterol—found that women who took the drugs for five years slashed their risk of chest pain, heart attacks, and sudden cardiac death by 46 percent.

And here's a well-kept secret: Those results look to be better than what men can expect from the drugs. In the Air Force study, statins cut men's risk by only 37 percent; a few other studies have also suggested a greater benefit for women. Yet research has found that doctors can be slow to put women on statins and that when they do, the dose is often too low to get cholesterol down.

"Just starting patients on statins isn't enough," Wenger says. What's needed, she says, is careful monitoring to make sure the dosage brings levels down.

Part of that monitoring involves periodic tests of liver function, because in rare cases, the drugs can harm the liver. On the whole, though, statins have proven to be quite safe. And if recent research 38findings are borne out, doctors will likely become more comfortable—heck, positively giddy—about prescribing statins for women. Last year, three studies appeared within one week indicating the drugs raise bone density and reduce fracture risk. Researchers suspect statins increase the rate of bone formation, while other osteoporosis drugs slow the bone destruction that is part of the normal "remodeling" of the skeleton. Such an effect would be a substantial bonus if it's supported by follow-up research.

Lynne Naeve started on cholesterol treatment in 1991, before many of the really impressive studies on statins were published. And initially, getting her numbers down proved a challenge. The first medication she tried was nicotinic acid (niacin), a B vitamin that's long been a staple of cholesterol treatment. Unfortunately, it triggered flushing and a rash. (Newer preparations, available by prescription, have eliminated these side effects.) As statins became available, Naeve's doctors prescribed several types before one brought her numbers in line. "On statins, I haven't had any side effects or problems," Naeve says. "I don't think of myself as high risk anymore."

the tests every woman should have

To lower your chances of heart disease, experts at the National Cholesterol Education Program advise getting a fasting lipoprotein profile at least once every five years. That means that you need to stop eating for 12 hours before the test, and the results you get include values for total cholesterol, LDL cholesterol, HDL cholesterol, and triglycerides. If a nonfasting test is done, only the values for total cholesterol and HDL will be usable. Here's what the numbers mean for healthy people, according to the most recent (May 2001) updates from the NCEP.

Total Cholesterol

LESS THAN 200 mg/dL *Desirable*
200 to 239 mg/dL *Borderline High*
240 mg/dL or ABOVE *High*

HDL Cholesterol

BELOW 40 mg/dL *Increases your risk for heart disease*
ABOVE 60 mg/dL *Lowers your risk for heart disease*

LDL Cholesterol

LESS THAN 100 mg/dL* *Optimal*
100 to 129 mg/dL *Near Optimal / Above Optimal*
130 to 159 mg/dL *Borderline High*
160 to 189 mg/dL *High*
190 mg/dL and ABOVE *Very High*

Triglycerides

BELOW 150 mg/dL *Normal*
150 to 199 mg/dL *Borderline High*
200 to 499 mg/dL *High*
500 mg/dL and ABOVE *Very High*

If you have heart problems, diabetes, high blood pressure, or a family history of heart disease, or if you are a smoker, then you should talk with your doctor about your LDL goals.

hidden risks: tests you may want to discuss with your doctor

HERE'S A CONUNDRUM: While experts agree that cholesterol is a crucial heart disease risk factor, many people who suffer chest pain or even heart attacks have levels that are perfectly normal.

This puzzle has prompted researchers to scour the body in search of other cardiovascular villains. In the past few years, studies have turned up new factors to consider: high levels of the amino acid homocysteine, for instance, or of a substance called C-reactive protein. What's more, you can now get tested for these troublemakers.

However, there have been no studies as yet showing that reducing your levels of homocysteine or any other novel risk factor will cut your chances of developing heart disease. Because of the uncertainty, many insurers won't cover the tests. But researchers say there's good reason to believe that high levels of such factors signal increased danger. And lowering them seems to be safe. If you're at high risk—because of, say, a strong family history of heart disease—ask your doctor if testing for these factors could give you a clearer picture of your vulnerability.

C-REACTIVE PROTEIN (CRP). This substance is a marker of inflammation in blood vessels, which may make plaque more likely to break off and clot. In a recent, attention-getting study, women with the highest levels had more than four times the heart attack and stroke risk of those with the lowest. Eating a low-fat diet, exercising, losing weight, and giving up smoking all lower CRP, as do taking aspirin and statins.

HOMOCYSTEINE. A few years back, this amino acid looked like the smoking gun in many cases of heart disease. In a study of 28,000 postmenopausal women, those with the highest levels had twice the coronary risk of those whose levels were lowest. Other potential culprits, particularly CRP, have since emerged as clearer danger signs, but high homocysteine shouldn't be ignored. It's simple to lower it with a diet rich in fruits, vegetables, whole grains, and fish, plus supplements of folate and vitamins B-6 and B-12.

LIPOPROTEIN(A). High levels of this hybrid creature—a molecule of LDL cholesterol hooked to a large protein—can triple the risk of heart attack and stroke. Lp(a) levels are not easily lowered, though taking the B vitamin niacin can help somewhat. If a test shows a worrisome amount, cutting LDL levels becomes crucial: Bad cholesterol multiplies the danger posed by Lp(a).

PARTICLE SIZE. The size of cholesterol particles can also affect risk. For instance, a mix of small HDL or LDL and large very low-density lipoprotein (VLDL) significantly increases the likelihood of disease. Diet, weight loss, and niacin pills can all improve particle size.

Her comfort no longer comes from an unfounded faith that her gender will protect her from a disease that kills half of all American women; instead, it comes from information and judicious action. "Every woman should know her numbers: total cholesterol, HDL, LDL, and triglycerides," says AHA president Robertson. "It's your responsibility to go to your doctor and get this information. Then make sure your levels are as close to perfect as you can get them." ✳

Dianne Hales is a writer in the San Francisco Bay Area and coauthor of The Mind–Mood Pill Book *(Bantam, 2000).*

DELICIOUS NEWS
Dark chocolate lowers cholesterol!
It's still laden with calories and fat. But the good news is that dark chocolate contains antioxidants that clear bad cholesterol.

how your emotions can be hurting your health

New research suggests that negative emotions—anger, depression, and anxiety—can damage your heart and even trigger a heart attack. There are ways to help protect yourself and be both healthier and happier.

BY INGFEI CHEN

When Angela Jackson had a heart attack three years ago, doctors no doubt blamed it on her high blood pressure and cholesterol levels. But if you ask the shy African-American divorcée, she offers a different explanation. At age 53, the St. Louis schoolteacher (whose name we've changed for this story) has known a lifetime of turmoil—from grief over her father's death when she was 10, to the stress of single-handedly raising a daughter with manic depression. Over the years, she grappled with bouts of depression. "I felt hopeless for a long time," recalls Jackson, a tall woman who keeps her hair neatly tied back with a bow.

In 1996, when her ailing mother died from a heart attack, Jackson spiraled into a mind-numbing gloom. Getting out of bed was a struggle; at school, her focus and patience deteriorated. Engulfed by dark feelings for so long, she feels it was no coincidence she wound up in the emergency room. Something had to give, and that something was her heart.

But is Jackson right? Can depression and anxiety really stir up an assault on the heart? Such a notion is gaining more credence. Traditional risk factors, such as high blood pressure, smoking, and obesity, explain only about 40 percent of heart-disease cases. Psychologists have long viewed a fiery temper as hazardous to the ticker, but lately they've been spreading the blame around: Anyone carrying too much negative emotional baggage—be it anger, sadness, or twitchy apprehension—is in danger, researchers now say.

"The news in the last five years or so," says Karina Davidson, Ph.D., a clinical psychologist at New York's Mount Sinai Medical Center, "is that depression and anxiety seem to put you at a much bigger risk of first

A fiery temper has long been seen as hazardous to your heart. But now psychologists are spreading the blame—too much of almost any negative emotion can be a danger.

developing heart disease, and then of having it worsen." Thomas Pickering, M.D., Ph.D., a heart-disease and hypertension specialist at Mount Sinai's Wiener Cardiovascular Institute, puts it more strongly: "Depression," he says, "is probably as important as blood pressure and physical inactivity as a risk factor for developing heart disease."

What's more, researchers are testing the idea people who learn to tame their emotional torment—by making simple changes in the way they think and behave—can ward off coronary problems, the number-one killer of women and men in the United States. Even for patients like Jackson, it may not be too late to prevent further cardiac trouble.

But wait a minute. Haven't we been down this path, into the jungle of human nature, before? Just 25 years ago, enthralled researchers declared the so-called Type A personality—think aggressive, white male executive—a risk factor for heart attack. Then the idea took an embarrassing nosedive: Better-designed studies failed to confirm the link.

Out of the wreckage, however, red-faced scientists found something still standing. Two aspects of Type A behavior—anger and hostility—looked toxic to the heart. Since then, research evidence has piled up supporting the theory that a short fuse leads to cardiovascular problems. (One recent study of 8,474 men and women with normal blood pressure found that a tendency to fly off the handle almost tripled the odds of a heart attack.)

How? Intense anger kicks the body's nervous system into fight-or-flight mode. It uncorks stress hormones that goad the heart into frenzied thumping. Some blood vessels dilate to ensure muscles get the nutrients they need, while others, such as those in the gut, constrict, driving blood pressure skyward. Platelets get sticky—ready to clot and stop the bleeding from any injury you might sustain. That's fine if you're faced with a band of thugs and have to run for your life. But if the system gets tripped every time you're stuck in traffic, for instance, look out. Over time, blood-vessel walls get battered and artery-narrowing plaques build up, until a wayward clot hits a bottleneck, and—bam!—you're having a heart attack.

> Depression is probably as important as blood pressure and physical inactivity as a risk factor for developing heart disease.

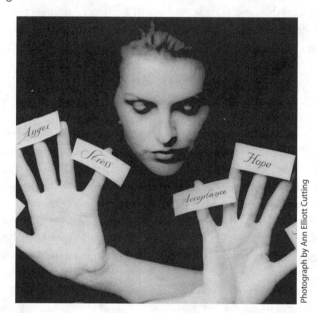

Photograph by Ann Elliott Cutting

Constant crankiness isn't the only emotional trigger scientists worry about, though. In the late '80s, other studies found clues linking depression and anxiety with heart disease. Since then, while the evidence isn't airtight, investigators have built a strong case that negative emotions directly affect heart health. Some of that evidence comes from St. Louis, where Angela Jackson was recovering from her heart attack.

Jackson was seriously depressed and withdrawn. She often found herself weepy over missing her mother. She was also very lonely. Painfully shy and convinced that no one could like her, she'd always kept to herself, holing up in her small apartment where she didn't even have a phone. At school, the teacher always ate lunch alone.

Jackson participated in one-on-one sessions with licensed clinical social worker Iris Csik. Then she went to weekly group counseling sessions at the Washington University School of Medicine. Slowly she came out of her shell. Csik asked her to try small experiments: sitting with other teachers at lunchtime, making eye contact, and saying "good morning" to folks in the hall. Jackson found these "homework" exercises terrifying, but to her shock, colleagues were welcoming and friendly.

Jackson also learned that when she was feeling bad, she needed to get busy. If she found herself misty-eyed over her mom, she tried to quit dwelling on the past and focus on present plans, such as going shopping with a friend from work. To ease stress, she began using relaxation techniques—and still does. "I close my eyes, take deep breaths, and start counting until I calm down. And I pray a lot," she says.

The treatment was aimed at easing more than just her angst—it was for her heart too. Jackson was part of a major clinical trial called ENRICHD (Enhancing Recovery in Coronary Heart Disease), the first large-scale test of whether reducing emotional distress can fight heart disease. At Washington University and seven other medical centers around the country, investigators tracked over 2,400 heart-attack victims who were clinically depressed or had few people for emotional support. All were under a physician's care, and the patients with the most serious depression were given antidepressants. Half the group, including Jackson, received up to six months of psychotherapy to treat their sadness and work on their social skills. The goal was to see if such counseling could lower their very high odds of dying from a second heart attack.

The rationale behind the trial was compelling. Over the past decade, research has found that in people like Jackson, who already have cardiovascular problems, depression boosts the risk of heart attack or sudden cardiac death, according to Robert Carney, Ph.D., study investigator and Washington University psychologist. About 40 percent of all heart patients suffer with the mood disorder. One sobering report concluded that in those who've had a heart attack, depression more than quadruples their chances of dying within six months.

But which comes first, the blues or heart problems? In the last five years, many newer studies have argued that chronic sadness can lead to heart disease or stroke. In one major study last year from the Centers for Disease Control and Prevention, 30-year-olds

how to soothe your inner crank

Anger can be awfully important to your defense system. How you handle it is the tricky part. Men tend to explode in rage; women typically fume in silence. Neither response is healthy, but fortunately there's a third way: "People who are really at ease with their anger can be gracious and polite—but they do not allow themselves to be trampled on," says Karina Davidson, Ph.D., a psychologist at New York's Mount Sinai Medical Center.

Constructive approaches like that might protect your heart. In a study of 22 male heart-attack survivors, Davidson and colleagues found that after eight weeks of group anger counseling, patients were less hostile, saw their blood pressure drop (by 8.5 points), and over the next year, spent fewer days in the hospital for heart problems. Davidson and Stuhr are studying 40 women to see if results are similar. In the meantime, here are the researchers' best secrets for resolving your anger.

RELAX. It sounds cliché, but it works. When you feel riled, take a few deep breaths—exhaling slowly—and count to 10. Is the situation really worth getting mad about? If it is, then. . .

TALK IT OUT. There are several steps you can take:
• Emphathize: Try to put yourself in your antagonist's shoes: Ask for her side of the story, or at least state your understanding of it. This is hard when you're royally miffed, but it's a disarming tactic that can help clear up misunderstandings. For example, a waitress brings your steak well-done instead of the rare that you ordered. If you'd normally either chew her out or say nothing but later stiff her on the tip, consider respectfully telling her, "I asked for a rare steak but this one is well-done. Maybe you can tell me what happened." It could be she picked up the wrong dish, and yours is in the kitchen.
• Assert yourself: State your point of view, "but do it in realistic terms, not 'You bad, me good,'" Davidson says. So if the waitress tells you she's new on the job, you could reply, "I know you're learning the ropes, but I prefer my steak rare."
• Problem solve: Seek a compromise so you can both walk away without bad feelings. In this example, the waitress ideally will either fix her goof or offer an alternative. If not, consider calling in the manager and calmly explaining, "Your waitress seems to be having a bad day, and we're having difficulties with my order. What can you do for me?" As you negotiate, remember that if the other party demands something unreasonable, you have a right to say no.

For more on how to defuse conflicts, take a look at *Lifeskills* (Times Books, 1999) by Duke University anger researcher Redford Williams, M.D., and Virginia Williams, Ph.D.

with many symptoms of depression were twice as likely to develop high blood pressure within five years as happier peers. In March 2001, doctors who tracked 2,847 elderly men and women in Amsterdam over four years reported these results: Among subjects who started out free of cardiac disease, the odds of later dying from heart problems were nearly four times higher in those suffering from major depression.

Moreover, people with depression often suffer from anxiety as well, which seems to wreak similar havoc and substantially hurt their prognosis. Here, too, studies have found that an ongoing case of nerves may harm even a healthy ticker. In a Harvard study of 34,000 men over two years, those who experienced sweat-inducing anxiety from fear of flying or other phobias were three times more likely to

> Chronic sadness can lead to heart disease or stroke. One sobering report concluded that in those who've suffered a heart attack, depression more than quadruples the odds of dying within six months.

suffer a fatal heart attack. More controversially, some research hints that chronic worrying of the garden variety can drive up blood pressure or worse. After following 749 women for 20 years in the Framingham Heart Study, scientists discovered the risk of having a heart attack or dying from heart problems was almost eight times more common in homemakers with any symptoms of anxiety than in those with none.

Scientists have a number of theories about what goes wrong between the brain and the heart. Depressed people may simply have poor health habits; they're more apt to be smokers, less likely to eat right, and may not stick to taking their medication, says Carney. But he and others think there's more. One key culprit seems to be the body's reaction to stress. Studies have revealed that perpetually nervous or saddened souls are stuck in the same fight-or-flight response that goes berserk in hotheads, though generally at a much lower gear. The hallmarks are there: excess levels of stress hormones, a quickened heart rate, and hyperactive platelets that may clump into an artery-clogging clot.

Another complication, says Carney, is that the hearts of depressed patients are less versatile at speeding up or slowing down in response to the body's demands. And that is known to make the heart prone to overly rapid or erratic beating that can trigger

sudden cardiac death. Meanwhile, depression also seems to run down the immune system. A weakened ability to heal injury to artery walls might foster inflammation and plaque buildup.

Still, figuring out what's gone awry is one thing; fixing it is another. The ultimate question is, can the best treatments for inner anguish protect your heart? The ENRICHD trial put a tried-and-true form of psychotherapy for depression and anxiety to the test. Called cognitive-behavioral therapy, it teaches patients to recognize and understand their emotional reactions (that's the cognitive part) and then to change them (that's the behavioral part). Depressed people tend to have a darkly distorted view of the world, Carney says. The counseling teaches them to see the light. "They start out taking small steps, but eventually people can make very significant life changes," he says. (See "Thinking Your Way Out of a Funk," page 36.)

Just ask 67-year-old Darlene Roja, who went through counseling in the ENRICHD study after her heart attack in 1997. She was worried about her husband, who has prostate cancer. But one trick she learned helped a lot. "I would just ask myself, if this were my friend with the same problem, what would I tell her?" she says. "I would say not to worry; his doctors are keeping a close watch on him, and he's doing fine now." She says the cognitive-behavioral therapy gave her back her life. "I feel I can handle anything now."

Jackson has had her own successes with therapy. Step by step, she moved out of darkness and is now on a more even keel. She's had a few bouts of chest pain, but has so far escaped anything worse. Whether she can thank ENRICHD for that is unclear. Results will be released soon, but the National Institutes of Health, which funded the study, is keeping them under wraps. The stakes are tremendous: If the findings are positive, Carney and other experts say, it would dramatically change the way doctors care for heart patients.

So what do mainstream physicians think about this? So far, they haven't paid much attention to the premise that bad feelings can hurt the heart. "Cardiologists take the view that they deal with the heart and psychiatrists deal with the head," says Mount Sinai's Pickering.

Burned once by the Type A fiasco, and with answers from ENRICHD still pending, negative-emotions researchers know they still have miles to go before convincing the skeptics. Yet anybody constantly adrift on the swells of resentment, sadness, or anxiety, they say, has nothing to lose and everything to gain by taking steps to quell those turbulent waters. Life would be smoother, happier, saner in the short run—and possibly a whole lot healthier down the road.

The potential is so great, in fact, that a few clinicians are already hedging their bets. At Mount Sinai's heart

thinking your way out of a funk

When it comes to crummy moods, we just can't help our emotions, right? Not so. In any given situation, judgments instantly race through our heads—and it's those automatic thoughts that ultimately color how we feel. Negative thinking fuels negative emotions, which can, in turn, stir up bellyaches, headaches, and other physical ailments, says Iris Csik, a clinical social worker at the Washington University School of Medicine in St. Louis. Indeed, research shows that people battling depression, anxiety, or hostility tend toward automatic thinking that's always pessimistic or cynical.

But one kind of psychotherapy, called cognitive-behavioral treatment, tries to stop the emotional chain reaction at its source. It teaches people to tune in to their overly negative thoughts, critically evaluate those, and replace them with more accurate and realistic thoughts. The treatment isn't a quick-fix personality transplant, though. "You have to continually work at it," Csik says. "You have to apply the things you learn to day-to-day life with real people and real problems. But the more you do it, it'll start feeling like the real you inside." Here are a few steps in the right direction.

KEEP A DAILY MOOD JOURNAL. Begin by paying attention to your innermost thoughts. Spend 10 minutes a day jotting down the following pieces of information about specific events that left you upset or blue. After a week, you'll start to see patterns in your thoughts and relationships. Follow these guidelines as you write:

1. Scene: Describe the distressing situation. Stick to the facts.
2. Thoughts: What were you thinking or imagining?
3. Feelings: Put them into words. Were you angry, ashamed, anxious, jealous, happy, sad, hopeless?

4. Symptoms: Did you have any unpleasant physical reactions, such as stomachache, headache, or feeling like your blood was boiling?
5. Actions: What did you do about the situation?
6. Result: What were the consequences?

GET A REALITY CHECK. The next move is to start scrutinizing—and then readjusting—your thought processes.
1. Check for distortions: Are you overgeneralizing or seeing your life in strict all-or-nothing terms? Jumping to conclusions? Ignoring the positives only to focus on the negatives? Blaming yourself for something that wasn't all your doing? Look for other possible interpretations. Instead of thinking, "I'm a total loser," try "I have good points and bad points, just like anyone." If you couldn't help organize the family reunion and it got canceled, rather than cry, "It's all my fault," be sure to give other factors their due—such as the fact that your sister's kids came down with mono.
2. Examine the evidence: Say you're anxious and fretting, "I don't have any friends. No one likes me." Stop and ask whether that's really true—nobody likes you? A closer look at the statement will, in all likelihood, prove it false.
3. Take a step outside yourself: When you're mired in self-criticism and feeling like a failure, ask yourself, "If my friend Jesse were in this dilemma, what would I tell her?" You'd never accuse her of being a failure. Give yourself the same supportive advice you'd give your pal.

FIND HELP. *The Feeling Good Handbook* (Plume, 1999) by Stanford University psychiatrist David Burns, M.D., walks through cognitive-behavioral techniques for everything from depression to social phobia to marital problems. But if you're constantly struggling, consider seeking professional help.

institute, Pickering has rewritten the rules for the way that doctors assess heart-disease risk. It's now become a matter of protocol to ask patients about their feelings, in addition to checking the usual vital signs. Whenever possible, those in emotional distress will get treatment. In a world dominated by EKGs and blood-pressure numbers, it's a gutsy move. But director Valentin Fuster, M.D., takes the long view. "I think 10 years from now, people will look back and say it was not so radical. That's how these things always start." ✳

Ingfei Chen is a freelance writer based in Santa Cruz, California.

FISH OIL
government-approved for fighting heart disease

Deservedly, fish has netted a healthy reputation. Scientists say the omega-3 fats abundant in salmon, tuna, mackerel, and fish oil supplements can lower the risk of heart disease. Now, even the government is on board. New Food and Drug Administration guidelines let supplement makers tout that health claim on their bottles. Don't expect to see big banner labels, though; you'll have to scan the jar to find the wordy pronouncement.

Tea—a proven treat for your heart

Teatime in England, with its buttery scones and cakes, may not seem like the healthiest custom. But if you pass on the rich treats and fill up on the tasty brew, your heart's arteries will thank you in more ways than one. A recent study found that drinking tea can improve blood flow in these vessels—within two hours. Boston University researchers say the key ingredients are antioxidants called flavonoids.

HOW TO IDENTIFY POSTPARTUM DEPRESSION

Maternal tears in the days that follow childbirth can be as common as dirty diapers, but knowing when the salty side effects signal serious complications can be tricky. A new study has revealed a simple and effective—and yet rarely performed—quiz for identifying the postpartum depression that is all too often swept under the rug.

The questionnaire asks women about such things as her ability to laugh, what makes her anxious, and whether she has any thoughts of harming herself. In a recent study at the Olmsted Medical Center in Rochester, Minnesota, the 10-question screening tool (known as the Edinburgh Postnatal Depression Scale) was believed to help catch cases of postnatal depression that would have gone undetected otherwise. When 342 women completed the questionnaire at their six-week postnatal checkups, the researchers found that those patients with abnormal scores were seven times more likely to be diagnosed with postpartum depression than those who scored in the normal range.

"There's no doubt in my mind that we are missing half to two-thirds of postpartum depression cases," says Michael Silverstein, M.D., an OB/GYN at the New York University Medical School. "I think this study demonstrates the intrinsic flaw in what we've been doing in the past. If somebody doesn't come in on the ground, hysterical, we assume they're well," Silverstein says. The study's authors estimate that postpartum depression strikes anywhere from 8% to 15% of new mothers, but Silverstein believes the figures are actually somewhat lower.

Postpartum depression is marked by frequent crying, lack of motivation, difficulty sleeping, and a loss of interest in normally pleasurable activities. In contrast, says Silverstein, women with a normal case of the baby blues are teary but functional.

The scope of postpartum depression extends beyond the mothers. "The biggest consequence is the huge impact it has on your family and ultimately on your ability to take care of yourself and your new baby," says Silverstein. This quiz may be the first step toward healing.

TEST YOURSELF
Beat the period before your period

"THAT TIME OF THE MONTH" can make you feel like a prisoner to your hormones. Take this test and find out how to break the vicious cycle of premenstrual syndrome (PMS).

1. If PMS hits with a vengeance, you should hit the gym.
   True or False?

2. Which of these eases PMS?
   - a) Magnesium
   - b) Calcium
   - c) Vitamin E
   - d) All of the above

3. With age, PMS gets worse.
   True or False?

4. To rein in your monthly urge to gorge, stick to three square meals a day.
   True or False?

ANSWERS
1. True. Working out helps reduce bloating.
2. B. Calcium—about 1,200 mg a day—can ease bloating by reducing water retention. Some claim that taking magnesium supplements assuage symptoms and that popping vitamin E diminishes breast tenderness, but the evidence is sketchy.
3. True. But the reason is a mystery. Unfortunately, discomfort slowly increases until menopause.
4. False. In fact, eating five or six smaller meals a day keeps you from bingeing when the cookie jar calls.

the most effective treatment for menstrual cramps

Grandma always said a heating pad offered the surest relief from menstrual cramps, and recent research confirms it. A study of about 90 women, ages 18 to 40, found that the good old heating pad was just as effective as ibuprofen, the over-the-counter drug of choice for women suffering from period pain. But severe cramps may need to be hit with both barrels, says gynecologist Mark Akin, M.D., principal investigator of the study. "The combination of ibuprofen and heat had a better result than either one by itself," Akin says. The researchers theorize that the heat softens and relaxes the muscles and reduces the painful effects of cramping.

Procter and Gamble supplied disposable heating pads for the study; they plan to market the thin, oval-shaped devices, which adheres to panties and fits across the lower abdomen. For now, a box of the heating pads can be purchased online at www.thermacare. com ($8.99 per box of three); the pads will be available in stores nationwide this year.

Moderate exercise benefits
you and your baby

Believe it or not, your pregnancy is a great time for you to get in shape—even if you've always been a total couch potato. Whether you're a neophyte or a fitness buff, moderate exercise (such as brisk walking) three or four times a week can decrease your risk of having a low–birth–weight baby, according to a recent study published in the *American Journal of Obstetrics and Gynecology*. But make sure you don't go overboard: Pregnant women who exercise too much are more likely to have problems than those who don't exercise at all. And check with your doctor if you're new to the workout world.

THE LINK BETWEEN ASTHMA AND MENSTRUATION

There's much more to women's health than Pap smears and breast exams. But when medical issues fall outside the gyno realm, sometimes women don't get the attention they deserve. Take asthma. Women are hit the hardest: From 1982 to 1992, the disease increased 82 percent among women, compared with a 29 percent increase among men.

Research into how the disease specifically affects women has been slow in coming, but some new studies have revealed important gender differences, such as a link between asthma and menstruation. Nearly 40 percent of asthmatic women suffer from aggravated asthma symptoms related to their monthly cycles. "Studies have shown that there's a fourfold increase in emergency-room visits (by asthma sufferers) depending on the phase of the menstrual cycle," says Eileen Hoffman, M.D., clinical assistant professor of medicine at New York University Medical Center.

In non-asthmatic women, research suggests there is an increase immediately after ovulation in the number of small receptors in the bronchial tube—receptors that assist in receiving air. These "air helpers" become more sensitive and more efficient during this time, enhancing a woman's ability to breathe.

Female asthmatics, on the other hand, do not have the same increase in the number, sensitivity, or efficiency of those receptors, which can make breathing more labored for them. "There is a unique physiological response here that's going unaddressed," says Hoffman.

She suggests that women with asthma reference their attacks to their menstrual cycles. "Look at a calendar and see if you can correlate a worsening of symptoms just before the start of your menstrual flow," Hoffman says. "If they relate, you need to be treated by a physician who can appreciate these variations."

laughter and your heart
It's no joke: Cardiologists say people who laugh easily are less likely to suffer heart attacks.

How Often Should You Have a Pap Smear?

With cervical cancer, the question isn't how to detect it—the Pap smear does a great job of that. The question is, how often should women have the crucial test? Recently, the suggestion surfaced—as it does now and then—that some women can get away with having a Pap smear only once every three years. But don't cancel your doctor's appointment just yet.

As part of the Heart and Estrogen/ Progestin Replacement Study, doctors at the University of California at San Francisco tracked 2,561 postmenopausal women who'd had a normal Pap result. Over the next two years, 110 of them showed abnormal readings. But in follow-up testing, only one had a true precancerous cervical lesion. That's a lot of false alarms. So the researchers concluded that if a postmenopausal woman has normal Pap smears three years in a row, she may safely switch to an every-third-year screening schedule after consulting her doctor.

This strategy isn't new: It's in line with what the American College of Obstetricians and Gynecologists (ACOG) has recommended since 1988. Here's the catch: According to William Creasman of ACOG, skipping yearly tests is safe only for women at particularly low risk of cervical cancer. Most of us don't qualify. When it comes to cervical cancer, low risk means you've had sex with just one man, and he's had sex only with you. It also means you've never had a sexually transmitted disease (STD), you're not a smoker, and you didn't have sex before age 18.

Most of us should still have a Pap smear every year. Just remember: If you test normal one year and get a red flag the next, don't freak out. It's almost certainly a false alarm.

melatonin
can this over-the-counter hormone prevent breast cancer?

Touted as a sleep aid and an anti-aging potion, melatonin's biggest promise may lie in its power against breast cancer.

BY CATHERINE DOLD

Smack in the center of your head, right about where your spinal column meets your brain, there's a pea-sized gland whose purpose stumped scientists for centuries. All anyone knew about the pineal gland was that it responded to light. Some speculated the pineal was a vestigial third eye. Philosopher René Descartes proposed that it was the seat of the soul. Finally, in 1958, researchers discovered that the pineal gland produced a hormone called melatonin. Since then, melatonin has been tried—with varying degrees of success—as a cure for jet lag, an all-purpose sleep aid, a libido booster, and a potion to reverse aging. In the spring of 2000, a group of cancer researchers meeting at the National Institutes of Health (NIH) considered the biggest, most surprising claim yet for melatonin: It may be useful in preventing and treating breast cancer.

The prevention part of this theory got its start in 1985 as the brainchild of epidemiologist Richard Stevens, of the University of Connecticut Health Center. Stevens knew—as, indeed, all epidemiologists know—that breast cancer is a disease of civilization: Women in industrialized nations have a five to seven times greater risk of developing the disease than women in underdeveloped countries do. Other researchers have wondered whether a high-fat diet might be to blame or modern women's leisurely path to childbearing and the breastfeeding that's known to protect against breast cancer.

But Stevens had seen studies in which rats had their pineal gland removed, only to become particularly vulnerable to breast-cancer-causing chemicals. He knew, too, that light—both natural and electric—is nearly as effective as surgery in stopping the flow of melatonin. Stevens says, "Melatonin is the chemical expression of darkness in our bodies." In societies with few or no electric lights, women produce melatonin from sundown to daybreak. By contrast, a woman who starts her day with Bryant Gumbel and ends it with David Letterman halves her melatonin-producing hours. That's a chronic disruption of the natural pineal cycle, says Stevens, and, theoretically, it could raise the risk of breast cancer.

Some researchers are asking a troublesome question: Could a habit of late nights and early mornings raise a woman's risk of breast cancer? **Good sleep habits might be the best prevention.**

Other researchers found Stevens's idea compelling but tough to investigate. In 1991, epidemiologist Robert Hahn (who went on to the Centers for Disease Control and Prevention) hit on a way to put the theory to a partial test. The optic nerves of profoundly blind women don't respond to light, so their pineal glands produce melatonin on a regular schedule. If melatonin protects against breast cancer, Hahn reasoned, then blindness should be somewhat protective as well. When he checked thousands of hospital records, he found the likelihood of a blind woman having breast cancer was about half that of women with sight.

Since then, epidemiologists in Norway and Sweden have analyzed their cancer registries, finding that the worse one's sight, the lower the risk of cancer. German researchers even investigated cancer rates above the Arctic Circle, reasoning that the long nights may boost melatonin production; again, results suggested that the hormone plays a protective role.

Start your day with Bryant Gumbel **and end it** with David Letterman, and you could be cutting your melatonin levels by half and may also be increasing your risk of breast cancer.

Exciting, no question about it. Other scientists at the NIH conference had even more surprising news: Doses of melatonin might radically improve the treatment of breast cancer. According to Steven Hill, an oncologist at Tulane University in New Orleans, petri-dish studies with human cancer cells suggest that melatonin blocks estrogen receptors on the cancer cells, starving the tumor of the hormone that spurs its growth. (About half of all breast cancers are estrogen-sensitive.) It doesn't take much melatonin to do the job, either. "The amount the pineal gland makes at night was enough to arrest cancer cells," says David Blask, a cancer researcher at the Bassett Research Institute in Cooperstown, New York, who has done related work.

Hill and others have also tested melatonin in combination with some standard anti-estrogen drugs. In test tubes, Hill dosed breast cancer cells with retinoic acid, a chemotherapy drug that causes vicious side effects. He had given some of the cells a melatonin bath beforehand. Those cells, Hill found, were more easily killed by the retinoic acid, suggesting that melatonin might allow patients to use lower doses of the debilitating medicine.

Worried about possible side effects, doctors aren't prescribing melatonin yet. Instead, they recommend a daily dose of sunlight and a good night's sleep.

Few studies have been done in humans. In Milan, Italy, oncologist Paolo Lissoni administered one of several powerful anticancer agents alone or alongside melatonin to 250 patients with metastatic cancer that had failed to respond to treatment. The patients getting the combo experienced fewer and milder side effects. Compared with patients on chemo-only treatment, twice as many getting melatonin survived a year or more. "Lissoni's clinical trials are small," says Blask, "but if you take all his studies in aggregate, melatonin looks promising."

Despite the good news, no one is ready to recommend melatonin for cancer patients just yet. "I get calls all the time from cancer patients who are looking for something new," says Blask. "I never recommend that they take melatonin. The only studies done in the United States have been on animals, so we really don't know what the proper dose would be."

And no one is suggesting the worried well use melatonin in hopes of breast cancer prevention, either. In fact, Hill advises caution. "It's a hormone, not an herb or a food. It could have all kinds of side effects," he says. Some studies suggest too much melatonin can interrupt menstruation, for instance. "You wouldn't take estrogen without a doctor's guidance," says Hill. "Melatonin is the same thing, a powerful hormone. My belief is, don't take it until we know more about it."

There are a few perfectly safe ways to get more melatonin. First, don't drink to excess. In recent research, Stevens has found that alcohol can depress melatonin production. "More than three drinks can do it," he says. And get outdoors every day. "Sunlight seems to reset your circadian clock, and that's key to maintaining a healthy hormonal rhythm." Of course, a good night's sleep is critical. Blask's work suggests it can goad the pineal gland into producing enough melatonin to prevent tumors from growing. Says Hill: "Go to bed earlier. Will that cure breast cancer? Probably not. But you never know—it may ward off some cases." ✳

A New Screening Option
for women with dense breasts

Although mammography remains the most useful test available to women for the detection of breast cancer, it does have a bit of an Achilles' heel: dense breasts. Researchers at the Mayo Clinic studied more than 16,000 women and found that as breast density increases, the ability of mammography to detect cancer decreases.

But there is hope: Women who have dense breasts should consider ultrasound (also called a sonogram) as an adjunct to mammography, especially if they're concerned about their breast-cancer risk.

Denser breast tissue appears white or gray on mammography X-rays, sometimes making tumors, which appear white as well, hard to detect. An ultrasound, though, is able to penetrate denser tissue for clearer views.

The majority of women under age 39 (about 80 percent) have dense breasts. But older women—particularly those with breasts smaller than B-cup or those who are on estrogen replacement therapy—may also have high-density breasts.

While ultrasound is not recommended for routine screening and does not replace mammography, internist Ruth Johnson, M.D., founding director of the Breast Clinic at the Mayo Clinic in Rochester, Minnesota, advises women with dense breasts to be aware of the ultrasound option as an additional test. "If there's a section of the breast that's very dense, or a question raised about whether a mass might be lurking in that dense breast tissue, then an ultrasound would be the next test of choice," Johnson says. "Any question of a lump, and an ultrasound is mandatory. A lot of people don't get that."

NO MORE EXCUSES:
better breast health is a click away

It's ALWAYS an ideal time to recommit yourself to practicing early detection. That means yearly mammograms for women over 40, monthly breast self-exams (BSEs), as well as annual exams by a doctor or nurse practitioner. Got a problem with that? Most women do. The Net can help solve your breast-care dilemmas.

DILEMMA: Feel like a misguided teenage boy when you perform your monthly BSEs?
PROBLEM SOLVED: Watch . . . and learn. Check out a video clip of an exam being given by a trained doc. She demos all three methods of self-examination: vertical strip, spiral, and wedge.
GO TO: www.thriveonline.oxygen.com/medical/medicaltests/breastexam_video.html

DILEMMA: Can't remember to perform your BSEs every month?
PROBLEM SOLVED: A waterproof card that hangs over your showerhead reminds you to check yourself when you lather up. Click your way to the resources section of this site to order the free, two-sided card that illustrates BSEs and describes them in both English and Spanish. Muchas gracias!
GO TO: www.breastcancerinfo.com/bhealth

DILEMMA: Can't remember to make your annual appointment for a mammogram?
PROBLEM SOLVED: Register on the National Alliance of Breast Cancer Organizations' site to receive an e-mail reminder to schedule your next exam. When you sign up, the organization will compile a breast-health fact sheet tailor-made for you.
GO TO: www.nabco.org

DILEMMA: Can't afford a mammogram?
PROBLEM SOLVED: If your insurance doesn't cover it, ease the pinch a mammogram puts on your pocketbook by learning about how to get low- or no-cost mammograms. (This site can also help you find a federally certified, accredited mammography facility that's close to home.)
GO TO: www.lifetimetv.com/health/breast_mammogram_lowcost.html

DUCTAL + LAVAGE
the new test that detects breast cancer sooner

FOR YEARS, MAMMOGRAPHY has been the only test that can tell if a woman has breast cancer. (And it's an imperfect one at best.) Finally, that may be about to change. Breast surgeon Susan Love has developed a new procedure, called ductal lavage, that can detect cancer earlier than a mammogram and, therefore, can potentially save more lives. *Health* spoke with Love recently to find out more about this exciting new development, which Love believes may lead to the "beginning of the end of breast cancer."

Q: What is the test and how does it work?
A: It's a nonsurgical exam that allows a doctor to sample cells in the lining of the milk duct, where all breast cancers originate. She applies a suction device to the nipple to determine if any of the breast's six to eight ducts contain fluid. If one or more do, she'll anesthetize the nipple and insert a hair-thin catheter to "wash" the ducts with a salt-water solution, collecting a sample of breast cells to check for precancerous changes.

Q: How is this procedure an advance over mammography?
A: The problem with mammography is that by the time we can feel or see a lump, it's been there for 8 to 10 years. That means it's all that much more advanced and harder to treat. With access to the ducts, we can find abnormal cells that aren't cancerous yet but are just thinking about turning malignant.

Q: Are you saying that precancerous cells may be stopped?
A: Yes. The evolution of cells from abnormal to cancerous is, to a great extent, stoppable—and maybe even reversible—through hormonal stimulation. That's what tamoxifen is all about. And it seems to be more effective the earlier you catch the cancer. In last year's prevention study, women at high risk for breast cancer who took tamoxifen reduced their chance of getting the disease by 50 percent. But for those who already had atypical cells, it cut the risk by 88 percent.

Q: If a woman gets an abnormal result from a ductal lavage, what should she do?
A: The recommended treatment is going to vary with the circumstances of the woman. In all cases, a mammogram should be done to see if there's cancer in the breast. If nothing shows up, the patient may decide just to go on tamoxifen. On the other hand, if she's from a high-risk family, she may opt for a mastectomy. And if the mammogram does turn up cancer, she'll consider the same range of options—radiation, lumpectomy, chemotherapy—that anyone with breast cancer would.

Q: Who should have a ductal lavage?
A: Right now, because it's relatively new and we're still working it out, we think women who are at high risk or have breast cancer in one breast would be the perfect candidates.

Q: Where can they have it done?
A: There are 20 centers around the country that participated in the trials and have trained doctors in the procedure. (For more information, check out www.susanlovemd.com.)

Q: How much does it cost?
A: It depends on the center, but the procedure should run less than $1,000. A mammogram is less expensive because a technician can do the X-ray. Insurance has covered lavage in several cases, but we can't guarantee that it will.

Q: Will women eventually get ductal lavages instead of mammograms?
A: Lavage should be used in addition to mammography, not instead of it. It's good at finding very early-stage cancers, but past studies have suggested that it's not as good at finding cancers later on that are bigger. I foresee a day in the not-too-distant future when we'll go in to get our Pap smears and get our ducts checked at the same time.

BREAST CANCER
after surgery, what's next?

When a woman is diagnosed with breast cancer, step one is almost always clear: Get the lump out, with either a lumpectomy or mastectomy. After that, things get complicated. Should she have chemotherapy? What kind? Radiation? When, and for how long? And is she a candidate for tamoxifen?

The good news is that new studies addressing these questions are being published all the time. But the unending flow of information can be overwhelming for women and their doctors, leading to care that is less than optimal. To the rescue: a panel of experts convened by the National Institutes of Health. The scientists reviewed the research and outlined the "gold standard" of what to look for in treatment after breast cancer surgery. Here are the panel's major findings, interpreted by LaMar McGinnis, a spokesperson for the American Cancer Society:

PROBLEM: Some doctors prescribe tamoxifen only for women who have not received radiation or chemotherapy.

GOLD STANDARD: Tamoxifen—given possibly in conjunction with radiation or chemotherapy—is recommended for most women whose tumors had hormone receptors. Suggested length of treatment with tamoxifen: five years.

PROBLEM: Chemotherapy regimens often consist of just one medication.

GOLD STANDARD: Chemotherapy is more effective when several drugs are used.

PROBLEM: Chemotherapy is often given only to women whose cancer has spread to lymph nodes.

GOLD STANDARD: Almost all breast cancer patients should get chemotherapy. Possible exceptions include women over 70 and younger women with very small (less than one centimeter) tumors.

PROBLEM: Chemotherapy treatment schedules are often inconsistent.

GOLD STANDARD: It is crucial that the course of treatment be completed and that no sessions are skipped.

PROBLEM: Radiation treatment is often reserved for women whose tumor was removed by lumpectomy.

GOLD STANDARD: A woman who had a mastectomy should get radiation if her tumor was large or if four or more lymph nodes contained cancer cells.

PROBLEM: Women with advanced breast cancer are sometimes given high doses of chemotherapy—high enough to be fatal if their immune systems aren't then rescued with a stem-cell transplant.

GOLD STANDARD: Because it's not clear that the brutal treatment lengthens survival, it should be used only in clinical trials. Also, Herceptin and taxanes are still being investigated; while these treatments are recommended for women with advanced cancer, other women should take them only in carefully controlled clinical trials.

To find out more about current clinical trials, log on to cancertrials.nci.nih.gov or call 800-422-6237.

How to Find the Best Surgeon for You—in 3 Steps

1. ASK LOTS OF QUESTIONS. What does this procedure involve? How often has the surgeon performed it? What are common complications and what is the likely outcome for a person of your age, gender, and health? What follow-up care will be needed, and will the doctor be available after the operation? If the surgeon dodges your questions, you may need to find someone else, says Michael Donio, of the People's Medical Society.

2. CHECK CREDENTIALS. You can contact the American Board of Medical Specialties (at www.abms.org or 866-275-2267) to learn if your doctor is a board-certified specialist in the field.

3. DO A BACKGROUND CHECK. Even great doctors get sued on occasion, but several lawsuits can be an indication of trouble. At www.docboard.org, you can find malpractice judgments from 17 states, as well as records of sanctions by participating state medical boards. For a fee of $10, www.docinfo.org lets you search sanction records in all 50 states. Another excellent resource to check out is www.searchpointe.com.

THE BEST CHOICES FOR BREAST RECONSTRUCTION

Women who had reconstruction at the same time as a mastectomy didn't have the dip in body image like those who waited.

For a woman who loses a breast to cancer, recovery means more than healing from the surgery—it means learning to feel good about her body again. To that end, more mastectomy patients are having their breasts reconstructed. But the decision brings an exhausting series of choices: Should it be done at the same time as the mastectomy or later? Should a woman use implants or her own tissue? These options are considered safe, but until now there has been little research on which contribute most to a woman's sense of well-being.

To find out, researchers at the University of Michigan questioned 250 women who'd opted for various forms of reconstruction. Just before each woman's surgery and one year after it, they queried her about her physical and mental health. It turned out to matter little whether patients got implants or not: After a year, most women were doing well either way.

Timing made more of a difference. On most measures, women who'd had reconstruction at the same time as the mastectomy had a slightly greater improvement than those who'd waited. The most striking finding was in the area of self-image: After a year, both groups felt just as good about their bodies after the surgery as they had before. But the "immediate reconstruction" group avoided the dip in body image scores experienced by those who waited.

"I'm amazed by that," says Edwin Wilkins, a plastic surgeon at the University of Michigan, who led the study. "I'm amazed we could do any operation that could negate the devastating effects of mastectomy on a woman's body image."

Faith Fancher, a TV news reporter in Oakland, California, chose immediate reconstruction three years ago. "When I woke up I didn't have the breast I had before, but I did have something there," she says. "I didn't have that feeling of loss."

Because some complications patients may suffer could take longer than a year to appear, Wilkins will continue to evaluate the participants. He's developed a Web site to help patients struggling to make decisions about reconstructive surgery. To learn more, log on to www.surgery.med.umich.edu/breastrecon.htm.

Chemotherapy:
reduce side effects with moderate exercise

A recent study reveals that women with early-stage breast cancer can diminish the fatigue and nausea caused by their treatments through low-intensity exercise. Patients told to walk three to five times each week felt less pain and had more energy than those who weren't as active.

How Optimism Can Motivate . . . and Backfire

What keeps breast cancer from coming back? A positive attitude, according to 60 percent of survivors surveyed by researchers at the University of Toronto. That opinion is a little worrisome, say cancer specialists: A can-do spirit certainly helps a woman make healthy lifestyle changes, but it might backfire in a sense of personal failure if the disease should return (and there's no evidence that attitude alone can keep cancer at bay). Interestingly, only 4 percent of the women credited the powerful cancer drug tamoxifen.

Is **iron-poor blood** stealing your energy?

If workouts are getting the better of you, here's an ironclad way to put the spring back in your step.

BY CHRISTIE ASCHWANDEN

Okay, we all know life isn't fair. But this seems a little harsh: A woman who rarely eats meat, munches vegetables like a ravenous rabbit, and has just added an exercise program to her salubrious lifestyle may find that exercise is sapping her energy, while the meat-and-potatoes gal sails through her workouts with vigor to spare. Can someone please call foul?

Cornell University nutritionist Jere D. Haas won't. Knowing that 7.8 million American women are low in iron, Haas wondered if their deficiency could be holding them back at the gym, turning their workouts into a brutal slog. So he recruited 42 healthy women who had low iron stores—but weren't anemic. Anemics don't have enough of the mineral to produce red blood cells, essential components in the delivery of oxygen to the body's tissues. Those who are iron deficient are just a step away from anemia, and often have anemia-like symptoms such as fatigue and decreased aerobic endurance, but in a milder form.

To see what would happen to a person's endurance level once she got an iron boost, Haas had half the women in his study take a supplement and the others a placebo. He then put all of them on a four-week exercise program that had them steadily cranking away on a stationary bike five times a week for 30 minutes. At the end of the experiment, the women in the supplement group had raised their iron stores to normal—and their energy levels followed suit. On average, they

pedaled nine miles 3.5 minutes faster than their time at the start. The sugar-pill poppers improved their initial times by a mere 1.5 minutes.

Haas says the message is clear. Women who are low in iron may get some benefit from exercise, but their deficiency is holding them back.

"Many women don't realize that they could be getting more out of their workouts," says Haas. "Even though they feel worn down, they see themselves improving and they think they're okay."

Rosalia Scalia discovered this on her own. Called "the grass eater" by her friends, the 43-year-old Scalia is vegan, eating no animal products. In addition to going for an occasional run, she walks 30 minutes to and from work every day. Years ago, when a test indicated she had low iron stores, Scalia began taking an

Iron's Best Friend: Vitamin C
More than just an antioxidant, vitamin C helps your body absorb iron. Swallow a C supplement or, better yet, add red bell peppers to your beans and toss some tangerines into a spinach salad.

iron supplement. After a few months she got lazy and stopped. As time went by, she began to notice that her friends had far more energy during their workouts. "I just wanted to fall asleep," she says.

She had no idea what could possibly be wrong until she read a news story about Haas's study. "It never dawned on me that my iron could be low again, but the study sounded an alarm," she says. She started taking a supplement again, and within a month was back to her old self.

Scalia's active lifestyle and vegan diet made her prime for iron deficiency. Iron is more difficult to absorb from vegetables than from meat, so vegans and vegetarians need to be extra vigilant. While red meat is one of the best sources because it's rich in heme iron, a type that's especially easy to absorb, other good sources of iron include beans, dried fruits, soybeans, tofu, spinach, and other leafy green vegetables.

What's troublesome about this type of deficiency is that even if your plate is chock-full of iron, you aren't necessarily in the clear. Women just starting an exercise program are also at increased risk.

Connie Weaver, a nutritionist at Purdue University, has found that women jumping into a fitness regimen experience a slight but significant drop in iron. In one study of formerly sedentary women, she found that even those exercising only a few hours a week saw an initial dip. Weaver says this seems to indicate that if women begin a new workout program with low to normal iron levels and aren't getting enough iron through their diet, they could be pushed into deficiency.

Scalia's daily dose of iron has her feeling better than ever, even though she can't be sure that low levels sent her into a slump. Her history of deficiency makes it likely, but Haas says it's impossible to credit her improvement to the supplements since she started popping iron before getting a test. Haas warns strongly against following her lead.

If you're unusually beat during and after workouts, says Haas, try eating more iron-rich foods. If that doesn't give you a lift, ask your doctor for a blood test. Don't get checked for anemia, since this test won't indicate if you're merely iron depleted. Ask for a serum ferritin test, which will measure your total iron.

Should you score low, take a supplement that contains the recommended daily allowance of 18 milligrams. Whatever you do, don't go straight for the supplements and skip the test. About 1 in every 250 Americans has hemochromatosis, a predisposition to store too much iron that can lead to serious problems, including arthritis, diabetes, and heart failure.

But for most women, the problem is too little iron, not too much. Haas admits it doesn't seem fair that those of us who are striving to be healthy are the ones derailed by low iron, but adds, "All it takes is a simple blood test to get yourself back on track." ✷

when it's not low iron,
what is sapping your strength?

You can rule out an iron deficiency with a blood test, but that's just one possible drain on your energy. Take a look at your life: What else might be to blame? Here are some possible culprits.

Sleep Deprivation
As an adult you need at least eight hours of shut-eye each night to keep your energy running on high, but most of us get less than seven hours during the workweek. Don't fool yourself into thinking you can make it all up on the weekend. Skip that last sitcom and get in the habit of turning in on time.

Too Much Stress
If you spend too much time worrying, you are wasting a huge amount of energy—energy that can be put to better use elsewhere in your life. Try releasing your tension daily by practicing yoga or meditation or going for a run. You may be surprised by how recharged you'll feel.

Depression
Fatigue and insomnia are common signs of depression. If your blues are lingering, don't be afraid to seek help. Counseling, medication, and exercise can help you feel better than ever.

Not Exercising
Just like a car that's been sitting in the garage, a body that's not regularly revved can run sluggishly. Get back in gear. First-time exercisers usually report a spike in energy levels, provided they aren't iron deficient.

Irregular Diet
Skipping lunch is just asking your body to bonk. Eat regular meals, striving to balance your carbohydrates, proteins, and fats. Remember that sugar and caffeine may give you a temporary boost but will quickly send you into an energy slump.

Illness
A whole slew of serious illnesses, such as thyroid disorders and cancer, can steal your strength. But fatigue may also be a symptom of a minor bug you thought you'd beaten. It's not uncommon to feel lousy for a week or two after recovering from a nasty cold or flu, even if other symptoms are gone.

counting on
CALCIUM
how to make sure you get enough to prevent osteoporosis

Think your bones are getting the boost they need?
Don't bet on it—even if you take a supplement.
Here's how to get a jump on the trickiest mineral of all.

BY BILL GOTTLIEB

Mary Lanier (her name has been changed) was in the bedroom with her husband when he told her he wanted a divorce. Dazed, she retreated to the bathroom, where in the mirror she saw a 43-year-old woman who a minute before had felt securely married. "Damn it," she said, and brought her right arm down on the sink. The pain was immediate and excruciating.

An X-ray at the hospital showed she'd fractured her wrist. The doctor set it with a splint, assuring her it would heal in three to six weeks. But a second X-ray three weeks later revealed no sign of fresh calcium knitting bone to bone, so the doctor ordered a bone density test. Then, Lanier—a small-framed executive who hates milk and manages to eat barely one meal a day—learned she has osteoporosis, a disease that leaves bones so weak they can snap as easily as twigs.

Osteoporosis afflicts about 10 million Americans, 80 percent of them women. Another 18 million have osteopenia, or low bone density, a possible prelude to the full-blown disease. That means one of every two American women will at some time in her life suffer an osteoporosis-related bone fracture, most likely of a wrist, vertebra, or hip. And—scariest of all—24 percent of those over 50 who have hip fractures will die within the year, often of pneumonia or other complications. That's as many as are killed each year by breast cancer.

Unfortunately, some risk factors for the disease can't be eliminated. If you're a thin or small-framed woman, are Caucasian or Asian, have reached menopause, or have any close relatives who've been diagnosed with the disease, your likelihood of getting osteoporosis runs especially high.

You probably know the risks—unless, of

> Calcium can help cut your blood pressure, shield you from colon cancer, and ease or end PMS symptoms. What's more, it can help keep you slim.

course, you've been hibernating for years. And you surely know how to head them off: Get more calcium. Mary Lanier thought she knew the basics too, yet she made a lot of mistakes as she set out to mend her bones. Chances are, you don't know how much calcium you really need, which source is best, what the right dose is, or when your body can use it most.

Admit you're falling short.

"Most women think they get more calcium than they actually do," says Connie Weaver, a nutrition professor at Purdue University in West Lafayette, Indiana. It's a nice round number—1,000 milligrams per day—experts say every adult woman under age 51 should be sure to hit; those older need 1,200. Either way, not many achieve this number daily.

"Except for girls under 11, there is no female population in America that, on average, takes in as much calcium as we know is necessary to prevent osteoporosis," Weaver says. In other words, whether you're 18 or 80, it's likely you're in what experts call negative calcium balance—that is, you excrete more calcium each day than you take in. Where does your body get the extra? Yup, from your bones.

Watch what you eat and drink.

You can lower your risk by exercising regularly, of course, and by swearing off tobacco. And you can strengthen your skeleton if you eat wisely—though that's easier said than done.

After her diagnosis, Lanier began eating two servings of cottage cheese a day. It was the only dairy food she liked, but little did she know it wasn't doing her bones much good. It turns out that cottage cheese isn't exactly a calcium blockbuster. Research shows that under some circumstances the high levels of salt and animal protein in foods like cottage cheese can actually force calcium out of bones.

Should we all give up cheese? Absolutely not, says Robert Heaney, a professor at the Osteoporosis Research Center at Creighton University in Omaha, Nebraska: "The negative effects on your bones from

Most women should take a calcium supplement with vitamin D in it since that nutrient promotes effective absorption of calcium. Beyond that, get your bone builders from vegetables, fruits, and whole grains.

how much calcium do you get?

You may think you're getting a lot of calcium in your meals, but you're probably not, says Connie Weaver, a bone expert at Purdue University. What's your daily total? Here's how to figure it out.

FOOD	MG
yogurt, low-fat (1 cup)	447
orange juice, calcium-fortified (1 cup)	350
sardines, canned (3 ounces)	325
milk, 1 percent (1 cup)	300
cheese, Swiss (1 slice)	272
spinach, cooked (1 cup)	245

If you typically eat one of the above calcium superstars every day, figure you average 300 mg. If you rarely do, give yourself a zero. (Sorry, but all the other calcium greats—ricotta cheese, whole milk—are loaded with artery-clogging fat.) Grant yourself another 300 mg if you generally eat several foods that are moderately rich in calcium every day. Some examples:

FOOD	MG
tofu, firm ($^1/_2$ cup)	204
white beans, cooked (1 cup)	161
figs, dried ($^1/_2$ cup, or about 5)	143
Parmesan cheese (2 tablespoons)	138
frozen yogurt ($^1/_2$ cup)	103
breakfast cereal, calcium-fortified	100
English muffin, toasted	98
broccoli, cooked (1 cup)	72
almonds (1 ounce, or about 24 nuts)	70
green beans, boiled (1 cup)	58

To see if you're falling short, subtract your total from your daily goal*—1,300 for girls ages 9 to 18; 1,000 mg for women ages 19 to 50; 1,200 for anyone older. If you can't manage to make up the difference with foods, take a supplement every day.
*Dietary Reference Intake set by the National Academy of Sciences.

Caffeine can chip away at the calcium stores of women who are already running short.

high intakes of salt and protein are only important at a low calcium intake." In other words, says Heaney, who has also served on the government panel that sets recommended calcium doses, you don't need to sweat that issue if you're getting plenty of the mineral. (See "How Much Calcium Do You Get?" page 49.)

In fact, recent scientific studies show that bone fracture risk may rise when you eat too little protein, says Bess Dawson-Hughes, a respected bone researcher at Tufts University. She also says the common claim that soft drinks rob your body of calcium is a myth. She does, however, urge women to drink no more than two cups of coffee a day. Downing a lot of caffeinated drinks—like imbibing more than four alcoholic beverages a day—can chip away at the calcium stores of women already running short.

Don't think only of antacids.

Okay, your goal is 1,000 milligrams (mg) of calcium a day—and you've figured out your meals furnish just 600 mg. How do you make up the difference? Supplements, naturally. But which ones?

They aren't exactly all the same. Best known are the calcium-based antacids, made from calcium carbonate—chalk, essentially. Fewer people are familiar with the ones made of calcium citrate, yet recent research suggests it's absorbed more readily, says

Howard Heller, an assistant professor of internal medicine at the University of Texas Southwestern Medical Center at Dallas.

In a study published last year in the *Journal of Clinical Pharmacology,* Heller and his colleagues gave 25 women a breakfast dose of 500 mg of calcium carbonate, checking every hour to see how much of the mineral they hung on to. On another day, the women took the same amount of calcium in the form of citrate; on still another, they took a look-alike pill. The result: When they took citrate instead of carbonate, they absorbed, on average, 94 percent more calcium. A published review of 15 other studies found that citrate beat out carbonate by an average of 20 percent. "That doesn't sound like much," says Heller. "But if you have a negative calcium balance of only 27 mg a day, you lose one percent of your bone mass every year."

Fine, says Heaney, but citrate's superiority is far from proved. He insists calcium carbonate works beautifully, and you should feel free to stick with it. Others point out that it's less bulky than citrate, so you can take fewer pills for the same dose of usable mineral (what scientists call elemental calcium), and it's usually cheaper—an added bonus. Just swallow the pills at mealtime, when your stomach churns out the acid needed to dissolve them.

Pop supplements around the clock.

Your body can absorb only so much calcium at a time and excretes the rest. So whichever supplement you pick, take it in divided doses. "Three doses a day are

Lots of foods, from beans to sardines, are rich in calcium. But few people eat enough to hit their daily goal.

better than two, and two are better than one," says Weaver. For example, she suggests, if you're going for 600 mg of supplemental calcium a day, take 200 mg at breakfast, 200 mg at lunch, and 200 mg at dinner.

Skip the bone-building complexes.

Some calcium supplements also include magnesium and boron, as well as vitamins D and K—all nutrients that research suggests aid in protecting bone. Are they helpful?

"Yes, the mineral magnesium is important for bone health," says Machelle Seibel, a professor of gynecology and obstetrics at Boston University School of Medicine. "But calcium and magnesium compete with each other for absorption, so these combination products make no sense.

"Women should take a calcium supplement with vitamin D in it," he says, "since that nutrient is so important for the effective absorption of calcium."

Beyond that, experts say, get your other bone builders from fruits, vegetables, and whole grains.

Turn it up at menopause.

Midlife, with its falling estrogen levels, is a critical time for bones. Estrogen acts as a "warden" that keeps calcium locked in the skeleton. When that hormone ebbs at menopause, the mineral escapes, and for five years bones rapidly lose density. (After that, for unknown reasons, the loss slows.) That's why at age 51 the daily calcium goal climbs from 1,000 to 1,200 mg.

Dawson-Hughes cites a study in which women getting 1,200 mg a day retained higher bone mineral density and suffered fewer fractures than women who got 600 mg or less. "But calcium alone will not prevent bone loss that occurs as a result of dropping - estrogen levels," she says. Another study tracked women who took estrogen, calcium, or both. "Estrogen and calcium together lowered fracture rates more than estrogen alone or calcium alone," Dawson-Hughes says.

Even the rare person with a near-perfect diet will almost certainly need extra calcium after age 60.

> One of every two American women will at some time in her life suffer an osteoporosis-related bone fracture.

Women—and men—who can't pump up the mineral in their meals should take daily supplements that include vitamin D (or calcium plus a multivitamin). Older Americans often run short on D, especially those living in northern states, where there's too little sunshine in the long winters to power the skin's vitamin D factory.

Think about your butt.

Calcium's benefits reach beyond your skeleton. Studies show the mineral can help cut your blood pressure, shield you from colon cancer, and ease or end premenstral syndrome (PMS) symptoms. What's more, it can help keep you slim. In a recent study in the *Journal of Clinical Endocrinology and Metabolism,* Heaney and colleagues report that a low-calcium diet prompts your body to secrete hormones that slow your metabolic rate. In essence, Heaney explains, the body responds to the shortfall as if it's starving and needs to conserve energy. This slowdown makes weight control just that much harder. Calcium may also keep your body from absorbing some of the fat in rich foods like chocolate.

"If you're trying to lose weight, one of the worst things you can do is cut down on dairy products," he says. "As long as they're nonfat or one percent, they'll help you shed pounds."

Remember what's most important.

Yes, calcium is crucial, but it does next to nothing for those skeletons that aren't subjected to some heave and ho, some push and shove. Perhaps you've heard the term "weight-bearing exercise"? That includes walking, running, dancing, step aerobics, serious yard work, and strength training—either using hand weights and resistance machines or doing push-ups and other moves on your own. When your bones are asked to deal regularly with added stress, they fight back by bulking up, drawing on—right!—the calcium that you take in. ✳

Bill Gottlieb is the author of Alternative Cures *(Rodale, 2000).*

A New IUD May Improve
hormone replacement therapy

"BIG IN EUROPE" may be faint praise for rock bands; oddly enough, the phrase also applies to the contraceptive IUD. Sixteen percent of French femmes use the device, as do a quarter of their Swedish counterparts. But as of 1994, less than 1 percent of American women chose that method of birth control.

Do continentals know something we don't? Maybe so. Last December, the Food and Drug Administration approved the first new IUD in more than a decade. Mirena, made by Berlex and already for sale in Europe, is an IUD with a difference: It may be good not just for contraception, but also for hormone replacement therapy (HRT). *Mais oui!*

Mirena is a small plastic T that is positioned in the uterus for five years at a time, where it emits a tiny daily dose of progestin, a synthetic version of the reproductive hormone progesterone. It is at least as effective at preventing pregnancy as having your tubes tied.

Mirena was approved as a contraceptive, but if the European experience is any guide, it may become popular as an HRT option too. Normally, HRT consists of daily pills containing estrogen—which cuts hot flashes and protects bones—and progestin, which offsets the risk of uterine cancer associated with estrogen. But some women are sensitive to progestin; it makes them moody and bloated and causes unpredictable bleeding.

Mirena offers a way to avoid these side effects by delivering progestin directly to the uterus. It doesn't seem to affect mood, and it reduces bleeding after about six months. (Progestasert, another IUD, works in a similar way but must be replaced yearly.)

If this sounds too rosy to be true, remember that all IUDs can have side effects. Some women's bodies simply expel the things. And, in the first month of use, IUDs may slightly raise the risk of pelvic inflammatory disease. But then again, maybe we've figured out the *quoi* in the *je ne sais quoi* of those mysterious French women.

HOW ETHNICITY AFFECTS MENOPAUSE SYMPTOMS

Ever since baby boomer women began approaching menopause, we've been deluged with information about what to expect and how to cope. But until recently, virtually all of that advice came with a caveat: It was based on research done only on Caucasian women.

That's finally changing: The first large-scale look at how menopause affects women of varying ethnic backgrounds turned up some striking differences.

In the Study of Women's Health Across the Nation (SWAN), researchers questioned more than 12,000 women ages 40 to 55, none of whom were on hormone replacement therapy. They found that African-American women reported more hot flashes, night sweats, and forgetfulness than other groups. Caucasian women had the highest incidence of sleeping problems and were the least likely to become forgetful, while Hispanics had a greater chance of experiencing vaginal dryness, urine leakage, and pounding hearts. For Asian-American women, the primary symptom was forgetfulness.

Epidemiologist Ellen Gold of the University of California at Davis suspects that the variations are related to diet, other lifestyle factors, and varying hormone profiles. The study's next phase will try to pin down the reasons. Ultimately, she says, the research could lead to more tailored treatments for women of different ethnicities. The study also turned up good news for any woman hoping to tame troublesome symptoms: Across all ethnic groups, nonsmoking women who exercised regularly were less likely to have them.

HRT: the choice made clearer

SHOULD I OR SHOULDN'T I? When it comes to hormone-replacement therapy (HRT), that's the question on every menopausal woman's lips. HRT has been shown to relieve menopausal symptoms such as hot flashes, memory lapses, and vaginal dryness, and some studies indicate it may reduce the risk of osteoporosis. But in some women, HRT produces such side effects as breast tenderness, bloating, and unpredictable vaginal bleeding, and it can raise the risks of breast cancer and heart disease.

Two new reports based on the national Women's Health, Osteoporosis, Progestin, Estrogen (HOPE) study may make the HRT decision easier. Both found that low doses of estrogen and progestin combined were as effective as the standard dose of HRT at relieving hot flashes and vaginal dryness, and were less likely to cause the side effects common with HRT.

"If you're just starting out on HRT, it may be best to begin with lower doses of the combination hormones to see if they are enough to relieve menopausal symptoms," says Wulf Utian, M.D., Ph.D., executive director of the North American Menopause Society and lead author of the study. The final word on the risks and benefits of HRT for healthy women may come when an ongoing study called the Women's Health Initiative is completed in 2005.

In the meantime, lower-dose combination pills, which could be available by early 2002, may offer an effective option to menopausal women, at the same time exposing them to less estrogen and progestin.

can natural remedies cool those hot flashes?

If you're suffering from menopause symptoms, you may want to consult Mother Nature. The American College of Obstetrics and Gynecology recently issued new practice guidelines on natural remedies, and while most of the botanicals were dismissed as ineffective, soy and the herb black cohosh were both touted as good short-term remedies for those annoying hot flashes. Just don't forget to tell your doctor about any herbs you add to your daily regimen.

THE CAUSE OF MENOPAUSE: *a new theory*

For years, scientists have blamed the onset of menopause on aging ovaries. But researchers at the University of Michigan School of Nursing now suspect another culprit: circadian rhythms, the body's built-in clock that, among other things, keeps you on a regular sleep schedule.

"It's been the conventional wisdom that women experience menopause because the ovaries get old and run out of eggs," says Michigan professor Nancy Reame, Ph.D., lead researcher of a government-funded study researching the causes of menopause. "We're testing the hypothesis that menopause starts in the brain rather than in the ovary." To do that, they have compiled a group of about 45 women, ages 40 to 50, and are tracking the presence of the hormone that controls reproduction. Through blood samples drawn every 10 minutes for 24 hours, the researchers are looking for patterns in daily hormone fluctuations to see if they correspond to circadian cycles.

"If we could figure out some of the mechanisms involved in normal menopause, we could perhaps apply this to the treatment of premature menopause or some of the infertility problems associated with normal aging," Reame says. Results of the study should be available in summer 2002.

women in *motion*

What got you moving in the right direction, healthwise? Real women share their turning points.

Mine came after a half-gallon of mint-chocolate-chip ice cream. I polished off the last third of the container left from the previous day's pig-out straight from the carton (yes, I used a spoon). This was nothing new for me: I had no self-control when it came to food—never had, never thought I would. But something happened that day. It was as if I had been in a pitch-black room, and someone had suddenly switched on the light. For the first time, I saw how out of control I was. And I had to do something about it.

That was my turning point, the "aha" moment that got me moving toward a healthier life. These are the moments when women realize that their health—emotional and physical—must become a priority. In 2000, we set out to discover what triggers these "aha" moments by commissioning our first Women in Motion study with polling and consulting firm Harris Interactive. We asked more than 3,000 participants when they began putting their health first, and why. The answers are intriguing:

The average age at which the "aha" occurred was 35, and the number-one reason was the discovery of a health problem.

More interesting than the numbers, though, were the women's own stories, in their own voices. So we decided to let them speak. You'll find some of their stories on the following pages.

As for my own story? I started to exercise. It was Jazzercise at first (this was the early '80s, mind you). Then I graduated to running, then cycling, then swimming, eventually competing in triathlons. I began to see food as fuel—never losing the pleasure I got from it, but learning how to find pleasure in the fresh flavors of vegetables, fruits, and meats, and weaning myself off junk food.

It isn't enough to say that I lost weight. It isn't important, even, to say how much. What I did was embark on an adventure that helped me discover who I really am: a confident, powerful woman who believes she can do just about anything, including pass up (or indulge in, if I feel like it) a dish of mint-chocolate-chip ice cream.

Lisa Delaney
Health executive editor

> "I embarked on an adventure that helped me discover who I am: a confident, powerful woman who believes she can do just about anything, including pass up (or indulge in) mint-chocolate-chip ice cream."
> — LISA DELANEY

Self-Amazed

"Last Halloween weekend, I had a reunion with four friends from college who live all over the country. Even though we rarely see each other, they're some of my best friends—things I could never say to other people I can openly say to them. We had a great time: All five of us crashed in the same room, and we went for walks and ate long dinners. Before we went out one night, we had an epic discussion about everything from politics to men. As we were talking, I was thinking, 'Here I am, surrounded by these women who are all so incredibly amazing. Why don't I feel that way about myself?' So, when I got home, I decided to treat myself like I was amazing too. I gave up self-deprecating remarks and started on an exercise regimen: I now run or walk five days a week, crank out 250 sit-ups and 30 push-ups daily, and go to yoga twice a week. The next time I saw my college friends, they couldn't believe what great shape I was in! That felt good, but the best thing is that I've created a healthy pattern for a lifetime."

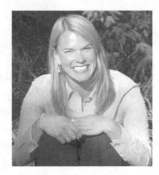

Alicia Brabazon, 29
first-grade teacher
Philadelphia, Pennsylvania

Smoking Up the Trails

"I was a gymnast in high school, but after I suffered a career-ending injury, I developed some poor health habits. I smoked about a pack a day, put on more than 30 pounds, and took a job working as a bartender. Then, when I was 21, a bunch of my friends convinced me to run a four-mile race. I didn't train for it at all—I just went out and ran it.

"It was so much fun, I stuck with it. I quit smoking, lost weight, and had a lot more energy. After a while, I began running marathons, and a few years later, I decided to try doing a 50-K (31-mile) trail race. I found I really liked distance running; I feel like I can go forever when I'm out on the trails.

"In 1998, I did my first 100-mile race, the Rocky

Raccoon, and set a course record. I've also won other ultramarathons. I love what I do, and I'm passionate about it, which pours into the rest of my life."

Amanda McIntosh, 36
personal trainer
San Antonio, Texas

Off the Meds and In Control

"Back in 1995, one of my doctors prescribed a very potent drug to help me battle insomnia. Although I didn't realize how strong the drug was at the time, I soon found out. After eight months, I looked like a walking skeleton (at 5 feet 8 inches tall, I had dropped to just 107 pounds). I was weak and terribly out of shape. Although I had been a runner, I had to give it up while I was taking this medication because physically I just couldn't handle it—I had absolutely no energy or stamina.

"That's when I realized that I had to retake control of my health. First, I changed doctors and got off the medication. By eating a healthy diet, starting to run again, and weight training, I was able to regain the weight I had lost and get back into shape.

"That scary experience made me realize that we can't take our bodies or our health for granted. We are in control of how we feel by how we take care of ourselves. Life is short enough as it is, and I want to do my part to be able to enjoy every minute of it!"

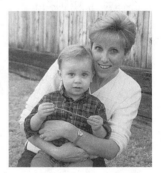

Kim Fisher, 41
insurance company vice president
Oklahoma City, Oklahoma

A Dog Tale

"A 2-year-old golden retriever named Spencer made me reconsider my commitment to health. I'm vision-impaired, and I met Spencer at seeing-eye school. During our daily training walks, I was embarrassed by my sluggish pace and out-of-breath state.

So I decided to turn my life around. I wasn't happy that I had failed myself; I wasn't happy about anything. In the three years since I brought Spencer home, though, I have lost 50 pounds, eat healthy foods, and continue to walk and investigate other fitness options such as Pilates and Spinning. My only health concern is Spencer: He's like a Sunday driver. He goes too slow. Now I think he's out of shape."

Cindy Ray, 54
self-employed
Leon, Iowa

Two in three U.S. women have reached a point in their lives where health and well-being is a priority.

—*Health* WOMEN IN MOTION STUDY, CONDUCTED BY HARRIS INTERACTIVE

Mountains. I was amazed: The trails scale dry mountain ridges and dip into green valleys, and are home to deer, mountain lions, and other wildlife. I was hooked. Soon I began trekking into the mountains on weekends and summer evenings. I began to sleep better, eat more, and care less about my ex-boyfriend and boss. The trails became the place I could lose myself, exercise, and reflect. Today I live in New York City, but I found an apartment near the park, because I still need a brisk walk every day."

Andrea Scharff
landscape designer
New York City

Sweatin' to the Oldies

"I didn't know it at the time, but I started making my health a priority back in the '60s, when I was just 3 years old. I would exercise with my mom to an exercise album—an old 33 LP. I loved it so much that I just kept doing it, even after she stopped. I still work out almost every day, even now—38 years later. In addition to running 25 miles a week, I also lift weights and practice Ashtanga yoga. Just for fun, I stand on my head every day. I figure that one day I might not be able to do it, and I want to know the exact day when that happens!"

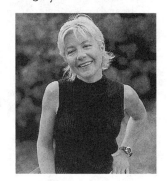

Nita Hughes, 41
graphic designer
Little Gap, Pennsylvania

Mother Nature, Therapist

"In January 1994, I lost all my possessions in the Los Angeles earthquake, dumped my boyfriend, and realized the only thing between me and the job of my dreams was a nightmare boss. I was anxious, couldn't eat or sleep, and was basically a mess. A friend suggested we go for a hike in the Santa Monica

Moved by the Spirit

"My brother was diagnosed with high blood pressure when he was 20, but because he didn't take his medication, he required a kidney transplant about five years ago. That was a real wake-up call for me. I went to the doctor and found out that I also have high blood pressure, as well as high cholesterol, and I decided to make some changes. I started eliminating salty foods from my diet and cut back on sweets. I eat a lot more vegetables these days—salads, spinach, broccoli—stuff I never used to look twice at! I try to walk each day at lunch for about half an hour; it really helps clear my head. I smile a lot, because it's important to have a good sense of humor about things. And I haven't lost my sense of faith: I pray every day. Ninety percent of good health is keeping a positive attitude. I look at everything my brother is going through. He still has such strong spirits, and he's getting along fine."

Stefanie Bryant, 37
administrative assistant
Newark, New Jersey

Putting Stock in Exercise

"In 1994, my job as a stockbroker had become entirely too stressful. I was never at home, always focused on work, and completely burned out. No matter how many successes I had under my belt, there was always someone who was opening a bigger account or getting more accounts than I was.

"That's when I decided to put myself first. So I left my job, went back to school to get my MBA, and started running again, which I had done only sporadically since 1985. Running makes me feel as if I've accomplished something worthwhile. So, first thing in the morning, I 'pay myself first' by getting out to exercise. It's a great way to start the day. I have a new job that I love, feel better about myself than I have in years, and have more energy to spend on doing fun things with my husband!"

Claire Cooney, 38
financial consultant
Portland, Maine

An Unexpected Gift

"I was diagnosed with multiple sclerosis in 1992: The diagnosis devastated me. I was working full time and caring for a young child while my husband was on the road. I wasn't eating right or exercising regularly.

"It wasn't until a relapse in 1998 that I started taking better care of myself. One day I woke up in excruciating pain and could barely move; the symptoms were related to MS. That was the defining moment for me. I had to make some changes in my life, and I had to start making my health a priority.

"Because stress can trigger MS symptoms, I cut back on my work hours. My part-time job allows me time to take care of my family. Before my relapse, I thought that taking care of myself was selfish. Now I realize that it's actually a very giving thing to do because I need to be healthy to be a good wife and mother. In many ways, getting this disease has been a gift—it is a constant reminder of my priorities: my health and my family."

Sandi Salera Lloyd, 38
book researcher
Allentown, Pennsylvania

"Before my relapse, I thought that taking care of myself was selfish. Now I realize that it's actually a very giving thing to do."
— SANDI SALERA LLOYD

You Betcha

"A few years ago, I told my sisters I was planning to run the Chicago marathon. They didn't believe I could, so I said, 'Wanna bet?' Michelle bet five bucks, Linda said she'd make my wedding cake, and Sandy bet $2,000 and said, 'No walking.'

"So I started training. At first, I couldn't go a mile without stopping. I called my sisters when I got up to five miles, and then 18, and they still said I'd never make it. None of them made good on their bets, but they did send me a pre-race care package. I finished Chicago in about four and a half hours, have run the Honolulu marathon, and hope to run New York this fall. Now, Michelle and Linda are marathon runners, but I'm sure Sandy never will be."

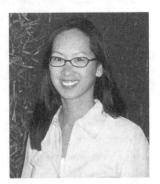

Jeannie Wong-Lin, 29
optometrist
San Francisco, California

Ready for Motherhood

"I started running in 1992 when I suffered a miscarriage and needed an activity to help me deal with my grief. Running helped prepare me for my second child by making me feel better about myself.

"A year after my second baby was born, I began running again. I realized I still needed it, but for a different reason: I craved time to myself. So I put on my personal stereo and listened to music, which really kept me going. Running recharges me, giving me the energy to keep up with my kids."

Patrice Deprey, 38
part-time bookkeeper
Frostburg, Maryland

A Healthy Legacy

"Three years ago, my healthy 60-year-old father had an emergency triple bypass. His doctors told us his clean lifestyle was the only thing that helped him survive: If my dad had been overweight, smoked, or drank, he would have died instantly.

"This made me dig up my family medical history. Turns out, both sides of my dad's family have chronic histories of heart and artery problems. I had to face the reality that I might suffer the same fate. So I began a huge lifestyle overhaul. Prior to my dad's operation, my diet consisted entirely of fast food, sweets, and soda. These days, I eat cereal and fruit for breakfast every morning and a healthy lunch and dinner. I did this all in stages—I did not change my life all at once. Each month, too, I tack on some new exercise. I get annual stress tests to monitor my heart, and I'm confident that while I may not be able to avoid a heart attack completely, I've increased my chances of surviving one."

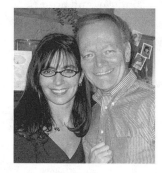

Christina Miranda, 31
public relations executive
New York City

A Life-Changing Remark

"I once overheard someone ask a colleague if I was pregnant. I wasn't, and the comment really hurt my feelings. And then I started thinking about it: I knew that I had been gaining some weight, and I certainly had not been doing anything about it.

"But hearing someone say that I looked fat jump-started me on a lifelong habit of exercise. That one comment—uttered long ago—made me vow to keep moving for the rest of my life!"

Lisette Roy, 46
librarian
Lehigh Valley, Pennsylvania

Running for Her Life

"At age 18, I was seriously depressed and contemplating suicide. I couldn't get out of bed in the morning and spent most of the day in a haze, so I decided to see a psychotherapist. She wanted to put me on an antidepressant, which would have been Ritalin (the only real option available in the early '70s). I didn't think medication was the answer for me. She also suggested exercise to get my blood flowing and to give my mind a break. I was willing to give it a shot, but I didn't really know where to start. So I headed to the track at Arizona State University and ran around once. That was a huge accomplishment; I was so proud of myself that I called a friend and told her, and she joined me the next day. After a month, I could run twice around the track, and before I knew it, I was running two or three miles twice a week. After about six months, the depression started lifting, and I realized that I'd found my cure. Running literally saved my life."

Sue Redding, 44
designer and professor of design
San Francisco, California

A Trip of a Lifetime

"Two years ago I decided to take my sons skiing for spring break. I went to the gym and told the trainers they had six weeks to make me strong enough to keep up with two teenagers on the slopes. The trip was a success: I kept up all four days. I still go to the gym

Discovering a personal health problem
is the number one reason women decide to
make health a priority, followed by having children—or being around
them—and the realization that they're getting older.
—*Health* WOMEN IN MOTION STUDY, 2001

> "I learned through meditation and yoga the level of commitment necessary to affect change, and that's what really made a difference in my life."
>
> — ANASTASIA LEVINSON

three times a week and work with a personal trainer. I also re-evaluated my eating habits: I limit desserts and try to fill up on fruits and vegetables. I'm more fit than ever, with lots of energy and focus."

Sharon Keys Seal, 47
business coach
Baltimore, Maryland

No More Quick Fix

"I was a product of the '80s—and you can read whatever you want into that—and I spent a lot of time lost and consuming everything in my path. About six years ago, though, I began taking some yoga classes, which pushed me both physically and mentally. Although I continued to eat Crunch Berries for dinner and drink six cups of coffee for breakfast, a four-month spiritual retreat to an ashram made me re-examine my attitude toward wellness.

"I came from a quick-fix approach: lose 10 pounds in a week, go to the gym for four hours every day for a month, put 18 carrots in the juicer and drink it all now. But I learned through meditation and yoga the level of commitment necessary to affect change, and that's what really made a difference in my life."

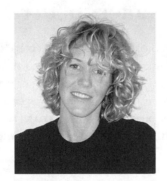

Anastasia Levinson, 35
yoga instructor
Miami Beach, Florida

Scoot for a Cure

"In August 2000, my spark plug of a mom was diagnosed with ovarian cancer. She died four weeks later. To honor her and get over my grief, I wanted to do the wildest thing I could imagine: I decided to ride my scooter 1,000 miles down the Pacific Coast, from southern Washington state to San Francisco over 48 days (during June and July 2001). On my way, I'll be raising money for the Lynne Cohen Foundation, an organization dedicated to finding an early-detection test for ovarian cancer. Although I was a gymnast in college and ran competitively in my 20s, I've never before taken on a challenge of this magnitude. But I'm serious about this, so I sold my car in September; for the past seven months, my scooter has been my sole mode of transportation.

"A week before my mom died, I told her about my adventure. Though normally overconcerned, she gave me an all-understanding smile and said, "Go for it!"

Ally Lecaux, 45
special projects coordinator
Eugene, Oregon

Who, Me?

"I'm pretty astute at picking up on heart problems in other people, but I never thought I'd end up having a heart attack at age 49. Just last year, though, I had indigestion for three days—and treated it myself with an over-the-counter acid reliever—before deciding to have an electrocardiogram. I wasn't experiencing any of the classic symptoms of a heart attack, and, besides, I was too young to worry about having one.

"I was wrong. I ended up in the hospital's coronary care unit and having angioplasty to open the blockages in two of my arteries. Because of my experience, I try to make more time for my family and myself. I think my attitude has changed too. If something doesn't turn out exactly the way I want it to, it's OK."

Deborah Beiter, M.D., 50
family practitioner
Little Gap, Pennsylvania

Whole Grains May Help Reduce Stroke Risk

FROM NUTTY WHOLE WHEAT slices to chewy quinoa to earthy risotto, whole grains bring a welcome richness to any meal. But the rewards go beyond taste: Grains may just save your brain.

In an early study, Harvard epidemiologist Simin Liu reported that the right kind of grains can greatly cut one's heart disease risk (see page 9 for more information). Could whole grain foods protect against strokes as well? He tapped into the Nurses' Health study, an ongoing project that has tracked 121,000 women for the last 25 years. After singling out 75,000 women with no history of cardiovascular disease or diabetes, Liu analyzed their eating habits over the past decade. Those who had eaten the most whole grains—2.7 servings a day—reduced their risk of ischemic stroke by more than 40 percent compared with women who consumed the least, less than half a serving.

Unfortunately, that's just what the average American gets—about a half-serving daily. Most people eat refined grains, such as white bread and pasta, that have been stripped of the nutrients that Liu thinks are critical—antioxidants; vitamins B-6, B-12, and E; and minerals like magnesium and potassium.

Getting more whole grains is easy, says Liu. "Try substituting foods," he says. "Replace white rice with brown, processed cereals with bran, and have some popcorn the next time you go to the movies."

New pill takes yuck factor out of colonoscopy

Does even hearing the word *colonoscopy* make you cringe? Then swallow this: Researchers at Georgetown University are testing vitamin-sized capsules equipped with miniature video cameras to film the entire intestinal journey, stem to stern. Patients just pop the pill, don a small waist pack with a recorder that captures two images per second, and let nature run its course. The gizmo could replace the more invasive procedure. Food and Drug Administration approval is expected soon.

the delivery room aide that guarantees better labor, drug-free

Wouldn't it be great if someone came up with a drug that reduced time in labor by 25 percent, and halved the need for cesarean sections, epidurals, and painkillers? That day is here, but not because of any pill or injection, according to a study from Cleveland's Case Western Reserve University School of Medicine.

Researchers point to the growing number of doula-assisted labors. A doula—derived from a Greek word meaning "woman in service to another woman"—is trained and certified by a childbirth-education organization, such as Doulas of North America (DONA), Birthworks, or International Childbirth Education Association. Unlike midwives, who are medical professionals, doulas don't make clinical decisions; they offer emotional support and manage pain with nonmedical techniques like massage, birthing positions, and acupressure.

John H. Kennell, M.D., the Case Western pediatrics professor who conducted the study, found that doula-assisted moms smile at, talk to, and stroke their babies more than those who don't use doulas. He attributes that to doulas' ability to reduce the stress and anxiety that can surround the birth of a child.

"If a deer is laboring in the woods and senses danger, she'll stop her labor and move to somewhere safe before she has her baby," says Jessie Levey, a childbirth-preparation educator at Elizabeth Seton Childbearing Center in New York. "Women also need to feel 100 percent safe for labor to progress smoothly. Having a doula provides that security."

Almost unheard of a decade ago, doulas were attending about 40,000 U.S. births a year by the late 1990s, DONA estimates. Their fees range from $300 to $1,500, depending on experience and location; insurance doesn't cover that cost in most states.

If you'd like to find a doula near you, ask your obstetrician or midwife, or check out the DONA referrals online at www.dona.com.

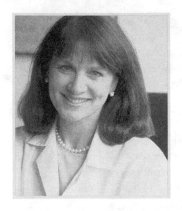

Good Question
about Women's Health

by Nancy Snyderman

Estrogen Creams: Are They a Safe Treatment for Vaginal Dryness?

My doctor suggested an estrogen cream to treat vaginal dryness, but I'm concerned about the breast cancer risk associated with hormone replacement therapy. Is a cream as dangerous as estrogen in a pill?

No one really knows, and anyone who says he or she does isn't telling the truth. I could easily make the case that the amount of estrogen absorbed through the vaginal lining is probably not high enough to raise your risk. Also, the estrogen dose in a pill is much higher than it is in a cream. But it's still more hormone going into your body than Mother Nature intended, and there's no conclusive evidence about the comparative cancer risks of each version.

Also, some experts are concerned that because the cream is absorbed close to the uterus, it could raise your risk of developing endometrial hyperplasia, which can be a precursor to endometrial (uterine) cancer. For this reason, they recommend that anyone with an intact uterus also take progesterone to cancel out any potential risks.

The bottom line? If my family had a history of any kind of cancer in which hormones play a role—and that includes breast, ovarian, uterine, or prostate cancer—I'd ask my doctor for an alternative. Astroglide, for example, is a wonderful lubricant, and it's a whole lot more fun than an estrogen cream that you put in yourself, long before you have sex. With Astroglide, your partner and you can use it together as part of your sexual play. But if you don't have a worrisome family history or a particular fear

of breast cancer, your doctor's advice may be perfectly reasonable. Only you can decide.

The Link Between HRT and Asthma

I'm thinking of going on hormone replacement therapy (HRT). Is it true that taking estrogen might worsen my asthma?

The therapy certainly seems to raise a woman's chances of developing the disease, according to a recent finding from the landmark Nurses' Health Study. The higher the estrogen dose and the longer the women were on the hormone, the greater the risk; those women who took it for more than 10 years were the most likely to develop the disease. And adult-onset asthma is certainly no picnic. Common symptoms include difficulty breathing, shortness of breath, and dry cough. If left untreated, it can even be fatal.

In adults, the disease hasn't become the epidemic that we've been seeing in children, but it's not uncommon; the rate has risen over the last two decades. And women are at slightly higher risk than men, especially those with a history of allergies or skin problems, such as eczema.

As for women like you who have asthma, it's not so clear whether estrogen will cause problems. The nurses' study didn't look at that question, and the link between HRT and regular asthma hasn't been clearly established. Still, there is some connection between asthma and a woman's hormones—many women experience asthma for the first time during puberty, pregnancy or menopause—and research continues on this point.

The bottom line on all this confusion? The HRT-asthma link is definitely worth being aware of, but it's not strong enough at this point to keep you off the therapy. Just watch out for any new symptoms and stay in touch with your doctor.

The Facts About Tubal Ligation and Menopause

I had my tubes tied when I was in my mid-30s, and now I'm about to hit menopause. Will the tubal ligation make menopause any easier?

Lots of women ask me this question, and the short answer is no. A tubal ligation—in which the Fallopian tubes are closed off to prevent eggs from meeting sperm—will not alter the normal course of menopause. The Fallopian tubes have nothing to do with the production of hormones, which is the main factor in menopause.

Nor will this procedure speed up the onset of menopause, as some women who experience post-tubal ligation symptoms, such as pelvic pain and painful intercourse, may think. These symptoms occur only in a very small percentage of women who have tubal ligations near the onset of menopause, but these women shouldn't assume the two are in any way connected. Even though doctors have had a difficult time explaining the precise reason for these symptoms, they believe the most likely cause is scarring or damaged blood vessels in the pelvic region caused by surgery.

The one way tubal ligation will make the onset of menopause easier: It eliminates worries about unplanned pregnancy as your periods become infrequent. And that's no small comfort.

The Test That Rules Out Cervical Cancer

I just got what my doctor called an ambiguous result on my Pap test. Should I consider the HPV test?

That's easy: Yes. But stay calm. Most women (90 percent) who get an ambiguous result don't even have a precancerous condition, much less cancer. Any number of benign problems, including yeast infections, can cause that kind of finding on a Pap

smear. That's why women are generally told not to worry but to get retested in four to six months. But who wants to wait up to six months to find out she doesn't have cancer? One alternative is to have a colposcopy, in which the doctor examines your cervix. Problem is, that test is expensive and uncomfortable, and it can lead to unnecessary treatment.

That's where the HPV test comes in. We know that HPV, or human papillomavirus, is a sexually transmitted virus that causes the majority of cervical cancers. Over the past several years, researchers have been trying to determine whether testing for it can tell us which ambiguous Pap results are truly worrisome and which are not. Now a recent study suggests that it can.

The study looked at 3,488 women with ambiguous Pap results. Only about 10 percent of the women turned out to need treatment, and the HPV test identified over 96 percent of them. Of the women with no HPV infection, 99.5 percent did not have cancer or precancerous cells.

The bottom line: If you test negative for HPV, you can be pretty sure you're home free. Even if you test positive, it doesn't mean you have cancer. In most HPV cases, the infection is transient and will disappear within a few months. Still, your next step should be to have a colposcopy. If there's an area that looks abnormal, the doctor can treat it right then by removing the cells or by freezing them, which kills them.

The Eye Ailment That Plagues Mature Women

I've been jogging more now that the weather's gotten nice, but I often find that my eyes start burning and itching. What's going on?

It could be allergies, but do you also experience this when inside, say, staring at the computer? If so, you might have a condition called dry eye syndrome (DES). It occurs when you don't make enough tears or they evaporate too quickly, leaving your eyeballs short on the lubricant they need. In addition to burning and itching, you may feel you've got sand in your eyes, and your contact lenses might be uncomfortable. In extreme cases, your eyes get so dry the corneas scratch easily, which can lead to vision loss.

About 1 million Americans suffer from severe DES, but about 10 million have a milder version. It's more common in women than in men, and it tends to come on around menopause, when declining hormone levels cause all sorts of membranes in the body to dry out. DES can also be the result of a rare autoimmune disorder called Sjögren's syndrome.

If you have severe DES, you may need to have a doctor insert tiny plugs into the ducts that drain tears out of the eyes. But for many people, eyedrops that are basically artificial tears can solve the problem. They come in a variety of formulas, so see an ophthalmologist if you have trouble finding one that works for you. Also, reduce your exposure to anything that speeds the evaporation of tears. Wear glasses or goggles when you're outside, and stay away from cigarette smoke and dusty environments. Jog in the morning, when the pollen hasn't yet been kicked up. And don't forget to blink. Staring leaves time for tears to dry up.

Where Wart Viruses Lurk—and How to Cure Them

I developed a wart on the bottom of my foot, and I'm wondering where it came from. How can I get rid of it?

Warts are so common. I don't know of any teenager who has escaped getting one. Warts that pop up on the bottom of the foot—called plantar warts—are one of the most common types.

Warts are caused by pesky viruses that live for a long time outside the body. These viruses love dark, moist areas, which is why toes are especially prone to getting them. It also explains why warts are so easy to get in areas like locker rooms and indoor pools.

The best thing to do about warts is prevent them. Keep your feet clean and dry. Avoid walking barefoot and wear flip-flops when you're in moist areas.

If I were to get an isolated wart, I would try any of the over-the-counter products first. Formulas with salicylic acid are terrific for treating warts, and most of the time they work. But if the wart is stubborn, if you have more than one, or if you're just worried, you should make an appointment with a dermatologist or podiatrist.

The two most straightforward ways a doctor treats warts are with liquid nitrogen or lasers. Liquid nitrogen freezes the tissue so that the wart falls off; lasers, which are likely your last resort because of the possibility of scarring, cut off the wart's blood supply. Unfortunately, whichever path you take, you may have to be persistent: Plantar warts tend to recur.

How to Stop Non-Stop Colds

I've had one miserable cold after another this year. Is there anything new I could take to treat them?

You might be interested in a study I saw recently about the medicinal power of chicken soup. No one's proclaiming it a wonder cure—nothing cures the common cold—but apparently old-fashioned chicken soup actually contains some substances that may ease your symptoms.

This won't come as a surprise to any good Jewish mother. You've heard the expression "Jewish penicillin?" Using chicken soup to treat a cold dates back to the Greeks, but in the 12th century, the Jewish physician Moses Maimonides gave it his professional stamp of approval. Now the "treatment" seems to have 21st-century science on its side.

Many cold symptoms are thought to be the result of an inflammatory response initiated by the virus (or viruses) that trigger the cold. When chicken soup was tested in the lab, it seemed to inhibit the activity of particular proteins that cause inflammation. And don't feel you have to slave over a hot stove. Several commercially prepared soups tested just as well as the researchers' homemade version. Five varieties even outperformed it.

While you're at it, you might also try taking zinc and echinachea at the first sign of a sore throat, achiness, or runny nose. They might lessen your symptoms or clear them up more quickly. With zinc, aim for a high dose: about 80 milligrams a day. For echinacea, try one dropperful of tincture in water four times a day.

Nancy Snyderman, M.D., is a medical correspondent for ABC News and author of *Guide to Good Health for Women Over Forty* (Harvest Book, 1996).

HEALTH BUZZ

THUMBS UP

the new gym

Hospitals across the country are opening fitness centers for those folks who might find the spandex-clad members of the neighborhood gym a bit intimidating. Hospital gown not required for membership.

mammograms

According to a recent study conducted by the American Cancer Society, women who get regular screenings reduce their risk of dying from breast cancer by 63%—about double what was previously thought.

safe sex

Planned Parenthood makes it even easier to plan. The famed abortion-rights organization now offers its own brand of condoms—at little or no cost to you—with its toll-free number printed on the wrapper.

THUMBS DOWN

forget the flashy kicks

A study of weekend athletes who wore sneakers with air cells—pockets of air in the heels meant to cushion hard landings—were more than four times as likely to sustain an ankle injury as those wearing sneakers without air-filled soles.

recess gets the bell

Because of increased academic demands and skittishness over playground fights, school districts across the nation have decided to reduce or even eliminate playground time.

petting zoos

The Centers for Disease Control and Prevention warns that thousands of children are exposed to the bacteria *E. coli* by touching farm animals in zoos and at fairs.

SELF-CARE
how to give yourself an effective breast exam

You probably think that doing a breast self-exam is one of the 10 commandments of health, along with schlepping to the gym and flossing. So you may be surprised to hear that there's little evidence showing that the exam helps detect early cancers. Still, many experts think self-exams are worthwhile because they familiarize you with normal monthly changes so you'll be better able to help your doctor distinguish run-of-the-mill lumps from troublesome ones.

A good rule of thumb is to examine your breasts when they are least swollen and tender (generally, a week after your period ends). If you're no longer menstruating, do the exam on the same day of every month. Here's what to do:

1. Lie down flat with a pillow or folded towel under your right shoulder. This spreads the breast tissue across the rib cage, making changes easier to find.

2. Raise your right arm over your head. Check for lumps in the right breast with your left hand. Use the finger pads (the most sensitive part of the hand) of the three middle fingers. Exert enough pressure to feel your rib cage beneath the breast tissue.

3. Move around the breast in either a spiral, an up and down, or a wedge pattern (as though your breast were a pie and you're feeling each piece). Don't forget the tissue that moshes toward your armpit; half of cancerous lumps are found in this area. Get to know your breasts by using the same pattern every month.

4. Put the pillow under your left shoulder, raise your left arm, and repeat the exam using the finger pads of the right hand.

5. Finally, stand in front of a mirror with your arms at your sides. Examine your breasts for any irregularities—such as puckering or dimpling that make the skin look like that of an orange—or changes in size or shape.

When to see a doctor

If you find a lump, thickness, or dimpling, or if you experience nipple discharge or redness, see a doctor right away. Otherwise, until age 39, women should have a doctor examine their breasts every three years. For those age 40 and over, an annual clinical exam and mammogram are recommended.

chapter 2

weight
loss

yes, you can!

from Atkins to the Zone

Which diet is right for you? Here's our verdict on the three most popular eating plans.

INTERVIEWS BY CASSANDRA WRIGHTSON

PHOTOGRAPHY BY DAN CHAVKIN

You've heard it countless times: All you have to do to lose weight is eat sensibly and exercise regularly. Problem is, most of us need a bit more guidance. That's why diets can be so appealing: They tell us what to eat and when to eat it. They make mindful eaters out of mindless feeders, order out of chaos.

As a nation, we apparently crave that structure. An estimated 50 million Americans will go on a diet this year. Type the words weight loss on Amazon.com, and you'll have over 1,200 books to choose from. Friends, relatives, coworkers—it seems like everyone is shunning fat or sugar or starches, while embracing fruit or protein or fiber. To help you through the maze, we've scrutinized dozens of weight-loss plans for the new book *The Diet Advisor* (Time Life, 2001). In this excerpt, we give you the goods on three of the most popular plans:

Weight Watchers, the Zone, and the Atkins diet. Each has its strengths and weaknesses (we tell you what they are), and each asks you to be disciplined, to make trade-offs and choices that may test your willpower.

But as the women here make clear, these plans really can help you lose, at least in the short term. There's no single approach that works for everyone; the challenge is to pick one that fits your life and doesn't harm your health. So assess the options before you choose. You *can* have the healthy body you want.

the plans at a glance

	CARBS	PROTEIN	FAT	CALORIES
Dr. Atkins*	5%	32%	63%	1,800
The Zone	40%	30%	30%	1,700
Weight Watchers**	55%	25%	20%	1,500

*percentages during the diet's initial weight-loss stage
**percentages vary slightly with the individual

the atkins diet

ROBERT ATKINS, A CARDIOLOGIST and the founding father of the low-carbohydrate movement, says you'll never go hungry on his diet. In his latest book, *Dr. Atkins' New Diet Revolution* (Avon, 1997), Atkins claims his plan has helped more than 20 million dieters lose weight and keep it off. Cut carbs to the bone, eat all the fat and protein you want, and watch the pounds drop away.

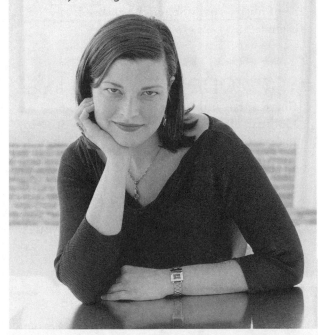

"I never was a big pasta fan, but I do miss bananas, cereal, and bread. And I would normally eat more vegetables than are allowed. But the Atkins diet is definitely working for me."

How Atkins Says It Works

Atkins believes that most people's weight problems stem from the way their bodies process carbohydrates. When you eat carbs, blood sugar rises and the pancreas produces insulin. In overweight people, according to Atkins, the insulin results in excess body fat. When you banish carbohydrates, he says, your body enters ketosis, a state in which you burn fat and your food cravings disappear.

What You Have to Do

Grab your carb counter and hold on. In the first stage of this diet, you limit carbohydrates to 20 grams a day (the average person takes in about 250 grams). During this two-week period, you may lose up to 16 pounds. In the next two stages you'll keep losing weight—albeit more slowly—and can add

Lauren O'Brien, 35, corporate caterer
Time on the Atkins diet: 5 months
Weight lost: 25 pounds

WHEN I CHANGED JOBS a year ago, I gained a lot of weight. Even though I'd never really felt fat before that, I'd tried every diet imaginable. I particularly liked the *Fit-or-Fat* series by Covert Bailey. It's a low-fat, high-fiber diet with a heavy emphasis on exercise. But that's time-consuming, and I wanted to lose weight fast. When someone gave me the Atkins book, I thought his plan looked kind of interesting. My roommate was just starting on it, so I decided to do it, too.

I try to stick to the prescribed diet as much as possible. I hold my carb intake to less than 35 grams. So obviously I never eat bread, pasta, cookies, sugar, or fruit. I like protein-rich foods a lot, so I have no problem eating meat all the time. I used to have oatmeal with wheat toast and a tall latte for breakfast, and I'd just crash a few hours later. Now I typically have a cheese omelet, three slices of bacon, and a cup of black coffee. And I don't experience that midmorning crash. I used to get sugar cravings every afternoon, so I'd always have a cookie. Then I'd just crash again. Now if I feel hungry between meals, I'll have a couple of slices of tomato and mozzarella or some tuna with olives.

I never was a big pasta fan, but I do miss bananas, cereal, and bread. And I would normally eat more vegetables than are allowed. But the diet is definitely working for me. For the first time in as long as I can remember, I'm not counting calories or fat grams, and I like that. I'm happy with my weight loss, but I'd like to lose a total of 30 pounds. I am getting sick of eating the same old things, though. I mean, how much tuna can a gal possibly eat?

a few grams of carbs a day. Once you reach your weight goal, you're in the lifetime maintenance stage. Now the trick is to figure out how many grams of carbohydrates you can eat without gaining weight back. For most people it's between 40 and 60 grams a day.

At every stage, you're allowed unlimited meat, eggs, and fatty foods. You will, however, have to stay away from whole grains, beans, breads, most fruits, and starchy vegetables. And it's farewell forever to ice cream, cookies, and anything else made with refined sugar.

What's Really Going On

Despite Atkins's claim that carbohydrates are to blame for obesity, the simple fact remains that it's calories that add pounds. Some people do lose weight on low-carb diets, probably because they're consuming fewer calories. Nutritionists credit water loss for the dramatic drop in weight during the first stage of this diet.

There is a biological state called ketosis, but there's no firm proof that it can curb appetite. And with side effects ranging from queasiness and bad breath to dehydration and weakened bones, ketosis is not the charmed condition Atkins makes it out to be.

Should You Try It?

Instant gratification is almost guaranteed: The dress you can't quite zip up today will fit perfectly next month. But the regimen is hard to stick with over the long haul, and the weight creeps back on as soon as your carb intake climbs back up.

If you don't dwell on the loss of noodles and baguettes, you probably won't go hungry. You can throw out the calorie counter and let yourself loose in the butcher shop. But there's a shadow over this picture: Any diet that offers unlimited saturated fat and cholesterol-rich foods is dangerous. Furthermore, the plan eliminates or drastically reduces foods known to reduce the risk of heart disease and some cancers, and it falls short on calcium and fiber.

Low-carb diets don't have to be this perilous. If you want to try one, go for a plan that restricts saturated fats and allows a more liberal daily helping of nutritionally beneficial carbs—fruit, for instance, or whole grain breads.

the zone

BIOCHEMIST BARRY SEARS, co-author of *The Zone* (Harper-Collins, 1995), has developed a high-protein, low-carbohydrate diet that he says will alter your hormonal balance and send you into a near-euphoric state called the Zone. Sears claims that once you're in the Zone, hunger-free weight loss is almost automatic. Eventually, he adds, your mind will be sharper and you'll be less bothered by common ailments such as colds and allergies.

How Sears Says It Works

According to Sears, eating carbohydrates raises the amount of sugar in the blood, which leads to high insulin levels and increased body fat. His theory of losing that fat rests on a series of interactions involving insulin, glucose, fat, and so-called super-hormones. The drama is directed by the foods you eat. Consume carbohydrates, protein, and fat in the right amounts at the right times of day, and excess body fat will be vanquished.

Getting to the Zone

Sears says that you must eat food steadily and in the proper proportions, "as if it were an intravenous drip." He lays out a system of carb, protein, and fat "blocks" with which you build three meals and two snacks a day. At each meal and snack, carbs are relegated to 40 percent of total calories and protein and

splenda:
A no-calorie sweetener that's just like sugar

Good news if you're looking to lighten up your favorite cookie and cake recipes: Splenda, a no-calorie sweetener that measures and pours just like the real deal, is now available in granular form for use at home. Unlike artificial sweeteners, Splenda—which is actually derived from sugar—stays sweet at high temperatures.

fat to 30 percent each. The diet weighs in at about 1,700 calories.

Sears recommends only low-fat protein, fiber-rich carbs, and monounsaturated fats. On the get-over-it list are most breads, rice, pasta, carrots, corn, peas, potatoes, bananas, raisins, papayas, fruit juices, ice cream, honey, and sugar.

What's Really Happening

Most experts say that elevated insulin levels do not lead to excess weight; in fact, there is no reason to pin obesity on a diet rich in carbohydrates, unless that diet is also rich in calories. Sears's complex theories of hormonally regulated weight loss have little scientific support. If you lose weight on this plan, it's probably because you're taking in fewer calories, not because you've taken a trip to the Zone.

Should You Try It?

If you're willing to spend time constructing Zone-favorable meals, cut back the bread, and crank up the protein, this diet will probably work for you. Despite a somewhat joyless approach to cuisine (remember that intravenous drip?), Sears recommends a plentiful pantry of healthy foods. You'll get to eat lean cuts of chicken and fish, abundant fruits and veggies, and oatmeal, if not pasta. Nothing is absolutely forbidden; if you do slip out of the Zone, you can easily re-enter.

Don't follow this diet if you have liver or kidney disease. If you have heart disease or diabetes, check with your doctor first.

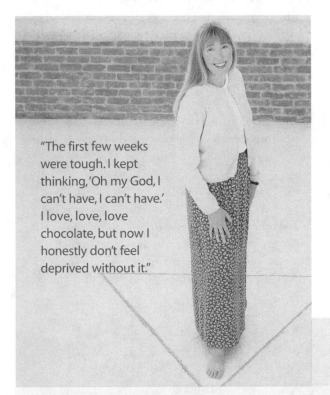

"The first few weeks were tough. I kept thinking, 'Oh my God, I can't have, I can't have.' I love, love, love chocolate, but now I honestly don't feel deprived without it."

Denise Howe, 32, teacher
Time on the Zone: 1 year
Weight lost: 20 pounds

FIRST TRIED THE ZONE three years ago because my girlfriends at work were on it. But when I left that job to go back to school, I also went off the diet. My eating habits really went to pot. I probably ate 18 out of 21 meals in my car commuting to classes. When I finally earned my teaching degree, I just felt crummy because of how unhealthy my eating habits had become. And, not surprisingly, I had gained 10 pounds. That's when I made up my mind to start Zoning again.

The first few weeks were tough. I kept thinking, "Oh my God, I can't have, I can't have." I love, love, love chocolate, but now I honestly don't feel deprived without it.

People think the diet sounds complicated, but you become more aware of what food combinations work. At first I was very particular. I weighed and measured everything. But then I got really good at eyeballing foods.

You do eat a lot, but it's low-calorie. My rule of thumb is no white food. I don't eat pasta, bread, or rice. Occasionally, I'll eat a whole wheat pita. A snack for me is an apple, an ounce of Cheddar cheese, and a few almonds. And that tastes great.

I need to eat every four to five hours, as Sears recommends, because if I don't I start feeling sluggish. But I don't have mood swings like I used to, and I feel more peaceful. My energy level is great, and I never have that ugh-I've-eaten-too-much feeling.

I feel so much better since I started back on the diet. We all pretty much fall into a pattern of eating the same things all the time anyway, right?

weight watchers

WEIGHT WATCHERS CLAIMS to have helped more than 25 million people trim down since its inception in 1963. Like most of the commercial company's programs, its current plan, *1-2-3 Success,* focuses on low-calorie, low-fat, high-fiber foods; regular exercise; and abundant support. For a fee, Weight Watchers will give you all the nutritional guidance and emotional inspiration you need to maintain a healthy weight.

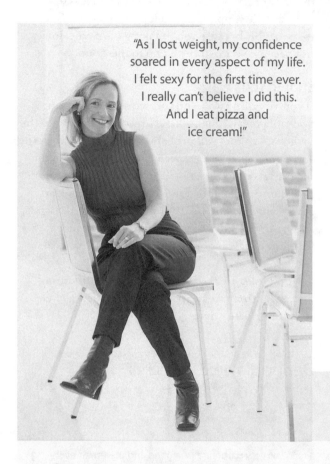

"As I lost weight, my confidence soared in every aspect of my life. I felt sexy for the first time ever. I really can't believe I did this. And I eat pizza and ice cream!"

How Weight Watchers Works

Unlike many fad diets, *1-2-3 Success* doesn't try to justify itself by way of intricate metabolic theories. At Weight Watchers, all calories are created equal, and each one you put in your mouth affects how much you weigh. The program helps you figure out what you need to eat, how you need to exercise, and how you need to think about food—and yourself—to reach your desired weight. It will then do everything it can to get and keep you there.

What You Need to Do

Under the plan, foods are assigned a point value based on calories, fat, and fiber content. You're allotted a range of total points each day, which you can "spend" however you like. The recommended food-group breakdown resembles the U.S.

Patricia Olsen, 42, asset manager
Time on Weight Watchers: 2 years
Weight lost: 31 pounds

I WAS ALWAYS CHUBBY growing up. But as desperate as I was to slim down, I didn't think I needed a diet. I just read nutrition books instead. When I turned 35, I felt like the clock told my body that it was going to fall apart—and my body listened. By the time I turned 40, I was up to 149 pounds, and I'm only five foot two. I told my doctor that I'd die if I saw 150 pounds on the scale, so he suggested that I try Weight Watchers.

The first three weeks I lost no weight. I was so discouraged that I cried my eyes out at a meeting one night. The holidays were approaching, and I didn't want to spend another Christmas wearing an apron all day because I couldn't button my pants.

At the next meeting the group leader said something that resonated with me. Shedding pounds on Weight Watchers is like learning a language or a musical instrument: You can't just attend the meetings and not do the homework. I'd never bothered to read the materials or learn the point system. It was only after that night that the weight started to come off. Those weekly meetings sure make a difference.

I really can't believe I did this. I haven't been under 120 pounds since I was 12. And I eat pizza and ice cream! As I approached my goal weight last year, my confidence level soared in every aspect of my life. I felt sexy for the first time ever. And coincidentally—or maybe not—I met Prince Charming, and now we're married.

government's food pyramid: About half the day's calories should come from carbohydrates, such as beans and whole grains, 25 percent from protein, and 20 percent from fat.

If points and percentages are the heart of Weight Watchers, then group support is its soul. You are urged to attend a weekly confidential weigh-in and take part in at least one group meeting a week. At these sessions, a trained leader will dispense advice, listen to your food foibles, and cheer you up and on.

The Facts of the Diet

There's nothing outlandish here, although transforming eating habits requires time and patience. The National Weight Control Registry, which tracks people who have lost 30 pounds and kept them off for at least a year, offers evidence that supports Weight Watchers' kind and gentle approach. Of the registry's 2,800 participants, more than half

reached their goals not by torturing themselves on a fashionable diet but by reducing fat and calories, eating sensibly, and exercising.

Should You Try It?

If you play by the rules, you'll lose weight safely on this diet. It combines calorie cutbacks with exercise, which is what most experts recommend, and while it gives you the freedom to indulge, it encourages you to eat sensibly.

Weight Watchers makes no promises as to how quickly or how much you'll lose; short-term miracles are not part of the program; even the long-term ones cost money. The one-time registration fee is typically $16 to $20, and the weekly fee is around $10; a year can cost $540. If the thought of others keeping tabs on your progress—or your backsliding—makes you shudder, or if you're turned off by support groups, Weight Watchers is not for you. ✳

THE DIETER'S SELF-TEST

Have you crossed the line between healthy dieting and dangerous obsession?

STEVEN BRATMAN, a physician and author of *Health Food Junkies* (Bantam Doubleday Dell, 2001), says anyone who is trying to make a major change in her life—such as losing weight or becoming vegetarian—will by necessity be a bit extreme at first. "But at some point you should loosen up," says Bratman, a reformed obsessive eater himself. "Otherwise, you'll wind up a fanatic. "He calls over-righteous eating orthorexia (*ortho* is Greek for correct). Whether a superstrict approach to dining is really an eating disorder may be up for debate, but there's little doubt that the consequences of such behavior can be grave.

Here's how to find out if you've crossed into obsessive territory:

Give yourself a point for each of the following questions that you answer affirmatively. Don't worry if you get a few points: It just means you're human.

If you score four or more, Bratman says, you may want to reevaluate your eating habits.

If you need a little outside assistance, consider seeing a nutritionist or a therapist. He or she can help you plan a reasonable

diet and tease out emotional issues that might be contributing to your problem.

• Do you spend more than three hours a day thinking about healthy food and planning or shopping for your meals?
• Do you often dwell on tomorrow's menu today?
• Do you care more about the virtue of what you eat than the pleasure you receive from eating it?
• Has the quality of your life decreased as the quality of your diet has increased?
• Do you keep getting stricter with yourself?
• Do you sacrifice experiences you once enjoyed to eat the food you believe is right?
• Do you feel an increased sense of self-esteem when you are eating healthy food?
• Do you look down on others who don't?
• Do you feel guilt or self-loathing when you stray from your diet?
• Does your diet isolate you socially?
• When you eat the way you are supposed to, do you feel a peaceful sense of control?

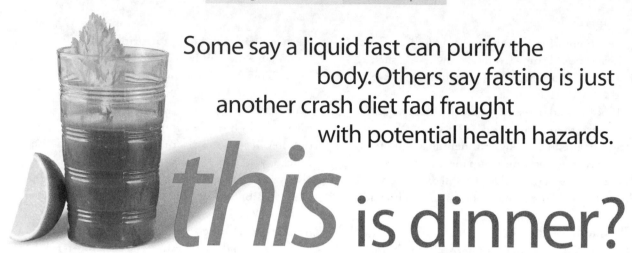

Some say a liquid fast can purify the body. Others say fasting is just another crash diet fad fraught with potential health hazards.

this is dinner?

BY LAURIE DRAKE

Yes, for a growing number of women on liquid fasts, it is. The long-discredited weight-loss fad, this time wrapped in promises that it can purify your body of modern-day pollutants, is finding new life across America. The result, then and now, is unchanged: It puts health in jeopardy.

Talk about reverse chic: One of the hottest spas in the country is on the wrong side of the tracks in Palm Springs, California. The We Care Holistic Health Center, a bougainvillea-shaded house surrounded by a fence in the desert, is about 8 miles north of the fancy resorts that give Palm Springs its upscale image. Here, there are no manicured golf greens, Olympic-size swimming pools, or Wimbledon-worthy tennis courts. The spa's "hiking path" is just a dirt road down to the main highway, but that's OK: No one comes here to exercise. They come to fast on vegetable juice, to drink teas they believe will rid their bodies of potentially dangerous toxic substances, and to lose weight. A lot of weight.

Women who come from New York, San Francisco, Tucson—anywhere the buzz has reached them about

We Care, which does no advertising—pay $750 for three days or $2,250 for a week, during which time they whittle down their diets to about 200 liquid calories a day and maybe rub shoulders with a supermodel or two. All ages and sizes, they hang out in the family room adjacent to the kitchen, where they drink one of 13 beverages they'll consume each hour from waking until just before bedtime; each beverage is checked off next to their names on a poster-sized chart tacked up by the refrigerator. When they're not downing a detox drink with psyllium (a natural laxative) or a shot glass of chlorophyll, or taking advantage of à la carte spa services such as massages and facials, they lounge around on big comfy couches and armchairs and talk in an informal kind of group therapy.

Of course, liquid fasts per se are not new. They were popular in the late 1950s and '60s, then again in the '70s when protein was added to the regimen. (Unfortunately, the protein used in one liquid diet, ironically named the Last Chance Diet, lacked an essential amino acid—not to mention vitamins, minerals, and electrolytes—and resulted in the deaths of 58 people.) What is new, and what makes today's fasts so alluring for so many women, is their promise of a detox. But are these newfangled fasts really the antidote to the pollutants and chemicals in the air we breathe and the food we eat? Or are they simply

While proponents believe these fasts purge the body of toxic substances, there is no evidence that fasting is a remedy. In fact, liquid fasts can cause a litany of frightening health consequences.

fad weight-loss regimens disguised as purification rituals in the name of personal health?

Ask a faster why she would submit her body to such a punishing regimen, and the ambivalence is obvious. "My naturopath told me I was a toxic time bomb," says We Care guest Janice (her name has been changed), a 45-year-old woman who admits to existing on Diet Coke, Big Macs, French fries, and Ding Dongs. But in the next breath, she mentions that she used to be thin when she was a high school cheerleader and that this is her seventh visit to We Care. Laetitia, an arthritic grandmother, came because her registered-nurse daughter sent her to lose weight. A beautiful young woman flips through a magazine, and only Laetitia has the nerve to ask, "Are you a model?"

Yes, she is: 24-year-old Michelle Behennah, who appeared in the 2000 *Sports Illustrated* swimsuit issue and can be seen on several Web sites created by devoted fans. "My model friends come here to slim down before fashion shows, but I'm here to rejuvenate my system and lose toxins," Behennah says. She's happy to reap the weight-loss benefits, though: In five days, she's shed seven pounds from her 5-foot-9½-inch, 145-pound frame. "I felt a little nauseous and light-headed in the beginning, but I've had more energy these last two days, and now I feel good; my brain feels clearer," she says. "I've never really been hungry, either. Every time I feel like eating, I have a sip of some juice or tea. I'm really happy I came, and I definitely want to come back in October for five days and then return for a week in January." On a wall at We Care is a gallery of runway regulars who, after their stays at the spa, send autographed photos of their sleek physiques, many bearing "We Care, we love you" or similar handwritten sentiments.

Admittedly, some of the guests can't wait to leave (and stop at the nearest Denny's). But others, like Behennah, get a high from juice fasting, and they are the ones driving this trend. They flock to supervised-fasting spas like the 15-year-old We Care, which is building more guest rooms. "We have a one-month waiting list to get in," says Susan Lombardi, one of the owners. Others head for the Optimum Health Institutes in San Diego, California, and Austin, Texas, which offer the "cellular detox program" and a three-day liquid diet of wheat-grass juice. More than

temporary loss

Sure, fasting will help you lose weight. But you'll gain it back—and maybe even more.

In 1996, 13 students participating in a hunger strike at California's Sonoma State University gave physicians at the university's health center a chance to see how starvation affects the body.

Eight of the protesters consented to testing, seven of them women. Their hunger strikes ranged from 5 to 11 days, during which time they drank only liquids: water, sports drinks, and fruit juices. Some also drank broth and milk, and most took vitamins. For some, the fast was a sort of mystical experience. Five of the students claimed that they gained spiritual insight through the trial. Several reported feelings of exhilaration, bursts of energy, and clarity of thought.

However, enlightenment wasn't the only result. Seven of the eight experienced an increased need for sleep. Six had fatigue and difficulty concentrating. Three suffered mild depression, which, for one student, continued after the strike ended. Two reported having difficulty driving a car.

But for women who are considering fasting, either at a spa or at home, one finding in the Sonoma State study stands out: While all of the students lost 5 to 8 pounds during the fast, six months later, all but one had gained back more than they had lost. This could be the result of a drop in metabolic rate that causes people on prolonged fasts to lose muscle tissue. Although this small study was preliminary, it should give prospective fasters reason to explore more healthful and effective options.

50,000 guests have stayed at the Institutes since 1976, and occupancy has soared in the last six months, says Judith Connelly, director of the Austin facility.

For around $800 a week, other fasting fans visit what we'll call "fast operators," private practitioners who take people into their own homes for juice cleanses, often including a colonic, an intensely uncomfortable process of flushing out the intestines with water. (Most fast operators shy away from the spotlight, attracting new clients strictly through word of mouth; when this writer called one such woman in Texas, the fast operator hung up as soon as she knew she was talking to a reporter.) Still others visit "fasting specialists," who operate out of clinics or retreat centers; the International Association of Hygienic Physicians lists 35 fasting specialists on its Web site.

Disciplined fasters do it themselves, buying ready-to-serve, imported plant juices (sold at such luxury retailers such as Nordstrom's) or adopting rigid liquid-diet plans outlined in books such as Dr. Jensen's *Guide to Better Bowel Care* (1998) which, according to Avery Publishing Group, has sold more than 1 million copies. Mark Stengler, author of *The Natural Physician's Healing Therapies* (Prentice Hall, 2001), says fasting is particularly hot in California because "it's such a health-crazed area." Stengler, a naturopath with a private practice in La Jolla, says, "A lot of my patients are women ages 35 to 40 who aren't necessarily sick, but their energy and skin could be better, and they have 4 or 5 pounds of cellulite or water retention they can't shake." He prescribes an "aggressive detox" home diet of fresh juices and green drinks, coupled with daily checkups and weigh-ins at his office.

The main drink of the day at We Care is a huge tumbler of vegetable juice served at about 1 p.m.: a choice of either a dark orange drink (a blend of carrot, beet, and tomato juices) or chartreuse green (wheat-grass, green cabbage, and parsley juice). The women drink what they can and stick it in the fridge for later. At 5 p.m., they get a mug of dark green pulverized vegetable soup that is downright savory (if lacking in salt). That's it, not counting the various capsules (enzymes, spirulina, acidophilus, fiber) taken throughout the day and washed down with herbal teas and little laboratory-like cups of blue-green algae. This meager menu of juice, soup, and pills makes the 1,200 calories per day recommended by the U.S. Department of Agriculture look decadent by comparison.

Such fasting regimens, proponents believe, cause the body to break down and purge tissue "diseased" from exposure to toxic environmental substances, which they think are responsible for all illnesses, from cancer to the common cold. But while it's true that environmental pollutants, even household chemicals, can collect in

your blood, there's no evidence that liquid fasts are the remedy. Indeed, what the women of We Care may think is a cure can actually cause a litany of frightening health consequences.

"There is no evidence that your body gets rid of old cells at an accelerated rate when you fast," says Janet Walberg Rankin, Ph.D., a professor in the human nutrition, foods, and exercise department at Virginia Tech in Blacksburg, Virginia. Rankin, who has studied the effects of fasting on healthy people, believes these kinds of fasts have the opposite effect of what some fasters are looking for. "Your body is always turning over old cells and old molecules. If anything, cellular turnover would slow down because when you fast, your metabolic rate declines," she says.

Under the kind of calorie restrictions proposed by many liquid fasts (200 calories a day or less), the body goes into survival mode, just as it would during starvation. Along with the drop in metabolism, body temperature, blood pressure, pulse, and breathing rate all fall. A healthy 35-year-old woman loses about $4\frac{1}{2}$ pounds of water in the span of a day or two, and her body begins to produce ketones, which make the blood very acidic, leaching calcium from her bones. She also loses muscle, can become constipated (thus the need for colonics), and burns off another 4 pounds of fat, bringing the total weight loss after one week to $8\frac{1}{2}$ pounds. That's compared with the 1 to 2 pounds per week most doctors recommend dieters.

And all this happens without medical supervision. There are no M.D.s on staff at We Care or the other fasting retreats, just disclaimers and liability waivers signed by each guest. (The We Care Web site offers this disclaimer on every page: We Care Holistic Health Center is not a medical facility. We do not give medical advice.) And few, if any, freelance fasting specialists have medical or nutrition degrees, even though they authoritatively dispense advice about what to eat (or rather, what not to eat), what to drink and when to drink it, and which supplements to take.

Thankfully, a faster's metabolic rate usually jumps back up to normal after a good meal, unless she has fasted for an extended period of time (from one to two

> Not all fasters spend big money at a spa. Some do it at home, drinking ready-to-serve plant juices and laxative teas.

weeks) and lost significant amounts of lean tissue and muscle, Rankin says.

Frequent fasting, though, can permanently reduce a woman's metabolic rate by causing a decrease in muscle tissue, which is more metabolically active than fat tissue. And, according to Rankin, a woman who fasts once a month "could be prone to the additive effects, over time, of loss of bone calcium and body protein." Unfortunately for a woman who undertakes "cleanses" in the name of thinness, the weight loss isn't permanent. As soon as she begins eating again, she will regain those initial pounds of water lost. Some evidence even suggests that fasters actually gain back more than they lose (see "Temporary Loss" on page 73).

So why do some women fast repeatedly? The attraction may be somewhat emotional, Rankin says. "Some people say they've never felt better on a very low calorie diet," she says. And even a cranky faster will smile at seeing her weight drop 4 pounds in a couple of days, even if it is caused by water loss. That quick weight loss motivates some women to suffer through their first fast and even return to fasting again and again, says Kelly Costello, Ph.D., a researcher at the Weight and Eating Disorders Program at the University of Pennsylvania School of Medicine. "But the large water-weight loss, which is regained quickly when you resume normal eating, can be very disappointing psychologically."

Marlene Schwartz, Ph.D., co-director of the Yale Center for Eating and Weight Disorders in New Haven, Connecticut, says that yet another reason some women fast repeatedly is the appeal of starting anew. "We live in a society where we love a quick fix, the idea that we can indulge and then somehow undo it all later," Schwartz declares. But that behavior can lead to an endless cycle of starving and overindulging. According to Schwartz, many repeat fasters are engaged in a process that is similar to bulimia, the disorder among women of normal weight who adopt over-restrictive diets and then go on food binges. Even a healthy woman could easily get caught up in a bulimic's binge-purge cycle after spending a week at a fasting spa. "You'll leave the spa literally starving, so that you overeat, which makes you feel bad about yourself because you've just been through this process of 'cleansing,' " Schwartz says.

Of course, some repeat fasters sincerely believe that they are protecting their bodies from the pollutants of the environment. Others simply use the "detox" label to legitimize what is essentially a crash diet. And some don't care what it's called, as long as they are able to drop a few pounds.

Losing those pounds is a gross exercise in self-denial at We Care, but it's a struggle repeat customers are willing to endure. Besides, they have an edge over the first-timers: They know a way to get more food. And that is to sign up for a cellulite treatment, an 80-minute scrub with fresh coffee grounds "to draw water from the tissues," followed by a shower, a massage, and a sauna. From there, customers are led to a bubble bath and handed potassium-rich pink smoothies to counteract the dehydrating effects of the sauna. The drinks are not rich—just ice, fresh strawberries, and whey protein—but customers sip them through straws like there's no tomorrow. Of course, as the brain gets back in gear, they are likely to realize that they have just paid $130 for a fruit smoothie.

To be fair, We Care does advise any guest who is experiencing migraines, headaches, or weakness to "come to the office for a drink that will raise your energy and ease your symptoms." But few do, because that would be admitting defeat among their fellow fasters. "I have a friend who came here and didn't even drink the evening soup, she was that competitive," Behennah says.

Psychologists call this powerful phenomenon "the group influence," and it exerts its pull in both healthy and unhealthy eating behaviors. It is the reason why Weight Watchers works, and it is why We Care works—for a short time, anyway. ✳

Laurie Drake is a contributing editor for Allure *magazine.*

> We live in a society where we love a quick fix, the idea that we can indulge and then undo it all later. But that can lead to an endless cycle of starving and overindulging.

HOLD ON TO YOUR TEACUP:
A recent study in the *New England Journal of Medicine* suggests that drinking green tea is not an effective way to prevent stomach cancer. Japanese researchers looked at the stomach cancer rates of green-tea sippers and found no improvement over those of folks who eschew the leafy brew. But that doesn't mean you've been left holding the (tea) bag: Another recent study in the *American Journal of Clinical Nutrition* found that green tea gives your metabolism a boost—and may help you lose weight.

ON THE WAY TO WEIGHT LOSS:
clothes that flatter your figure

LOOKING GOOD in your clothes while dieting is one of life's great fashion dilemmas. The best approach, says Cyndie Washburn-Nester, the senior fashion director for Casual Corner and August Max Woman, is to purchase a few select items that will flatter your figure until you hit that magic number.

In terms of tops, you might believe baggy is better, but think again. Formfitting knits or cotton-Lycra-blend T-shirts accent your silhouette and present a polished look. "Sweater sets are a smart choice because they offer a body-hugging shell and the camouflaging comfort of a cardigan," says Washburn-Nester. She recommends finding a pair with darts, to ensure a more tailored fit. Another way to get the same effect is with a collared men's-style shirt over a sleeveless shell or T-shirt.

Elastic waistbands are a simple way to avoid getting stuck with pants that look two sizes too big. "A pair of black wide-legged pants with a drawstring or elastic waist is an essential for every woman on a diet," she says. And, of course, dark colors do make you look thinner.

Finally, pick up the accessory of the season—a chain belt. Slung loosely around your waist, the belt can be adjusted to fit your slimming waistline. A geometric patterned scarf or pair of sexy high heels can also help jazz up your look—that is, until you're ready to ditch it all for a bikini.

rating the meal-replacement milkshakes

Frankly, we'd rather have some real food. Nonetheless, scads of dieters are popping open a meal-replacement shake and calling it lunch. So we decided to see what all the gulping is about. Here's how the top chocolate drinks stack up.

BRAND	CALORIES	SATURATED FAT	CARBS/FIBER	TASTE TEST
Ultra Slim Fast	220	1 g	40 g/5 g	Creamy, with a true cocoa flavor. We couldn't get one taster to stop drinking it. Our favorite.
Boost	240	0.5 g	41 g/0 g	The malty flavor brings back fond memories of Ovaltine. Too bad the consistency is more like chocolate milk than a shake.
Atkins	170	2 g	5 g/3 g	Painfully sweet, more fruity than chocolaty, with an artificial aftertaste.

Ephedra
Dieter's Miracle . . . or Menace?

Get the scoop on this popular herbal diet aid.
Supporters say the herb is safe and effective;
opponents say it's a dangerous drug that can kill.

BY TIMOTHY GOWER

Denise Brown was desperate to lose a lot of weight—no less than 40 or 50 pounds would do. So she didn't ask questions when a co-worker told her she was able to shed 25 pounds with the help of an herbal diet potion in the form of liquid drops. "I raced out and bought the stuff," Brown says.

Instead of losing weight, however, the 48-year-old nurse and mother of two teenagers from Northbrook, Illinois, found herself in serious trouble. After taking the drops daily for about four weeks, Brown suffered a stroke that paralyzed her left side. She's finally able to walk again, thanks to months of physical therapy. But her left arm is still so weak that she hasn't been able to return to her job working with severely disabled children. "I've lost my purpose in life," she says. "I feel like I lost part of my soul."

While still recovering in the hospital, Brown discovered that the diet drops she'd been taking contained

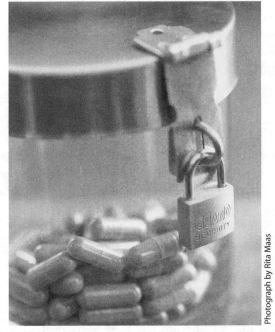

Photograph by Rita Maas

extract of a Chinese herb called ephedra, which she believes caused her stroke. She's now suing the company that manufactured the drops, and she's not the only one who's taking action. In February 2001, a jury in Alaska awarded more than $13.3 million to a woman who also suffered a stroke after using a similar ephedra product. That case appears to have opened the courtroom floodgates, with lawyers all over the United States reporting that they're hearing from clients who claim that supplements containing ephedra either sickened them or killed a loved one.

The combination of lawsuits and heightened media coverage has made the once-obscure herb one of the most controversial consumer products in the country. On one side are the many dieters and athletes who see ephedra as simply an easy way to lose weight and boost energy. On the other is a growing chorus of doctors and scientists who believe it is a potentially lethal drug that should be pulled from the market—an unlikely outcome, given that the federal government has so surprisingly little control over the sale of medicinal herbs. But despite claims of ephedra-related death and disability, this much is certain: The herb remains incredibly popular, with Americans buying an estimated 2 billion doses every year. And with that kind of consumer interest, this is a debate that won't end soon.

Ephedra, also known as *ma huang,* is a heart and brain stimulant. Its active ingredient is ephedrine, a synthetic version of which is sold in over-the-counter drugs used to treat asthma. Because ephedrine increases the heart rate, and some evidence suggests that it can cause the body to burn more calories, the herb ephedra is packed into a variety of "natural" diet and pep pills, powders, and other products.

Any reputable herbalist will tell you that ephedra can cause annoying side effects such as nervousness and insomnia, and at high doses, it may even increase blood pressure. In recent years, however, the U.S. Food and Drug Administration (FDA) has also received reports of at least 70 deaths and more than 1,400 "adverse events" involving people who had taken supplements containing ephedra. Those events included strokes, heart attacks, seizures, and psychotic episodes.

Despite those reports, companies can still legally sell products containing ephedra and other medicinal herbs without first proving they're safe to use, thanks to a law that Congress approved in 1994. While drugs like aspirin must undergo rigorous safety testing before they can be sold, ephedra and other herbs are considered safe unless the FDA proves otherwise.

Even in the face of that legislative obstacle, in 1997 the FDA proposed setting tough restrictions on the way ephedra is sold and manufactured, citing the numerous alarming reports it was getting regarding the herb. But that effort was blocked by the General Accounting Office (GAO), Congress' investigative arm that monitors government spending, among other things. Although the organization did find the long list of ephedra-related adverse reactions troubling, the GAO said that those allegations alone did not effectively prove that the herb is unsafe. After all, GAO officials reasoned, while some of the reports had been filed by doctors, others had come from consumers, who are encouraged to contact the FDA even if they're not sure

it was an herb that made them sick. In 1999 the FDA withdrew its 1997 report.

Despite the uncertainty of ephedra's safety, many Americans are willing to ignore what they read in the papers because they like what they see on the bathroom scale. Although research is limited, there is evidence to suggest that the herb helps some people lose weight. Nutritionist Carol Boozer of the New York Obesity Research Center led a study—sponsored by a consortium of supplement companies—in which overweight people who were otherwise healthy took a daily dose of ephedra and kola nut (the latter herb is a natural source of caffeine, which seems to heighten the effects of ephedra). On average, people in the ephedra group lost nearly 12 pounds, while those in a comparison group—who did not use the herbal concoction—lost half as much weight.

Some subjects in Boozer's study who took the herb experienced modest increases in blood pressure and heart rate, but none suffered life-threatening symptoms. "We found no evidence that ephedra is unsafe," she says. Boozer is quick to add, however, that more research is needed on short- and long-term use of ephedra.

While drugs like aspirin must undergo rigorous safety testing before they can be sold, ephedra and other herbs are considered safe unless the FDA proves otherwise.

In addition to funding Boozer's work, the supplements industry hired a team of Canadian consultants to review all the existing studies on ephedra and its main active chemical, ephedrine. That team concluded that healthy people can safely take up to 90 milligrams of ephedrine per day, roughly the maximum dose recommended by many manufacturers.

But ephedra's critics don't believe this research proves the herb is safe. Christine Haller, M.D., a medical toxicologist at the University of California at San Francisco, says most existing studies on ephedra have been small, while a large group of users would be needed to determine whether the herb poses a health risk. "You need to study thousands of people if you're looking for a rare event," Haller says.

Despite the uncertainty surrounding ephedra's safety, many Americans are willing to ignore what they read in the papers because they like what they see on the bathroom scale.

what's in that pill?

MEDICAL COMPLICATIONS may not be the only problem with ephedra supplements. According to a study published in 2000, ephedra users may not be able to trust the dosages listed on package labels.

University of Arkansas researchers analyzed 20 different brands of ephedra supplements and found that the amount of ephedrine and related active ingredients frequently did not match the amount listed on the label. One product had no ephedrine at all, for example, while the amount in some brands varied by as much as 260 percent from one lot to the next.

Still, Bill Gurley, Ph.D., professor of pharmaceutical sciences and the study's lead author, believes ephedra isn't the whole problem. Most diet and energy supplements that contain the herb are also laced with other herbs and natural compounds. Many, including ephedra, have druglike qualities—and like drugs, they may be dangerous when combined. "The more chemicals you have in there, the more chance there is for them to interact," Gurley says. "You're creating a pharmacological Pandora's box."

Haller and a colleague recently analyzed 140 reports of adverse effects the FDA received between 1997 and 1999. Their findings, published in December 2000 in the *New England Journal of Medicine,* suggest that about one-third of the cases were "definitely or probably" caused by ephedra, while another third may have been. The cases included 10 people who died and 13 who were permanently disabled.

Supplement-industry defenders suggest that the timing of some of those deaths and bad reactions may have been coincidental—that is, people died of another cause while they happened to be using ephedra. Cardiac pathologist Steven Karch, M.D., a consultant to the supplements industry, points out that several people listed in the *New England Journal of Medicine* article had serious health conditions that might have killed

them, including a teenage girl with a congenital heart defect. "It's a lethal malformation," Karch says. "This was a very sick child."

Others, Karch says, may simply have exceeded the recommended dose of ephedra. But Haller says she turned up a number of people who had no health problems when they began using ephedra, yet became seriously ill after taking small amounts of the herb—far less than the standard daily dose.

What's more, even people who know they should avoid stimulants such as ephedra are still at risk, because the law doesn't require these products to carry warning labels (some companies attach them anyway). Other consumers may have undiagnosed conditions such as hypertension that could make using ephedra deadly. In fact, about a third of the 50 million or so Americans who have hypertension don't realize it; when symptoms arise, they're often mild and progress slowly. And hypertension is common in people who are overweight—the largest group of ephedra users.

A long list of other conditions, including thyroid disease, diabetes, depression, and recurrent headaches, makes ephedra a dangerous way to lose weight. But Haller and others believe that some people who have none of these conditions may respond badly to the herb for unknown reasons. That's why Haller believes ephedra should be banned until it has been proven safe in tests involving large groups of people. In general, health experts recommend talking to a physician before taking any dietary supplement, especially if—like ephedra—it contains stimulants.

So the debate over ephedra continues. The herb seems to help some people lose weight, and legions take it without keeling over. Yet some people who use it get sick and even die, and there's no way of knowing who will be among the unlucky few. In Haller's opinion, the risk far outweighs the potential benefit. When people ask her if they should try ephedra, she responds with a question of her own: "Do you want to lose 10 pounds that badly?" ✳

Contributing editor Timothy Gower is co-author (with Robert S. DiPaola, M.D.) of A Doctor's Guide to Herbs and Supplements, *(Henry Holt and Company, 2001).*

step-by-step
WILLPOWER

Even marathon runners and personal trainers
can be putty in the hands of temptation.
We take a hard look at willpower
and help you hold fast to your resolve.

BY DOROTHY FOLTZ-GRAY

As the holidays approach every year, my mental spine goes limp. Yank myself out of bed and head to my strength-training class? It ain't gonna happen. Reach for a piece of fruit instead of the reindeer sprinkle cookie? Not a chance. In short, for 11 months a year, I'm blessed with a decent dose of what I call willpower. But in December, forget about it. I'm holiday's putty. By January, my soul needs the metaphorical equivalent of a shower and a shave. I'm bummed out because I bummed out—and I'm as bewildered as the next guy about this evaporated resolve.

What is this mysterious, elusive force called willpower? And where does it come from? Is it something that you're born with or something that you learn? And how come some people have a steely resolve, while others are merely temptation's puppet—especially around the holidays? And why is it possible to exert so much self-control about some things and so little about others?

I am not the only one perplexed by these questions. Scientists are rigorously plumbing the subject as well, although most of them eschew the term "willpower," uncomfortable with its moral implications. Instead, they delve into the origins of motivation and self-regulation, perseverance and restraint. And what they've come up with is a complex set of factors—some biological, some psychological, some environmental—that together determine the force responsible for getting you out of bed, helping you bite your tongue, pushing you to lace up your sneakers five times a week.

Most experts agree that willpower is not a magical resource. Rather, it is the ability to tackle challenges to meet particular goals—an ability that can be learned. Paul Karoly, Ph.D., a professor of psychology at Arizona State University in Tempe, says that one of the reasons willpower is so elusive is that sometimes a person's goal—exercising regularly, eating healthfully, or controlling her temper, for instance—is competing with other goals.

Failure to stick with a goal isn't the result of flimsy character, but an expression of priorities.

"Let's say you decide to start exercising," he says. "Exercise is now like the scrawny puppy fighting for milk among all the stronger puppies—your older, more valued goals. It's hard for the new goal to get a foothold." Failure to stick with one goal isn't the result of flimsy character, but an expression of priorities: Exercise may not be as important to you as, say, socializing or studying.

Even well-established habits have a hard time keeping their perch when routine is turned on its head, the very definition of a holiday. You may have every intention, for example, of sticking to your diet, holiday parties be damned. But after several such parties where food is the focus, your resolve may begin to sputter. As Karoly explains, your environment is at odds with your psyche, and absent the usual props a routine provides, environment may win out.

The biology behind this rumba of will and temptation is tough to unravel. But David W. Self, Ph.D., an associate professor of psychiatry at the University of Texas Southwestern Medical Center, offers one explanation. "We know that habit is based on learning and that the brain is organized in a way that reinforces habit," he says. "When an animal happens on something that it needs—food, water, a mate—a part of the brain called the dopamine system is activated so that the animal will remember how to find that thing. Humans have the same system."

The problem is that modern life—in which you don't have to forage for berries—leaves people plenty of time to form bad habits. And once you have learned a habit, such as lying around splat on the sofa every afternoon or munching on potato chips while you watch TV, it can't easily be unlearned. All you can do is overlay new learning on top of it. When you feel the urge to sink back into the cushions, for instance, you have to summon what Self refers to as "executive control"—the ability of the conscious brain to control the urges of the subconscious. That can be done, but it may require dogged focus until the new behavior becomes as ingrained as the old habit.

Complicating matters even further is that willpower is a limited resource. In several studies, Roy F. Baumeister, Ph.D., a professor of psychology at Case Western Reserve University in Cleveland, found that people have only so much self-control that they can expend. In one study, for example, Baumeister and his colleagues asked subjects not to think about white bears for five minutes. Of course, once the subject of white bears was introduced, it was difficult for the participants to think about anything else. To size up how much the task had taken out of them,

Whether your weakness is Krispy Kreme or a comfy couch, the good news is that you can conquer it.

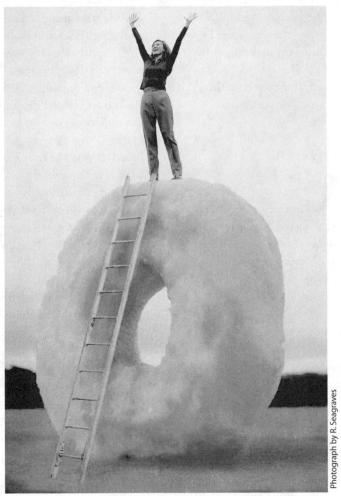

Photograph by R. Seagraves

Baumeister tested the subjects' stamina and perseverance by giving them hand grips and measuring how long they could squeeze them before and after the "white bear" task. The study participants typically released their grips faster the second time around.

The bad news: People have only so much self-control to expend.

Fortunately, you can increase your cache of willpower. Although everyone is born with an individual temperament, even those least drawn to discipline can pump up. For example, when Baumeister asked participants to focus for two weeks on improving their posture, most performed better on standard measures of self-control (such as willing themselves to keep their hands submerged in ice water) after the posture exercise than before. "How much better they did depended on how diligently they did the posture exercise," Baumeister says. "Exercising self-control every day over something they did not particularly want to do seemed to strengthen those capabilities."

Willpower is really about self-care.

So where does that leave you in December when you're on the verge of forgetting the "shoulds" and immersing yourself in holiday cheer? With decisions to make—not helplessness. Maintaining goals during the holidays is within your power—if you prioritize and plan. Here's how.

Decide what you want. It's tough to have willpower unless your priorities are clear. If you want to keep exercising over the holidays, for example, get out your calendar and schedule workouts around family events.

Publicize your plan. "Let people know in advance that on Monday, Wednesday, and Friday, you're going to be running at 9 a.m., and you may have to skip the pancake breakfast," suggests Robert Schleser, Ph.D., professor of psychology at the Illinois Institute of Technology in Chicago. "That way, you remain in control of what you're doing, and you can maintain who you are." And by telling others your plans, you enlist their help. Their knowledge of your goals adds the extra spark of a little outside pressure, what psychologists call extrinsic motivation.

The good news: Even those who are the least disciplined can learn new behaviors and increase their cache of willpower.

Don't up the ante. Holidays are not the right time to add on any new pressures. "Who needs to go on a seven-mile run Christmas Day?" Schleser asks. "Holidays are designed because humans need a break. Step back and evaluate what you need. If you are disciplined year-round, it may take a certain amount of discipline just to slack off." Karoly agrees: "Some people raise their standards over the holidays. But that only increases the likelihood of failure. Don't worry so much about being perfect."

Reward yourself. Sue Curry, Ph.D., director of the Health Research and Policy Centers at the University of Illinois in Chicago, tells the story of an ex-smoker who had suddenly begun experiencing cravings. Curry asked him what he had been doing to treat himself well. "'Nothing,' he said. He was feeling deprived in general," Curry says.

So when you're next tempted to skip your weekly Spinning session, promise yourself a massage after class. If you are determined to ignore chocolate over the holidays, don't fill up your days with hectic shopping. Skip the crowded mall and buy yourself some flowers instead, or go home and take a nice, long soak in the bathtub. That way, you won't feel like curling up with a candy bar later on in the day. Says Curry, "Willpower is really about self-care." ✳

Dorothy Foltz-Gray is a Health *contributing editor.*

CELLULITE SOS

There's nothing cuter than dimples on a baby (or Brad Pitt). But for the 85 percent of women who have some degree of cellulite, dimples are far from darling. What to do?

Cosmetic companies continue to introduce products that promise to shrink cellulite with ingredients such as herbs, eggs, and caffeine. Some experts question the effectiveness of these ingredients, but they suspect that massaging creams into the skin may produce temporary results. (A few to try: Darphin's Body Profile Complex, L'Avenir Cellutone, and Té Tao Toning Gel.) "Studies need to be done, but in theory it seems like there would be an improvement because massage can help move fluid out of the area, making cellulite less prominent," says Marsha Gordon, M.D., of the Mount Sinai School of Medicine.

For the same reason, hosiery may be temporary fix. Such products as Cellu-Lite Fashion Hosiery feature an ingredient that metabolizes fatty tissues. The company claims the panty hose reduce cellulite by 30 percent but must be worn all day for eight weeks to reap the full benefit. And at 16 pairs for $199, the hosiery is nearly as expensive as Endermologie, a cellulite-reduction massage treatment.

But remember that the cheapest—and most effective—cellulite-buster is still a healthy diet and aerobic exercise.

how about a broccoli sundae?

You weren't born hating Brussels sprouts—and Elizabeth D. Capaldi, Ph.D., professor of psychology at the University at Buffalo, contends that it's never too late to teach taste buds to like foods that are good for you.

Called "flavor-flavor" learning, Capaldi's theory involves attaching a yummy taste to a not-so-yummy food. A bit of sugar sprinkled on broccoli, for example, gives the palate the eat-more sign. The sugar can be gradually reduced until all that remains is the veggie—and your lifelong devotion to it.

the sure way to their hearts

Two-thirds of women show their love to people by cooking for them.
—*Health* WOMEN IN MOTION STUDY, 2001

THE LATEST FAT BUSTER—LICORICE

Giving in to candy cravings might not be such a bad thing for your hips after all. In a small study, Decio Armanini, M.D., and his colleagues at the University of Padua in Italy gave a group of men and women unsweetened extracts of licorice every day for two months. Though none of the volunteers lost weight—the licorice spurred water retention—they did shed fat. Women dropped 2.5 percent of their body fat, while men reduced their body fat by 1.5 percent. Armanini isn't sure why licorice encouraged fat loss, but he says that its active ingredient, glycyrrhizic acid, blocks an enzyme involved in fat storage and could send your body into a desirable fat-burning mode.

Before you indulge your sweet tooth, know this: Eating as little as 50 grams of licorice a day (about the size of a few jelly beans) has been shown to cause an increase in blood pressure. Also, most licorice sold in the United States does not contain real licorice root and is loaded with sugar. For the real deal, look for herbal teas and imported candy.

10 snacks to tame your appetite

These snacks aren't just delicious. Research shows they can actually keep you from gaining weight.

BY BILL GOTTLIEB

Appetite. It's like a wild creature living inside you, demanding to be fed. It doesn't even seem to speak the same language you do. Certain words with which you're only too familiar—fat, thin—mean nothing to your insistent hunger.

So just how do you tame that creature to avoid gaining weight? Well, you could drug it with an obesity medication that alters brain chemical levels so you feel full when you're not—and risk side effects like dry mouth, headaches, and fatigue. You could try to overcome it with willpower—just saying no to the high-calorie foods you tend to overeat—and end up feeling deprived. You could cage it for a while by adapting to an artificial eating pattern—that cruel and unusual regimen called a diet—until your appetite seeks its revenge, putting the pounds right back on your hips. Or you could do what's been proven to work. Don't try

to defeat your appetite, the latest scientific findings say. Satisfy it instead.

Nutrition scientists who conduct studies on dietary patterns have discovered that people tend to eat close to the same amount of food day after day, no matter how many calories or how much fat, protein, and carbohydrate the foods contain, says Barbara Rolls, professor of nutrition at Pennsylvania State University and co-author of *The Volumetrics Weight Control Plan: Feel Full on Fewer Calories* (Quill, 2000). It's volume—the mass of food you eat—that creates what these scientists call satiety, the feeling of fullness at the end of a meal, the sensation of not being hungry anymore. If you eat "low-energy-density" meals—plenty of substance but relatively few calories—you'll satisfy your appetite without gaining weight.

Not only do you stop eating when you feel satiated, you wait longer before you eat again, and you eat less at your next meal. Satiety, says Rolls, is the missing ingredient in weight management. Put it to work day in and day out, and there's a good chance you won't gain any extra pounds or regain the ones you've lost.

So what are these low-calorie, high-volume, appetite-busting foods that can help keep unwanted pounds at bay? You'll be surprised by how familiar and tasty they are. Here are 10 of the best.

The broth in chicken soup—with carrots, celery, peas, rice—makes it more filling than many dishes with the same number of calories.

chicken soup

"Soup creates satiety in just about every way a food can," says Rolls. Your eyes see a big portion. The steamy aroma generates sensory stimulation. The large volume of liquid fills your stomach. Plus, an ingredient-rich soup takes time to digest, keeping you full.

The ideal soup is typically a "low-glycemic-index" meal—producing a steady level of blood sugar, rather than a sudden rise and a hunger-triggering fall. "Fifteen studies have shown a beneficial effect of low-glycemic-index foods on hunger, satiety, or food intake," says David S. Ludwig, director of the obesity program at Children's Hospital in Boston.

But the main reason soup works so well may be its high water content, says Rolls. In a study published in the *American Journal of Clinical Nutrition* in 1999, Rolls and her co-researchers at Penn State fed 24 women lunch in the lab once a week for four weeks. Before each meal, the women were served one of three 270-calorie "pre-loads" (that's a first course to you and me): a chicken-and-rice casserole, the casserole plus a glass of water, or a chicken-and-rice soup with the same ingredients as the casserole and water. Of the pre-loads, the soup had the biggest impact, trimming what the women ate by an average of 100 calories. And the soup eaters didn't make up the difference by eating more at dinner.

Of course, chicken soup isn't your only choice. "You want a well-flavored soup that has real vegetables or whole grains or beans in it—a soup with some chunks to chew," says Phyllis Roxland, a New York nutritionist who works with physician Howard Shapiro, author of *Picture Perfect Weight Loss* (Rodale, 2000). The book touts the appetite-satisfying power of soups such as black bean, Chinese vegetable, and curried pumpkin. For her part, Rolls recommends light versions of soups like minestrone, potato leek, corn chowder, mushroom barley, and gazpacho; any of them make an appetite-taming first course or snack. Watch out for cream-based soups, Rolls warns; they're loaded with fat and calories.

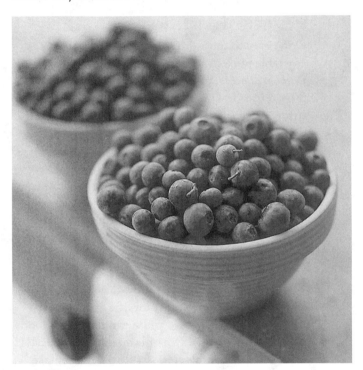

berries

With their appealing sweetness and juiciness, berries and other fruit may be the smartest snack of all, says Rolls. Along with a high water content, berries have lots of fiber, so they're filling with few calories. Picture these 100-calorie snacks: 10 jelly beans, 18 fat-free pretzels, and 2³/₄ cups of fresh strawberries. That's not enough jelly beans or pretzels to put a dent in your appetite. But the berries or fruit will—and that satisfaction can make a big difference.

In a 10-year study of heart disease risk factors published in 1999 in the *Journal of the American Medical Association*, David Ludwig and his colleagues analyzed

One of the easiest ways to outsmart your appetite is to eat a good breakfast, a weight control expert says, especially one that's high in fiber.

diet and weight-gain patterns in 3,000 people. "Dietary fiber had a strong protective effect against weight gain," says Ludwig. The amount of fiber people ate was more important in determining who did or didn't add pounds than the quantity of fat they ate.

vegetable juice

Don't want to start with soup? Have a big glass of vegetable juice instead. In a study published in the journal *Appetite*, men who drank a 14-ounce, 88-calorie glass of vegetable juice before lunch took in an average of 136 fewer calories at the meal than did men who didn't get the drink.

Probably any kind of vegetable juice will do, says Rolls. (The study used V-8.) At first, she and her colleagues thought the drink's salt or temperature might have done the trick. But further research showed these attributes made no difference. What worked, Rolls says, is most likely the juice's low energy density and modest dose of fiber.

bran flakes

Bran flakes, of course, are a terrific fiber source. Along with juices, soups, and stews, fiber-rich foods may be your best ally. Not only do they give you a lot to eat for very few calories, says Roxland, they take the edge off your appetite for longer than many other foods.

An easy way to get your fiber is to eat a good breakfast, says Rolls. "One study shows that people who eat a high-fiber breakfast take in fewer calories right then and at lunch, totaling about 100 fewer calories for the day." What's more, she adds, research reveals that daily breakfast eaters are most successful at losing weight.

Rolls herself usually eats a high-fiber cereal like Fiber One or All-Bran mixed with bran flakes. "Plain bran flakes are a little too much for me," she says. She adds nonfat plain yogurt and skim milk. When the weather turns chilly, she mixes oat bran flakes into hot oatmeal.

smoothies

Bran cereal with strawberries isn't to your taste? Reach for the blender and make yourself a smoothie. Gene Daoust, a certified nutritionist in San Diego and coauthor of the book *40-30-30 Fat-Burning Nutrition* (California Bill's Automotive Handbooks, 1997), recommends an "appetite-suppressing" fruit-protein breakfast smoothie made with a scoop of protein powder, $1/2$ frozen banana, $1/2$ cup of frozen strawberries, $3/4$ cup of water, and 2 teaspoons of almonds. The meal knocks out hunger because it's "nutrient dense." Like all meals that balance protein, fat, and carbohydrates, it has a low glycemic index, he says.

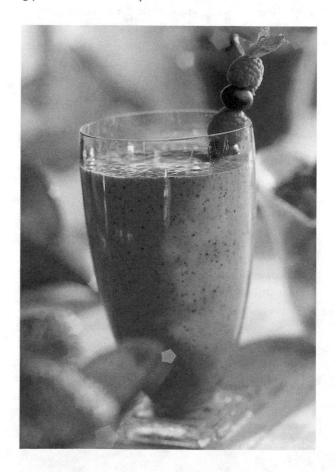

tuna

Studies from all over the world have shown that protein—the kind in a forkful of albacore or chunk light tuna—may be more filling, bite for bite, than carbohydrate or fat, says Angelo Tremblay, chief of the kinesiology division at Laval University in Quebec, Canada. In an unpublished study, Tremblay and his colleagues served overweight men meals that were either high in protein (30 percent of calories) or moderate in protein (15 percent) for six days, allowing them to eat as much as they liked. The men eating the high-protein meals felt the fullest, consumed the fewest calories—and lost the most weight.

Rolls cites a study in the *Journal of Nutrition* in which men were fed high-protein meals featuring beef, chicken, or fish. In the next three hours, fish produced the greatest sense of fullness. When Rolls ranked the energy density of various meats and seafoods, tuna canned in water scored about the lowest, delivering the fewest calories per forkful.

salsa

Tremblay is keen on protein, but he's hot on something else: the fiery chemical in red pepper called capsaicin. In experiments published in the *British Journal of Nutrition*, he and his colleagues added the spicy stuff either to breakfast or to "pre-load" appetizers at lunch, then measured how much people ate afterward.

They found in a test of 13 women that adding red pepper to a breakfast markedly cut the women's hunger between that meal and lunch and reduced the number of calories they ate at midday. When he tested 10 men, he found that a pepper-spiked appetizer held down calorie intake at lunch and in a snack a few hours later.

Tremblay says that red pepper acts as a "non-pharmacological stimulant," boosting the activity of the sympathetic nervous system. When that happens you feel less hungry, though no one's sure why. As a bonus, he found that the hot stuff in red pepper slightly upped the calories burned (a physiological process called thermogenesis), particularly after high-fat meals. How to put this to work? Serve omelettes with hot sauce and warm tortillas or toast. Or top baked potatoes with fresh salsa.

low-fat milk

Drinking milk before or with a meal helps you feel full sooner and eat less the next time, says Rolls. The lighter the milk, the greater the effect. That is, fat-free milk works better than 1 percent, and both work better than 2 percent (she's not sure why). Going low-fat also takes a load of calories out of your diet. "Studies show that nearly every successful strategy for cutting fat from your diet includes drinking lower-fat milk," says Rolls.

rice

"Rice has been a staple in cultures that have been thin for millennia," says Rolls. In her review of bread and grain products, Spanish rice (with its moist tomatoes), long-grain brown rice, and wild rice got the lowest energy-density scores. "Fiber-rich whole grains should be at the core of your diet," she says. It's not hard to do: Suppose you go to a Chinese restaurant but want to keep your meal around 400 calories. That permits you one egg roll. Or one small serving of spareribs. Or a small bowl of crispy noodles. Or—if you're wise—a filling 400-calorie meal of 4 ounces of spicy shrimp, $2/3$ of a cup of rice, $1^{1}/_{2}$ cups of broccoli in hoisin sauce, plus a fortune cookie.

low-fat frozen desserts

"Many people keep eating until they've had something sweet," says Rolls. Fortunately, that doesn't have to be bad.

"Frozen desserts are a good way to satisfy a sweet tooth without piling on calories," says Roxland. A Creamsicle weighs in at just 100 calories; a Tofutti Cutie vanilla or wild berry sandwich tickles the palate for only 120 calories. A half-cup of chocolate frozen yogurt adds a modest 115 calories to your dinner.

Of course, Rolls says, people who've gotten used to her approach can take another tack. "Have a satisfying amount of low-energy-density food at your meal—and then for dessert eat one piece of the most delicious chocolate you can find!" ✳

Bill Gottlieb is the author of Alternative Cures *(Rodale, 2000).*

Delicious Low-Fat Cheese? Yes, it *does* exist.

Even the makers admit it's a challenge. But you can enjoy some lightened old favorites—if you know where to look.

BY JONATHAN F. KING

I don't own a cell phone, download music from the Web, or ride a scooter on city streets, but I am a trendsetter in one arena of modern life. Because of my deep affection for pizza, double cheeseburgers, bleu d'Auvergne, and nachos—as well as for any crispy, salty, and cheesy food that comes in a noisy plastic bag—I'm doing my part to help the overall consumption of cheese in the United States continue its upward surge. And it is an impressive climb: At nearly 30 pounds per person in 1999, cheese chomping in this country rose a full 5 percent over 1998—the largest annual increase in almost two decades.

Alas, I've also been doing my part to contribute to the well-publicized increase in weight among Americans. Is there a causal relationship here? Common sense says "Duh!" even if the number crunchers haven't yet provided conclusive evidence. So it's occurred to me that I could possibly cut some pounds and some grams of artery-clogging saturated fat by converting to reduced-fat cheeses.

bone up

Fat or none, cheese is a great source of calcium. An ounce of Swiss gives you 272 milligrams; a tablespoon of Parmesan almost 70. But think twice about cottage cheese, which contains enough sodium to actually harm your bones.

There's certainly no shortage of these products in the dairy case; nearly 75 percent of America's cheese makers feature at least one reduced-fat item. Many make several, in a heady variety of low-fat and nonfat products based on such old favorites as Jack, Cheddar, and Swiss. On the face of it, it's smart marketing: Combine two deep-seated American obsessions—our love of mozzarella-laden pizza, Cheddar-slathered burgers, and cheese-based snacks on the one hand, and our concern about weight and the detrimental effects of fat on the other—and you've got a niche market to die for.

Or so a shrewd cheese maker might think. But there seems to be a level of fat below which consumers, by and large, just will not go. Most professional cheeseheads agree that the threshold lies around 50 percent—that is, when no more than half the fat is removed from a full-fat cheese. Go much further and consumer resistance kicks in. "Demand for non-fat cheeses has fallen off sharply," says Bill Haines, a marketing executive with Dairy Management, an industry association dedicated to promoting dairy products. "Consumers are finding that nonfat products just aren't acceptable." Why? A headline in a

Is your favorite cheese sharp Cheddar, mild Jack, tangy chèvre, crumbly Parmesan, or creamy Brie? With a little savvy, you can enjoy all of them without guilt.

recent trade magazine summed it up: Number One Obstacle to Consumers Trying Low-Fat Dairy Products Is Taste.

Accordingly, palatable low-fats are a prime objective of dairy-food researchers—many of whom work in states such as Wisconsin and California that like to grace billboards with pictures of cheese. But it's a formidable challenge. "Cheese is a complex product," says Lynn Kuntz, a former food scientist who's now the editor of *Food Product Design* magazine. "With no fat, it's a sort of Twinkie-like thing. It would be cheese made out of Jell-O."

For starters, fat enhances a cheese's natural beauty: The sheen of a full-fat Cheddar could never be confused with the plastic gloss—did someone say Jell-O?—of its low-fat or nonfat counterpart.

More profoundly, fat makes cheese taste like cheese, serving as a "carrier" of desirable flavors while muting some that could be objectionable, like bitterness. Fat coats your mouth, prolonging the time it takes for yummy flavors to dissipate. It contributes to both the texture of cheese and what food wonks call its mouth-feel. When fat is cut back, proteins come to dominate, making some reduced-fat varieties firm and rubbery. These cheeses stay true to form even when you melt them, whereupon, as they say in the industry, they "exhibit limited shred melt and fusion, followed by excessive browning and scorching."

The cheese labs' strategy so far has been to develop substitutes that provide some or all of dairy fat's renowned sensory pleasures, minus its equally pronounced nutritional shortcomings. This is a more complicated business than it might seem, for no single fat replacer can cover all the bases.

"The Holy Grail for cheese makers is a reduced-fat product that's as good as the full-fat," says Haines. "It hasn't been done yet. Whether or not it ever will be is uncertain."

So if the industry can't make low-fat cheese taste like the real thing, and the full-fat version is too, well, fatty, what's a cheese-lover to do?

First, learn which cheeses are relatively low in fat to begin with. Feta and goat cheeses are more flavorful than most domestic cow's milk cheeses and lower in fat than some. The Impastata brand of creamy goat cheese from Vermont Butter & Cheese Company, with 4.5 grams (g) of fat (3 g saturated) per ounce, is slightly lighter than soft goat cheese. It's loaded with flavor but not as sharp as feta or some of the stronger imported chèvres. Several cheese makers produce versions of fromage blanc, a ricotta-like cheese with negligible calories and zero fat. It's delicious with fruit and a stellar substitute for ricotta in cooking.

Next, make peace with some low-fat cheeses. Several taste okay, and a few are real winners. A favorite is the 50% Light Cheddar made by Vermont's Cabot Creamery; it's not just edible but downright enjoyable. An ounce has 4.5 grams of fat, 3 g of it saturated—half that of full-fat Cheddar. A similar product from Horizon Organic Dairy tastes even better, but it's slightly fattier, at 6 g of fat, 4 g of it saturated. I'd happily turn to either

Buy full-flavored cheeses, and you won't crave those second and third servings. "We're more likely to be satisfied if we eat smaller amounts of ones we enjoy," says a cookbook author.

Rethink your pizza.
A light sprinkle of finely grated Parmigiano-Reggiano delivers less fat and far more flavor than a shower of shredded mozzarella.

to meet my seven-year-old's—and my own—orange cheese requirements.

Third, learn to use full-fat cheeses to good effect. "People get discouraged by the lack of flavor in low-fat cheeses, so they end up eating more of them," says food writer Sam Gugino, author of *Low-Fat Cooking to Beat the Clock* (Chronicle Books, 2000). "We're more likely to be satisfied if we eat less of the ones we enjoy."

That means rethinking pizza, for example. A light sprinkle of finely grated Parmigiano-Reggiano delivers less fat and far more flavor than a shower of shredded mozzarella.

Full-fat cheese-lovers can always make room for it by cutting back elsewhere. Wine-and-cheese party tonight? Forgo the bacon cheeseburger at noon and top your salad with sunflower seeds, not Cheddar. Snack on some fruit instead of cheese puffs. Then, when the brie beckons, step right up with no shame. ✳

a cheese-lover's choices

Saturated fat is what you need to watch for in cheeses; experts okay up to 18 grams (g) a day (a 4-ounce hamburger patty has 8 g). How do some favorites rate? See the chart below. (Unless noted, portions are 1 ounce—a serving about the size of two dominoes.)

	CALORIES	TOTAL FAT (GRAMS)	SATURATED FAT (GRAMS)	
Sandwich cheeses				
Monterey Jack, 2% milk	80	6	4	These reduced-fats are worth a try. They're a bit drier than the full-fats, but melt (yes, they melt) or tuck them between two slices of bread, or grate them into a quiche or a casserole, and you'll hardly taste the difference. Most weigh in with about half the calories and fat of the full-fat versions.
Cheddar, reduced-fat	70	5	3	
Swiss, low-fat	80	4	3	
American, 2% milk, 1 slice	45	3	2	
Spreadables				
Brie	95	8	5	You could opt for nonfat cream cheese, but the low-fat cuts fat and calories by about a third and is barely distinguishable from the original; the same goes for ricotta. The secret for all these cheeses is to spread them thin.
cream cheese, low-fat	70	6	4	
goat, soft	76	6	4	
ricotta, part-skim, 1/4 cup	86	5	3	
Toppings				
blue	100	8	5	There's no need to smother pizza, salad, or pasta with cheese when you're using one that's full of flavor and texture. Try replacing full-fat mozzarella with a tastier alternative—a little will deliver a lot of satisfaction.
feta	75	6	4	
mozzarella, part-skim, 1/4 cup shredded	72	5	3	
Parmigiano-Reggiano, 2 tablespoons grated	46	4	2	

Watching what you eat? Bring a brown-bag lunch to the airport

Avoid the airport food courts' Hall of Shame

What's the essential carry-on for health-conscious frequent fliers? Brown bags. No, it's not the latest trend in luggage—it's a reaction to the grease-laden offerings at airport food courts.

If you're flying through Detroit, for example, you'll be eating hot dogs and Cinnabons if you don't pack an apple. In a survey of meals at the 10 busiest airports in America, the hall of shame award went to Detroit's Metro Airport, according to the Physicians Committee for Responsible Medicine, a national nonprofit organization that promotes preventive medicine.

Researchers from the committee evaluated menu choices, seeking at least one low-fat, cholesterol-free, veggie-heavy dish that did not have to be specially ordered. (For example, requests for a Cobb salad without the ham, cheese, or eggs didn't count.) Although the group did not conduct nutritional analyses, study leader Brie Turner-McGrievy, R.D., points out that most of the food was likely to be high in sodium as well, a one-way ticket to swollen legs on a flight.

Detroit's ranking, however, shouldn't suggest a Midwestern fat belt: The Minneapolis-St. Paul and Chicago airports scored second and third best, respectively. San Francisco landed in the top spot, with 24 out of 25 restaurants offering quick, healthful meals, including such Cal-Mex bites as vegetarian burritos. During a recent revamping, some of San Francisco airport's fast-food places were replaced with local restaurants, a trend that Turner-McGrievy hopes will continue. In the meantime, bring along an extra bag—packed with nutrition.

Preflight Bites Report Card

(ranked by percentage of airport restaurants with healthy options)

★★★★ 80% to 100%   ★★ 40% to 60%
★★★ 60% to 80%   ★ Less than 40%

San Francisco ★★★★   Atlanta ★★
Minneapolis-St. Paul ★★★   Phoenix ★★
Chicago ★★★   Las Vegas ★★
Denver ★★★   Dallas-Fort Worth ★★
Los Angeles ★★★   Detroit ★

Q+A
Don't let a diet steal your energy

I've lost a lot of weight in the last 18 months by eating right and exercising three times a week, but I still need to lose 10 pounds. The trouble is, I get so tired that it's hard to stay motivated. Any ideas to help get my energy back?

No wonder you're frustrated. After 18 months of huffing and puffing, you're entitled to be feeling a surge in energy, not the reverse.

That's because as your body gets more fit, it increases the number of microscopic energy factories, called mitochondria, in your muscle cells. One study found that people who'd worked out regularly for seven months ended up with 120 percent more of these power plants. That's good for weight loss, because the more mitochondria you have, the more easily you tend to burn fat rather than carbohydrates when you need energy. And now that your muscles are packed with these energy factories, you should be feeling more get-up-and-go.

So what's going on? Since we don't know how hard you're working out or what you're eating, we can only speculate as to why you're pooped. Fatigue can be a symptom of over-training; other signs are fitful sleep, a consistently rapid heartbeat, feeling depressed, or a drop in athletic performance. But since you're only working out a few days a week, that's probably not the problem.

Instead, you may not be eating enough protein to stay energized. While low-calorie diets are often recommended for weight loss, they can sap your strength, especially when you're working out regularly. Add a little more lean meat or tofu to your meals—or some beans—to stay revved during strenuous routines. Also, be sure you're getting plenty of fruits and vegetables. They not only offer important nutrients, but also help you stay hydrated; many people get tired when they're low on fluids.

DON'T LET
your marriage
make you fat

We know it sounds retro, but it just might be true:
MARRIAGE CAN MAKE YOU FAT.
If, that is, you eat like your husband. Here's how to take control
of your weight–and make dining together a pleasure.

BY JULIA CALIFANO

If Madeline Powell (her name has been changed) had her way, she'd eat strictly vegetarian. Dinner would be a simple salad or a rib-sticking bowl of oatmeal. But Powell, 39, of Warrenton, Missouri, has her family to consider. "My son is picky with vegetables," she says ruefully. "My husband is a meat-and-potatoes guy." She can't even serve chicken breasts with the skin peeled off; her husband would be appalled. "He doesn't understand why anyone would want to eat chicken without the skin!"

Dinner always includes enough for leftovers–or seconds. "Today I bought chips and dip for my 17-year-old son," Powell says. "He eats some and works it off playing football. Guess who eats the rest?" Exercise, too, has fallen by the wayside during her 21 years of marriage, and between them she and her husband have gained more than 100 pounds. Powell's glad her mate loves her the way she is. Yet she's frustrated that he doesn't support her weight-loss efforts. "I think, 'Golly, why should I care if he doesn't?' "

For many women, that's the 64,000-calorie question, and it highlights a thorny real-life issue that nutrition experts hardly ever discuss. On one hand, support—lots of it—is critical to shedding pounds and keeping them off. Research dating to the 1980s shows that women slim down more when their partners participate in their diets; in one study women who joined a weight-loss program with three relatives or friends were three times more likely to stick with it and lost 35 percent more weight than those who signed up solo. But far from helping their partner eat better, many husbands and boyfriends can be "a huge hindrance," says Karen Miller-Kovach, lead scientist for Weight Watchers International. In one survey of thousands of women, respondents gained an average of 25 pounds over 13 years of marriage. Unhappily wed women gained 42 pounds.

Not that men are bad guys, of course. They just tend to have a different relationship to food and weight than we do. For one thing, they can eat more than we can without adding an ounce: 2,200 calories a day for a sedentary man, versus 1,600 for a woman with the same lifestyle. Men are also less apt to care when they see the scale creeping up. In a survey of more than 100,000 Americans, 60 percent of moderately overweight women were trying to diet, versus only 36 percent of men.

The Mars-Venus differences extend toward attitudes about how to slim down. Men are more liable to rev up on exercise and women to cut back on fat, the same poll found. Research also shows that women are far likelier to overeat for emotional reasons and to blame themselves when they don't lose weight.

What does it all mean? Simply, when it comes to love handles, the man in your life may cut himself—and you—more slack than you do. Or he may have no idea how to give you the support you need to change how you eat and exercise. Or both.

Sometimes, though, the disconnect is trickier. "It's assumed that when a woman wants to lose weight, her mate is thrilled," says Seattle psychologist Barbara Jacobson Stuart, coauthor (with husband Richard B. Stuart) of *Weight, Sex, and Marriage: A Delicate Balance* (Guilford Press, 1994). "But very often, that isn't so." In one poll of more than 200 doctors treating obesity, 90 percent said sabotage happens all the time between couples. A man may fear that if his wife looks more attractive, she'll find someone younger and fitter than he is. He may worry that if she gives up junk food, she'll expect him to do the same. Or perhaps her cellulite has been the scapegoat for their lousy sex life. "He may unconsciously interfere with her diet so they don't have to confront other issues," says Edward Abramson, a psychologist and author of *Marriage Made Me Fat!* (Kensington, 2000)

Add kids, busy schedules, and other factors to the mix and—wham—it's no wonder the Stuarts call marriage and motherhood "the most fattening jobs in the world." But it is possible to modify your own patterns—and transform your mate into a real support system. The key, experts say, is to use the same communication skills you rely on to resolve other sticky issues. Following is advice on some of the most common, and most dicey, weight-mate scenarios.

THE PROBLEM
you match him portion for portion

"Many women serve themselves the same amount of food as their husbands without even thinking about it," says Mary Lou Klem, an assistant professor of psychiatry at the University of Pittsburgh School of Medicine and a researcher with the National Weight Control Registry. But this is one area of your relationship where you shouldn't strive for equality. Because men tend to be bigger and have more muscle mass, they can consume 12 calories for every pound of body weight without gaining a pound, versus 11 calories for women. This may not sound like much, but it adds up fast: If you and your mate each weigh 150 pounds and eat 1,800 calories a day, by year's end he'll be holding the line at 150—and you'll be nudging 165.

> If your mate makes a sumptuous dinner, **go ahead and enjoy it.** Then cut back on calories and fat at some other meal to compensate.

Fortunately, the solution is simple. Dish out less food to begin with (using a smaller plate than his can help) and eat slowly. "It takes at least 10 minutes for your brain to register fullness," says John Foreyt, who directs the nutrition research clinic at Baylor College of Medicine in Houston, "so try to prolong the meal—put your fork down between bites, pause midway through your entrée, and focus on the conversation." You'll finish at the same time your mate does (or after)—which means that you'll be less likely to go back for seconds. Another strategy: Start with a cup of low-fat soup and sip lots of water. Not only does this slow down the meal, it makes you less hungry.

THE PROBLEM
he cooks the way he likes

Of course, it's a lot easier to watch what you eat when you prepare the meals. But many busy couples divvy up the cooking. When Melissa Coventry of Pacific Grove, California, quit her job and went back to school for a business degree, her husband, David, an aspiring gourmet, took over—and she gained 10 pounds. "I asked him once how much cheese he'd put in the risotto and he said, 'Oh, not too much.' Later, I found out that by 'not too much' he meant the entire block."

Many women would rather **spend time with their families** than go to the gym.

One solution: Make your mate your exercise partner.

The key to solving this problem is to use honey instead of vinegar. Raise the issue at a neutral time and place—not during a meal or in the kitchen. Tell him how much you appreciate his cooking, then explain you're worried about your weight. Ask him to make just a small change: say, adding a low-fat recipe or two to his repertoire.

To gain some control over a meal's calorie count, volunteer to prepare the veggies or salad while he tackles the main course, suggests Joan Salge Blake, a nutrition professor at Boston University. Serve yourself, making the veggies your "entrée" and his dish the "side." You could also try Coventry's strategy: teaching by example. "He's seen me use Pam instead of gobs of butter and oil, yet still put out these incredible dinners."

THE PROBLEM
he tries too hard

"I know perfectly well what I should and should not eat," Schuster says. "When my boyfriend tells me not to pick before dinner, I get pissed off." Not only does this kind of "helpful" behavior make a woman feel like she's living with the chief of the food police, it actually increases the chances that she'll break her diet just to rebel, experts say.

The solution: Have a heart-to-heart. "Men often monitor their partner's food intake simply because that's the kind of help they think they would value if they were the ones trying to lose weight," Stuart says. Let him know that you appreciate the fact that he's looking out for your well-being but that this isn't the kind of coaching you need. Then tell him exactly what would be helpful. "This is a golden opportunity, so give the matter serious thought before you begin the discussion," Miller-Kovach says. Perhaps you'd like to celebrate each five-pound loss by going away for the weekend together. Maybe you want him

to bring home only sweets that you dislike. Perhaps you'd take more walks if he went with you.

On days when you'd like to indulge without so much as a raised eyebrow, make it clear in advance, she advises. "Tell him you plan to take the evening off and that you'll get back to your healthful eating tomorrow. Then you can both relax."

THE PROBLEM
you eat out a lot

"My boyfriend and I love going to restaurants because it's one of the few opportunities we have during the week to talk without all the distractions of home," says Randy Schuster, a 33-year-old food service director in San Francisco. The downside: In the first year of their relationship, she gained 10 pounds. "When we go out, I end up eating foods, like nachos, I never would have at home or if I were with a girlfriend."

Sound familiar? An obvious solution is to stick to places that offer healthful fare like sushi or grilled chicken. "You can eat pretty much anything, anywhere, and still manage your weight," says Miller-Kovach. "It's a matter of portion control." Her tactics: Start with a noncream-based soup, salad, or shrimp cocktail. Order an appetizer as a main course, with a baked potato and veggie to round out the meal. Or ask the waiter to halve your entrée before he brings it to the table and put the rest in a doggy bag.

THE PROBLEM
you eat like a kid

Madeline Powell isn't just married—she's a mom. Not only does she have to buy foods her son will eat, but also she has to deal with what he won't eat. "Moms tend to be human garbage disposals," says Pam

Ascanio, 41, a part-time teacher and mother of two in Reedley, California. "You convince yourself that kids' crusts and broken cookies don't count, when if you put it all on a plate, it would add up to a huge amount of food."

It may be unrealistic to expect these to be your thinnest years, but they needn't be your heaviest, either. The road to redemption starts at the grocery store. Ask your kids to help pick out produce and healthful snacks for the week. "They're much more likely to eat something they selected," Blake says. And though you hate to waste food, make it a rule: No kids' leftovers—ever. Ask them to help you resist temptation by clearing the table, scraping plates, and loading the dishwasher. "You may be surprised by how supportive your kids can be," Miller-Kovach says. "Since they're not threatened in any way by your desire to lose weight, they may be even more helpful than your spouse. All you have to do is ask."

Start buying the foods you want instead of what you think your kids will like. To keep them happy, allow just one special treat per shopping trip.

THE PROBLEM
he wants to lead you into temptation

Okay, let's give him the benefit of the doubt and assume he simply wants to reward your efforts by treating you to a box of Godivas. But if you ban candy from the house and he still brings you bonbons, something else is going on. To get at the root of his resistance, Stuart suggests, ask him how he feels about your losing weight. While he's unlikely to come out and admit he's racked with insecurity, offer reassurance anyway: "Explain that you're making eating and exercise changes to feel better, be healthier, and have more energy—not to attract the opposite sex."

If he complains about the inconvenience, do not apologize—or feel guilty. Instead, Abramson advises,

say something like, "I realize it's a pain for you when I get home late from the gym, but I appreciate the efforts you're making to help me improve my health." If your mate has his own weight or health issues, ask if he wants your support to improve his eating habits. If he'd rather be left alone, agree not to put any pressure on him.

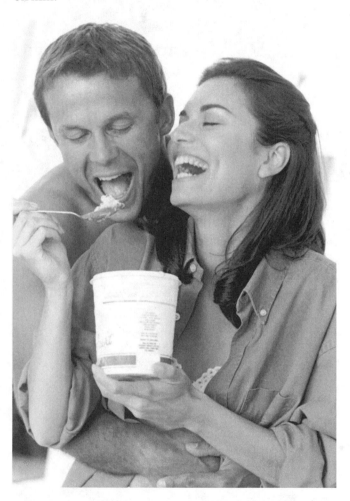

If you still don't get the cooperation you need, look for encouragement from friends, colleagues, neighbors, other family members, or a weight-loss program. "This doesn't mean you have a bad or nonworkable marriage," Blake says. "He may be a wonderful partner in other areas. This just isn't one of them." ✳

Julia Califano is a freelance writer based in Montclair, New Jersey.

the no-stress
Weight-Loss Plan

**No, an afternoon nap won't melt off the pounds.
But new research says you can keep inches off your middle
by learning to be more laid-back.**

BY DOROTHY FOLTZ-GRAY

Some days just don't go well. I'm behind on two deadlines, last night's dishes are still in the sink, I've fought (again) with my teenage son, and I have a headache. In short, I feel underappreciated, overworked, and bleak. On such evenings, all I want to do is slump on my couch and slug back some M&M's. Noshing—especially at night—is how I deal with stress. And I'm not the only one. Many women say that when they're anxious or overburdened, they find themselves reaching for food instead of doing any of the virtuous things, like exercise or meditation, that might actually help them more.

For years experts have been spinning theories about why we engage in this behavior. We eat for comfort, they tell us, to "self-soothe," to cope. We eat because we're insecure and we want to bury our feelings. To some extent, that all makes sense. (Sometimes, I really do feel better after chowing M&M's.) But such assessments can also be frustrating. Not only is our anxious overeating out of control, it's our fault. Worse, any solution seems hopelessly out of reach. To keep ourselves from heading to the kitchen at the first sign of stress, we would need a massive personality overhaul, requiring tons of therapy, a fairy godmother, or both.

But hold the M&M's. Finally, new research may absolve us. According to studies at the University of California at San Francisco (UCSF) and elsewhere, it's not just underdeveloped willpower that drives us to eat when we're stressed; stress may actually make us hungry. And, certain hormones released by stress can cause us to gain weight in a particularly annoying spot: our waists.

> Hormones released when we're stressed can cause us to gain weight, particularly around the waist.

And more than our vanity may suffer. In recent years, experts have identified excess weight around the middle as a risk factor for several serious diseases, including diabetes, hypertension, and heart trouble. That doesn't mean a thick midsection is necessarily a one-way road to disease. There are ways to tame stress and slim down that can put you back on the road to health. But first, here are some key facts.

Stress Makes You Hungry

Your body has a built-in response to stress that may work to your disadvantage when it comes to maintaining your weight. Let's say you're stuck in traffic. As you begin to stew about being late to work, a hormone in the brain signals the adrenal glands to release other hormones, including cortisol, that help the body deal with stress. Cortisol works by causing glucose and fatty acids, which provide energy to the muscles, to be released. Once the stress fades, however, cortisol stays high, and one of its aftereffects is an increase in your appetite to ensure your body replaces the fuel it's burned off.

The problem is that 21st-century stresses are more cerebral than ancient ones, so you don't expend much energy managing them. Think of the calories you would have burned fleeing from a lion or a spear-throwing enemy. After that kind of exertion, you might have been able to eat a hunk of hyena without gaining weight. But when you're late to work, you probably just sit behind the wheel and fume, so whatever calories you devour under cortisol's influence are pure excess.

The stress of modern life undermines our willpower in yet another way: It keeps cortisol levels unnaturally high at a time of day when they're supposed to be way down. Under calm, controlled conditions in a lab, cortisol levels peak between 5 and 6 a.m. as the body prepares to wake up, then fall during the day and begin a slow rise around 2 a.m. When they're low late in the day, we shouldn't feel the need to eat. But the 21st century doesn't allow for afternoon slackers. There's a package to mail by 5 p.m., kids to retrieve from school and ferry to soccer practice, dinner to prepare. That means just when your cortisol should be low, stress causes the hormone—and consequently your appetite—to rise. The next thing you know, you're filling up on snacks an hour before going on to eat a full meal.

Some research even suggests that eating when you're stressed may help you handle the pressure better, says Mary F. Dallman, a professor of physiology at UCSF who has studied stress hormones and eating patterns. In experiments with rats, subjects allowed to eat a high-calorie or high-carbohydrate diet during periods of repeated shocks released fewer stress

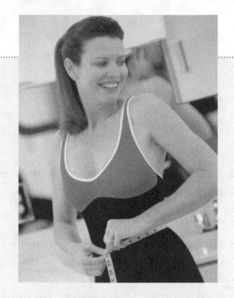

are you at risk?
To find out if your belly poses a threat, see how you measure up.

Check your hip-to-waist ratio. Divide your waist measurement by your hip measurement. Researchers have found that women with a waist-to-hip ratio greater than 0.85 are at increased risk of "metabolic syndrome," a constellation of conditions including high blood sugar, high cholesterol, and high blood pressure.

Measure your waist. If it's 35 inches or more, you're at risk.

Do the floor test. Lie on your back and press on your abdomen. You should feel soft, pinchable fat, and the abdominal muscle should lie relatively flat across your pelvic bones. If, instead, your stomach is round and hard (as if you were pregnant) and arches well above the pelvic bones, you have too much central fat.

hormones than unfed rats. Other studies revealed a similar change in humans: Those who ate lots of carbohydrates before being subjected to certain stressful tasks released less cortisol and were less depressed when the experiment was over. "It may be that when you

Don't stress out trying to determine which diet to pursue or what's the best workout.

Sitting still and relaxing may be just as important for controlling your weight.

Eating when you're stressed may help you handle the pressure better.

The idea of comfort food may be real.

overeat, you're cooling off your central stress system," says Dallman. "The idea of comfort food may be real."

Stress Gives You a Big Belly

It's not hard to see why overeating would make you gain weight. But Elissa Epel, a researcher in psychology at UCSF, confirmed a particular pattern. She and her colleagues asked 59 premenopausal women to engage in a series of stressful tasks involving arithmetic, puzzles, and public speaking over a period of several days. Women with the most belly, or "central," fat, which lies behind the abdominal muscles and is packed around the organs, were the ones who found the tasks most threatening. They reported more day-to-day stress, and they secreted significantly more cortisol than did women with less fat around their middles.

What's the link? When cortisol hits any fat cell, it activates fat-storing enzymes that cause the cell to plump up. But because central fat cells are designed to act as a source of quick energy during stress, they are covered with more receptors for cortisol than the other fat cells in our body. Cortisol is drawn to those particular cells, increasing fat there. "We now know that chronic psychological stress can shape the body by changing fat distribution," says Epel.

A Big Belly Can Be Dangerous

Excess central fat puts more at peril than our vanity; it also drives up the risk of heart disease, hypertension, and diabetes. Why? Again, cortisol.

Central fat is close to the liver, which controls a variety of metabolic functions in the body, including blood pressure, insulin, and cholesterol levels. During stressful times, rising cortisol triggers a release of fatty acids into the bloodstream; the acids eventually pour into the liver, taxing it and causing insulin, cholesterol, and blood pressure to shoot up.

To add insult to injury, the process is self-perpetuating. Any fatty acids the liver doesn't use return to the central fat cells, plumping them up even more. And as central

fat increases, it starts dumping fatty acids into the bloodstream all the time, not just during stress. "The constant presence of fatty acids in the bloodstream is what puts people at risk for diabetes and heart disease," says Raymond S. Niaura, the author of several studies on hostility and fat at Brown University, in Providence, Rhode Island.

Not All Belly Fat Is Worrisome

Most women over a certain age know the squeeze of too-tight jeans. But that doesn't necessarily mean you have the type of fat that can put you at risk for disease. To gauge whether yours is a problem, see "Are You at Risk?" on page 97.

Keep in mind that you don't have to be heavy overall to have a lot of central fat. In Epel's studies, lean women who carried their relatively small load of fat around their waists had much higher cortisol levels than did women who were well-padded all over. They also had the hardest time managing and adapting to the stress of difficult tasks.

Does that mean generally full-bodied women are at less risk than lean women with midriff bulges? Maybe. "Overweight women who carry most of their extra fat in their hips rather than their bellies—the 'pears' as opposed to the 'apples'—should not be at greater risk of disease," says Epel. "If they have a relatively small waist, their fat is not the type that is floating around in their bloodstream. Rather, it stays securely enveloped in the peripheral fat cells."

At the same time, not all midriff bulges are a problem, particularly the ones that some women develop in their peri- and postmenopausal years. That soft pinchable flesh, which lies on top of our stomach muscles, is relatively benign because it doesn't release fatty acids into the blood the way central fat does.

However, women at midlife also experience considerable stress. The combined pressures of aging parents, demanding careers, and marital strife hit many of us at about the same time as perimenopause. Most women over 40 carry at least some stress-induced fat, says Pamela Peeke, assistant clinical professor of medicine at the University of Maryland School of Medicine and author of *Fight Fat After Forty* (Penguin, 2001).

That doesn't mean every forty-something woman is headed for a life-threatening disease. The beauty of acknowledging that stress is a threat to your health is that there's a relatively simple solution: Learn to calm down. "That's not to say we won't respond to stressful situations," says Niaura, "just that we need to be able to recover quickly when they occur."

Alas, there's no measuring cup to tell how much stress is too much or how quick recovery has to be. As Epel's studies and others have shown, heredity and psyche affect our sensitivity—and our bodies'

responses—to stress. Nor do scientists yet know exactly how much central fat is too much.

The point is this: Don't stress out trying to determine exactly which diet to pursue or what's the best workout for burning calories. Eating less and exercising can help. But sitting still and relaxing may be just as important for controlling your weight. For once, cut yourself some slack. Living at 120 miles per hour, chasing deadlines and perfection, isn't living. It's a slow, dangerous burn that's literally weighing us down. So instead of reaching for the M&M's, face your stress head-on. Peeke's advice? "Give yourself 10 seconds to bitch, moan, and whine, and then move along, girlfriend." ❋

Dorothy Foltz-Gray is a contributing editor.

the laid-back weight-loss plan

ONLY A ZOMBIE could live in America and not be stressed from time to time. But that doesn't mean we have to end up with a bellyful of dangerous fat. Below are proven ways to get control of your stress—and your waistline.

Chill out. Vegging in front of the TV with a bag of chips isn't the solution. Numerous studies suggest that people actually feel less relaxed and happy after watching TV than before. Instead, try to work some sort of regular relaxation into your life, whether it's yoga, meditation, massage, or deep breathing. In a three-month pilot study by Elissa Epel, men with diabetes who meditated or did muscle relaxation exercises every day to control stress lost significantly more central fat than the control group that did nothing.

Feel the burn. "When you exercise, central fat is the first to be burned off," says Epel. By increasing brain chemicals called endorphins, exercise also calms us and drives down the cortisol levels that cause hunger. And working out accomplishes what a brisk skirmish with a tiger once did: It burns up the fatty acids released during stress so they're no longer a health risk. For women over 40, Pamela Peeke advocates what she calls a "non-negotiable" three-pronged exercise approach: a goal of

45 minutes of moderate aerobic activity five to six times a week, strength training twice a week, and daily stretching.

Practice portion control. The last thing you want to do when you're stressed is go on a strict diet; depriving yourself is bound to sabotage your efforts to lose weight and stay calm. Instead, focus on eating healthily—lots of fruits, vegetables, and grains, with smaller amounts of protein and fat—but eating less. Use a kitchen scale, plus measuring cups and spoons, to learn the size of reasonable portions. Then, serve yourself less by using smaller plates, and dine slowly so you don't go beyond the point when you're naturally full.

Nix nighttime noshing. For many women, stress is at its peak at the end of a long day, raising cortisol levels—and your appetite—just as they should be dropping. If you still find yourself on the prowl for goodies at night, reach for low-calorie snacks like veggies and fruit. Also, try attacking your stress directly by doing those relaxation exercises at night.

Go to bed earlier. Sleep too little, and you produce less growth hormone. That's bad because growth hormone coaxes fat from fat cells to be burned off, helping to counter the fat-storing effects of cortisol.

VITAL STATS

__60 million__
Number of chocolate bunnies made each Easter

__16__
Percentage of employees who have physically assaulted a coworker, computer, or chair

__13__
Percentage of employers with meditation rooms

__115,000__
Distance, in miles, that the average person walks in a lifetime

__17__
Percentage of stay-at-home moms who read the business section

__4__
Percentage who read the food section

__40__
Pounds of skin the average person sheds in a lifetime

Unless otherwise noted, statistics apply to the United States.

Q+A
trick your body into losing weight—drink more water!

I know that drinking water is a good idea. But does the temperature matter? I'm trying to lose weight and have heard that cold water's best.

Let's call that one an old husband's tale. It's good to drink water, of course, but forget the temperature. While your body does use up a few extra calories to warm the cold water to body temperature, the amount is negligible. Drinking ice-cold water to drop pounds is like sitting in a chilly room shivering to lose weight.

Water helps you shed weight by tricking your body into feeling full with fewer calories. Lots of studies have shown that people who up their fluid intake over time drop pounds. Interestingly, some practitioners of Chinese medicine preach that drinking cold water hinders weight loss. According to the theory, cold beverages are worse than warm because they slow the body's inner workings. Water or tea, these traditionalists say, should be lukewarm.

We might not go along with that—most of us like coffee and tea piping hot, water and beer ice cold. But on this much, Western and Eastern healers agree: Whatever the temperature of the drink, try to down at least eight glasses a day—even more if some of that liquid is alcoholic or caffeinated.

The Skinny on Variety—*a Little Monotony is Good for the Waistline*

A review of diet studies in *Psychological Bulletin* finds that a diverse diet (such as a multi-course meal) keeps you from tiring of the taste of the food, so you tend to eat—and weigh—more, explain the study authors.

In one study, participants who were given a four-course meal of sausages, bread and butter, chocolate dessert, and bananas ate 44 percent more than those who were limited to the same food—in one case yogurt—for each course. But before you restrict your diet to muesli, know this: Diversity does have some advantages. Eating a variety of foods offers a broader range of nutrients and may prevent deficiencies.

Still, even a very small decrease in diet variety can help your waistline. "Instead of having potato chips, ice cream, cookies, and candy in your house, pick one," suggests study co-author and registered dietician Hollie A. Raynor. Just don't go overboard: After all, the monotony of a tuna sandwich for lunch every day might just drive you back to buffet-style overindulging.

chapter 3

fitness

fun ways to firm up

exercise:
the best boost
for your brain

Dumb jocks aside, new research suggests that exercise can build your brainpower.

BY NINA WILLDORF

My boyfriend, Mike, thinks I'm crazy. Every morning at 6:30, my alarm clock blares, and I peel myself out of a cozy bed—an hour before it's necessary—just to go for a run. At 6:35, I often agree with him. But after a half-hour jog, my behavior no longer seems so nutty. My bleary eyes are clear; my pale, pillow-rumpled skin is pink and smooth. Stress? Low. Energy? High. Tush? Not tight, but a bit closer to being toned. And no, I'm not losing my mind, I tell a groggy Mike at breakfast. In fact, I may well be picking up a few new brain cells while dashing through Boston's wakening streets.

Researchers have known for several years that our supply of brain cells does not inevitably dwindle as we age. But recent studies go further: Not only do we actually generate new brain cells over time, but we may also be able to accelerate the process. All we have to do is get moving.

The first neurologist to poke a hole in the "no new human brain cells" doctrine was Fred H. Gage, a professor at the Salk Institute in La Jolla, California. In 1998, Gage reported finding newborn neurons in the brains of five terminally ill cancer patients. The new cells appeared in the hippocampus, that part of the brain associated with learning and memory.

Gage then proceeded to show that the number of brain cells in mice increases, too—but only when they run. In early 1999, Gage and his colleagues reported that mice that regularly used an exercise wheel had twice as many new brain cells in the hippocampus as did mice that just hung out. (Swimming mice failed to show any such increase, a finding attributed to the limited amount of time they spent in the water and to the mitigating factor of extreme stress: Swimming can be traumatic for mice.) Those new brain cells translated to additional smarts, as

keep your head
Lifelong exercise may lower the risk of getting Alzheimer's disease, suggests a study from Case Western Reserve University. People who ran, swam, skated, or otherwise powered through the decades were less likely to be stricken by the mind-robbing disorder.

well. When competing with their sedentary kin, mice that ran were more skilled at navigating mazes.

Why does exercise stimulate the growth of new brain cells? An earlier study led by Carl Cotman, director of the Institute for Brain Aging and Dementia at the University of California at Irvine, suggests one possible answer. In 1994, Cotman put running wheels in the cages of some of the rats in his lab. The researchers monitored the rats' activity by computer and, after several workouts, measured their levels of brain-derived neurotrophic factor (BDNF), a substance Cotman calls the brain's wonder drug. "It's like plant fertilizer," he says. "When applied to neurons, BDNF encourages their growth and protects them from injury."

Cotman's findings were striking: Rats who put in the most time on the wheel had one-and-a-half times to twice the amount of BDNF as did rats who declined to run. In light of Gage's work, Cotman now believes that BDNF may be more than mere fertilizer. "Neurogenesis, the making of new brain cells, was unknown in 1994," he says. "But now we think that one of the functions of BDNF may be to promote the growth of new neurons."

This is all well and good for Mickey and Minnie, but animal studies aren't always applicable to humans. Still, while noting that it's important not to expect too much, Gage is cautiously optimistic. "As a brain scientist, I'd always thought that the brain controlled behavior," he says. "Now we see that behavior can change the structure of the brain."

In fact, research with humans seems to support Gage's enthusiasm. In a study published in 1999, Arthur F. Kramer, a professor of psychology at the Beckman Institute at the University of Illinois, put 124 older, healthy adults to the test. For six months, half the group took three 45-minute walks a week, while the other half focused only on stretching and toning. The aerobic volunteers improved their performance on cognitive tests by 15 to 20 percent; the stretchers saw no gain.

These new brain cells might do more for us than simply improve our test scores. Kramer says that exercisers could develop better short-term memory, recall, and response time. "You might find it easier to locate your car in the parking lot, remember a phone number, or maneuver a car more quickly when a cat runs into the road," he says.

All it takes to generate those new cells is an aerobic workout three or four times a week. According to Kramer, any exercise that pumps up your heart will pump up your brain. Jogging, brisk walking, and swimming—waterphobic rodents notwithstanding—all qualify.

As a result, many of Gage's colleagues have been moved—literally—by the compelling nature of his lab's results. "People take a look at the data," says Gage, "and then they take off for a run." ✳

exercise your mind

Working up a sweat isn't the only way to build mental muscle. According to Lawrence Katz, a neurobiologist at Duke University, a fit mind has webs of tendril-like branches of cells that form when you challenge your brain, say, by learning something new. In *Keep Your Brain Alive* (Workman, 1999), Katz explains "neurobics," exercises that can help you stay sharp. Here are a few of his techniques.

Rearrange Your Routine

If you usually log miles on the treadmill, take advantage of the season and head outdoors. Once you've hit the trail, don't just go on automatic pilot: Explore different routes on your walks or runs, and your brain will get a workout drawing new spatial maps.

Be a Beginner

Learning almost anything new puts brain cells to work, so try your hand at a sport you've never done before. If you're a swimmer, learn to play tennis. Check out that evening salsa-dancing class instead of your usual step aerobics.

Change Your Scene

Instead of lounging at the beach on your next vacation, go backpacking or car camping. It's a sure way to experience the unexpected. You'll need to read maps, pitch a tent, and cook meals in the open air.

Bring a Buddy

If nothing else, convince a friend to exercise with you. Studies show that an active social and intellectual life is critical to mental well-being. "Social interactions can have a huge effect on brain health," says Katz. "Running with a partner is much better than going it all alone."

custom fitness:
creating an exercise program that's
right for your body type

Tired of not getting the results you want?
The key is finding the right program.

BY KIMBERLY WONG

PHOTOGRAPHY BY CATHERINE LEDNER

Jennifer Carton Wade had loathed her pear shape ever since high school. "I hated my butt," she says. She ran for years, but the miles she put in did little for her shape, and the extra weight she carried on her hips ended up causing pain in her knees. Looking for a less jarring way to work out, she happily accepted a friend's invitation to a spin-bicycling class. She assumed the class was for novices, but it wasn't. "I was tricked," says the 31-year-old occupational therapist from San Francisco. "When I got there, I realized the only 'beginner' thing about the class was me."

To Carton Wade's surprise, she managed to keep pace with the group. Biking, it turns out, tapped her body's natural strength—her legs and rear. "Something clicked inside of me when I started cycling," says Carton Wade. "It was much easier than going for a long run. By accident, I found something that I'm actually pretty good at."

All that pedaling held another reward: Her rear slimmed down, and she gained definition and tone in her thighs. "Everything just feels firmer," says Carton Wade. "I love that my legs look muscular and strong." These days, there's no getting her off a bike. In the two years since she was duped by her friend, she's barely missed a cycling class.

Sounds like the impossible dream: a workout that comes naturally and gives you the aesthetic results you're after? Well, pinch yourself—it's not just wishful thinking, according to the experts, even though few of us ever figure this out. "People beat themselves up over the fact that they're not good at something," says Leigh Crews, a personal

Figuring out your body type isn't too tough, though you will have to stand naked in front of a mirror.

trainer and spokesperson for the American Council on Exercise, "or that they work really hard but don't seem to get anywhere. They could be fighting their body type." Some people are just made to be runners, say, while others have a build that favors swimming or weight training. If you haven't found the right workout for your body, you probably know firsthand the frustration exercise can cause. But once you identify your body type, you can tailor your workout to your abilities, Crews says. What's more, you can start working on ways to balance your figure; you may even find, as Carton Wade did, that doing what comes naturally will give you the shape you've always wanted.

Body typing was developed in 1940 by psychologist William H. Sheldon. He had a theory that body shape determines personality. After scouring thousands of photographs, he came up with three basic shapes. The personality link didn't pan out, but the

differences he charted turned out to be useful to nutritionists and exercise physiologists.

Sheldon's three body types have unwieldy scientific names, but their characteristics are easy to grasp: ectomorph (thin), endomorph (round), and mesomorph (muscular). Often, a person falls mainly into one of the three categories, but some people are an even mixture of two types.

You can either thank or curse your parents for your shape; for the most part, genetics determine body type. But knowing Mother Nature's no-exchange policy up front has an advantage: "Accepting that you're stuck with your body type helps you set realistic goals," says Alan Mikesky, an exercise physiologist at Indiana University–Purdue University at Indianapolis.

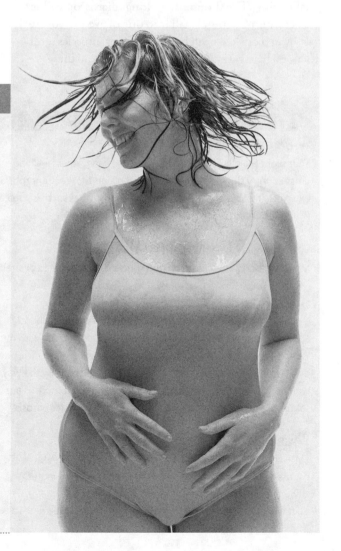

endomorph

WHAT COMES NATURALLY
Pear-shaped women don't carry just fat on their lower body; some of that extra heft is pure muscle, which can power you through activities such as in-line skating, swimming, dancing, and snow skiing. Also, short- to middle-distance fitness walking is good, but go longer and you're risking injury. Endomorphs tend to be more buoyant because of their padding, an advantage while swimming.

WHAT YOU MAY FIND FRUSTRATING
Sports that involve running or jumping.

HOW TO IMPROVE YOUR SHAPE
Your goal is to do long-distance, low-impact exercise to burn off extra fat and slim your hips. Adding a little upper-body strength training can help balance out a bottom-heavy endomorph.

YOUR IDEAL REGIMEN
• Skate, swim, walk, or cycle; 30 to 45 minutes; three to five times a week.
• Lift weights: 8 to 12 repetitions, one to two sets, two to three times a week.

"You may not be able to change your genetics, but you can certainly do the best with what your genes have dealt you."

How to know which category you fall into? Figuring it out isn't too tough, though you will have to stand naked in front of a mirror. If your parents passed down ectomorphic traits, chances are you're not harboring too many bitter feelings toward them at this moment. Ectomorphs have lean bodies; they're built like sticks. Picture Gwyneth Paltrow, with her willowy arms and narrow frame. They can even have a hard time gaining weight. (Crocodile tears, everyone.) Look in the mirror and flex your biceps and calves: An ectomorph's muscles, if visible at all, are long and thin.

For these string beans, it's building muscle that's challenging. The thousands of long microscopic fibers that constitute a muscle fall into one of two categories: fast-twitch or slow-twitch. Ectomorphs' muscles tend to have a high ratio of slow-twitch fibers, and these

fibers simply don't thicken in the same way fast-twitch ones do, no matter how much work they get. However, the slow variety use energy and oxygen conservatively, and that translates into plenty of stamina. (Marathoners tend to be ectomorphic.)

At the other end of the scale are voluptuous endomorphs. Their bodies hoard fat, favoring the hips and thighs as storage sites. They often look like a pear, though they can have an hourglass shape—think Marilyn Monroe. In the mirror test, endomorphs may not be able to make out their muscles, since body fat can conceal definition. But if your build is pear shaped, or you store weight in your hips, you're endomorphic.

Although endomorphs constantly battle the bulge, their muscles tend to be a more even mix of slow- and fast-twitch muscle than ectomorphs'. That means exercise can give endomorphs the best of both worlds:

ectomorph

WHAT COMES NATURALLY
Your slight build lends itself to distance running, fitness walking, cross-country skiing, snowshoeing, and hiking. Most ectomorphs are extremely flexible, so you'll find stretching activities such as yoga and Pilates rewarding.

WHAT YOU MAY FIND FRUSTRATING
Most ball sports; anything requiring sudden bursts of speed or strength.

HOW TO IMPROVE YOUR SHAPE
If ectomorphs complain, it's about their lack of curves. Full-body activities such as swimming or rowing can round you out with muscle. Weight training can also provide the definition you may crave, but don't overdo it; use weights you can lift 12 to 15 times. By the way, weight-bearing exercise is a must, because most ectomorphs are small boned, which can put you at a higher risk of osteoporosis.

YOUR IDEAL REGIMEN
• Walk or jog, 30 to 60 minutes, two to three times a week.
• Cross-train on a rowing machine or swim, 30 to 60 minutes, two to three times a week.
• Lift weights: 10 to 12 repetitions, two sets, two to three times a week.

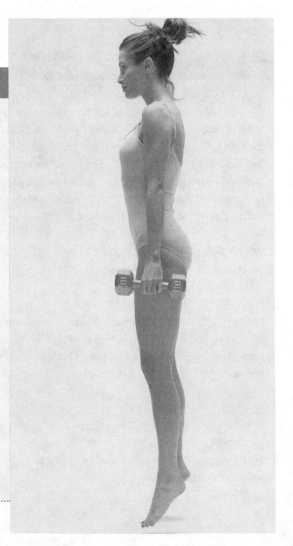

nice results from strength training and satisfaction from aerobic work, says Dixie Stanforth, an exercise physiologist at the University of Texas. Endomorphs can also use their powerful lower bodies to advantage in skating and cycling.

Lucky mesomorphs are born with the ability to build muscle quickly and burn fat easily. A mesomorph's muscular build makes her a natural athlete. Think of Olympian Marion Jones with her muscular arms, broad shoulders, and narrow waist and hips. Anything that calls for strength and short bursts of energy is going to favor the mesomorph, since her muscles have lots of fast-twitch fibers to provide the quick spark

needed for explosive sports like racquetball and tennis.

Because these muscle fibers get thicker in response to any work—be it swinging a racquet or pumping iron—a sharply defined bicep or calf is a giveaway that you're mesomorphic. So is a V-shaped build and a proclivity for tossing around bales of hay.

As you read more about your type (mesomorphs below, ectomorphs at left, and endomorphs on page 105), you'll learn which activities suit you and which you might not find as satisfying. The prescribed work-out falls within the recommended range of 20 to 60 minutes of aerobic exercise, three to five days a week. But each combines activities that come naturally with moves that will help balance your shape. If you happen to love something that isn't recommended for your body type, don't panic. It may be that you're a combination of two types or that you've simply overcome some inherent limitations. Combos such as ecto-endo or meso-endo are common. If, from the mirror test, you think you're a mixture of two types, read both sections and follow the advice that addresses your needs. ✳

mesomorph

WHAT COMES NATURALLY
Muscular mesomorphs are good at just about everything they try. You'll enjoy tennis, basketball, and soccer; your build is also great for kickboxing or martial arts.

WHAT YOU MAY FIND FRUSTRATING
Because of mesomorphs' preponderance of fast-twitch muscle fibers, endurance activities may prove to be a challenge.

HOW TO IMPROVE YOUR SHAPE
Be careful when weight training; you could easily over-develop specific muscle groups, making you look out of proportion. And even though you burn fat easily, if you don't watch your diet and exercise, you could pile on the pounds.

Mesomorphs should stretch out regularly, since all that muscle can make you stiff. "Mesomorphs need to balance high-energy activities with something more mellow like yoga, Pilates, or tai chi to help with the flexibility," says Crews.

YOUR IDEAL REGIMEN
* Choice of aerobic exercise, 30- to 45-minute sessions, three to five times a week.
* Regular stretching, such as yoga.
* Lifting weights isn't as crucial for mesomorphs; strength-train as needed to reach your goals.

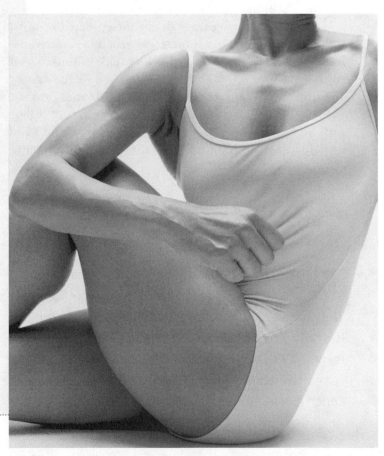

Q+A
Treadmill Tips

I recently purchased a treadmill and love the convenience. But I've started having pain in my shins. What am I doing wrong?

It's hard to say exactly what's happening, because shin pain can have dozens of causes. My guess, though, is that your zeal for your new fitness toy has caused an overuse injury. If you've boosted your exercise time or intensity since getting the treadmill (that was the whole point, wasn't it?), your muscles may not have had time to adjust to the demands you've been making on them, and the connective tissue that attaches the muscles to the bone might have torn. It's likely that that's what's smarting.

Many treadmill owners experience the same type of leg pain you're having. The machines are convenient, no doubt about it. But they're harder on your legs than an outdoor track or trail.

If you've been overdoing it, take a few days off and see if the discomfort goes away. Taking ibuprofen and applying a cold pack ought to help you feel better. (If the pain is severe and doesn't lessen after three days, contact your doctor.)

Once you're back in action, try alternating your treadmill workouts with a visit to a track a couple of times a week. Also, make sure your shoes fit snugly, support your arch, and don't allow your ankles to lean either inward or outward. You should replace running shoes every 250 miles or so. The next time you're shopping for a pair, spend a little extra for a pair with lots of cushioning; they'll be kinder to your shins.

Men Are from Couches, Women Are from Treadmills

The effect that pounding the pavement has on you, PlayStation has on him. A recent study published in *The Journal of Pain* discovered that a 10-minute run lessens a woman's sensitivity to pain. What does the trick for men? Video game competition. So the next time you have a tension headache, head for the treadmill. Leave the couch to him.

GOOD VIBRATIONS
Feng Shui and Exercising at Home

Who hasn't heard of the ancient art of feng shui that has folks nationwide moving beds and potted plants, even busting walls so positive energy can flow through their homes and spirits? But can you get the chi moving in a home gym?

Consider these basic feng shui principles and your workout space. Who knows—you may be attacking that treadmill with extra ha-cha-chi next time.

BAD FENG SHUI

- StairMaster in a dingy bedroom corner
- Treadmill doubles as a clothes hanger
- Workout room in windowless basement
- Black workout outfit

GOOD FENG SHUI

- Move workout area to center of room.
- Clean up: no clutter in your workout space.
- If you can't move equipment above ground, keep fresh flowers in the room.
- Switch to colorful workout clothing, even if it doesn't slenderize.

AND WHY

- It's hard to capture positive energy in corners.
- Clutter brings bad feng shui; you want clean lines.
- Light is a feng shui cure, as are flowers.
- Color plays an important role in positive feng shui.

CREATING YOUR HOME GYM: A COMPLETE GUIDE

Feel like being a homebody? With the right equipment, you can still work out.

HOME IS YOUR HAVEN for relaxing, socializing, dining, and sleeping. There's no reason you can't add working out to the list—especially on those days when the weather keeps you indoors or you don't have time to head for the gym.

Here you'll find everything you need for an at-home gym—tools for stretching, strength training, and aerobic routines. The basic gym (on the left) meets all your needs for about $435. The upgrade (on the right) provides more variety and runs about $880. Remember that in order to maintain health, experts recommend aerobic exercise at least three times a week for a minimum of 20 minutes; strength training two days a week, doing 8 to 10 moves; and stretching regularly. By having all the right gear at your fingertips, those recommendations should seem less like barking orders and more like invitations.

BASIC

Unwind at the end of your day or unknot after a tough workout using a Living Arts Mat ($22) and Strap ($7). The cushioned, nonslip mat is perfect for yoga, and the strap will help you hold positions longer. Call Gaiam: 800-869-3446.

Stretch to Develop Flexibility

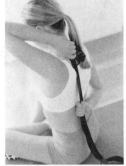
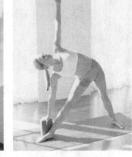

UPGRADE

Use Living Arts Bricks ($20 a pair) to get into just the right yoga position. Then take your stretching (and strengthening) to new levels with the Balance Ball ($27), which is not shown here. Call Gaiam: 800-869-3446.

BASIC

Tone muscle and preserve bone with Xertube Resistance Bands ($5 to $7). Curls, kick-backs, squats—with a little creativity you can mimic any weight-lifting move. As you get stronger, you can graduate to thicker and thicker tubing. Call SPRI: 800-222-7774.

Lift to Develop Strength

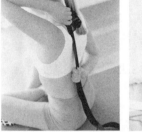
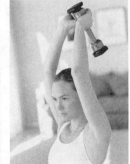

UPGRADE

Do your curls and presses with the Cap Solid Dumbbells ($14 for a 5-pound pair), available at sports retailers. When you're ready, pick up a set of Playmates magnetic weights that clamp to the ends of your weights ($20 a pair). Call 800-877-3322.

BASIC

The Wellness Machine ($399) gives you a stair-stepper workout anywhere you want it. You can exercise in front of the TV, in the bedroom, or even on the back porch. The smooth hydraulic canisters offer three levels of resistance. Call Gaiam: 800-869-3446.

Train for Aerobic Fitness

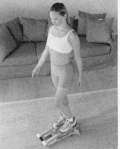
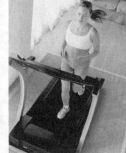

UPGRADE

Try the ProForm 785PI Treadmill ($799). Its wide belt, power incline, and preset programs will keep your walks or runs safe and provide variety. And the pulse sensor helps you maintain the optimum pace throughout your workout. Call 800-727-9777.

PHOTOGRAPHY BY DAVID MARTINEZ

exercise
your right to
bare arms

Why should rowers be the only ones with such strong and sexy arms?
Here's how to build beautiful biceps and toned
triceps—in and out of the water.

BY CAROLINE KNAPP

PHOTOGRAPHY BY DAN CHAVKIN

Behold the human arm, a thing of beauty and paradox. Lean lines of bone contrast with gentle swells of bicep and shoulder. Arms can bend, stretch, flex, wave, lift, hug, power a punch. They can also tell a story.

Mine tell a story about transformation and victory. They are strong arms: I am a relatively petite person—5 foot 4, small of frame—but I have been known to whup men in arm-wrestling contests, and that pleases me deeply. Once, I bench-pressed my own weight, which made me feel Amazonian. A friend refers to me—only half in jest—as "La Brutita," the Little Brute. And just the other day, my boyfriend called to ask me for a favor: He needed help moving a steel table. In the grand scheme of things, these may not sound like major triumphs, but they are to

me. My arms embody a hard-won confidence and autonomy that's as personal as it is physical; they are the one part of my body in which I have come to delight unequivocally.

That in itself is a statement of triumph. In the 80s, when I was in my mid-20s, I didn't know a bicep from a tricep, I'd never even heard of lats, and my sense of my physical self—arms included—was almost pathologically negative. Actually, it *was* pathologically negative. I was young, scared, and confused, and I did what a lot of young, scared, and confused women do—I developed anorexia. At my lowest weight—83 pounds—I was a waif, fragile as a wren, a mere line drawing of a woman, but some deluded part of me felt supremely strong-willed. Strange how

I have been known to whup men in
arm-wrestling contests, and that pleases me deeply.

My arms embody a hard-won confidence and
autonomy that's as personal as it is physical.

110

the ability to deny appetite provides a seductive illusion of power.

I remember quite clearly how this twisted logic was reflected in my view of my arms. At night, I'd lie in bed with one skeletal arm, stretched out in front of me—the sight would fill with a perverse sensation of mastery.

That feeling, of course, was disembodied and false—it had to do with the shape of my body, not the state of my soul—and, ultimately, the scrap of pride it gave me was about as sustaining as a saltine. And so, after much desperation, many fits and starts, and lots of therapy, I began to crawl toward a livable relationship with my body.

My arms were key to that effort, and I mean that quite literally. In 1985, I spent an exhilarating autumn on the Charles River in Cambridge, Massachusetts, learning to scull. I'd grown up near the Charles, and I'd always admired the sight of its community of rowers—so elegant and strong as they skimmed across the surface. I suspect some part of me wanted what they had, a level of control that wasn't illusory.

As it turns out, I had picked exactly the right sport. Maneuvering a single shell is like trying to stay upright on a giant knitting needle. As athletics go, sculling is like aquatic tightrope walking, requiring both enormous precision and guts. I was terrible at it for years—flailing and teetering, I held the oars in a death grip that caused them to slap the water at every stroke. But from the start, I was determined to master the craft. The beauty of rowing—the symmetry, the steady whoosh of water against hull, the marriage of strength and grace—captured me, and that first season I wandered around like a teenager giddy with love, aware that I'd found something to conquer besides the shape of my own body. This was something that would transform me.

I rowed and rowed. I rowed on stormy days and calm days. I struggled and hacked my way up and down the river. I developed patience, then (more slowly) I developed confidence, and then (finally) I developed a bit of skill.

Along the way, I developed arms—strong, capable arms. My forearms grew firm and sinewy. My upper arms became toned, then defined. My shoulders grew round and strong. Technically, rowing is considered a lower-body sport, because much of the stroke's power comes from the large muscles of the butt and thighs. But the changes in my upper body were more visible to me—and in many ways more important: Each sign of physical strength fueled a new sensation of internal strength. That summer I often slipped into the ladies' room at work and secretly flexed my biceps in front of the mirror. Muscles! What a concept! The little thrill this gave me was utterly distinct from the thrill I'd once felt at my emaciation, as different as self-care is from self-destruction, as giving is from withholding.

Like a lot of women, I've undertaken most of my efforts at physical transformation in the service of beauty and slenderness. Bad perms to make straight hair wavy, lotions and potions to smooth the complexion, stultifying exercise regimens (jogging, step aerobics) for weight control.

But arms are often exempt from this paradigm, blessedly immune. Arms offer a bit more wiggle room on the self-acceptance front

> In arms we get the pairing of **sexuality with strength** instead of frailty, with power instead of passivity.

than most of the female body, which makes them a bit easier to love than, say, hips or thighs. In arms, we get the pairing of sexuality with strength instead of frailty, with power instead of passivity: Think Linda Hamilton in *The Terminator;* Brandi Chastain, pumping her fist in the air after scoring the winning goal; Marion Jones, whose arms played as much of a role as her legs did in propelling her across the finish line.

I got on the water this morning, headed up the river under a cool and brilliant sky, and lost myself in the rhythm of the boat, the sparkle of the sun against the river's surface, the feel of the blades rushing through water. I felt strong and competent.

Most of the time, my arms are hidden from view, cloaked under sweaters or long sleeves. I don't show them off; instead, the satisfaction I take in them comes from a passion and a set of skills. Beauty from the inside out—this, I believe, is the definition of liberation. Arms like wings. ✳

Caroline Knapp is a writer in Cambridge, Massachusetts.

Five steps to great-looking arms

YOU NEEDN'T HAVE the Charles River in your backyard to get a rower's strong, sinewy arms. A simple routine like this one can prepare you for the tank tops and bathing suits that are de rigueur for summer trips to the shore.

While vanity may be motivation enough, having strong arms will make everyday tasks easier—from gardening to lifting your kids or groceries, says Petra Kolber, Reebok master trainer and *Health* contributing editor. "Women tend to get quick, satisfying results from resistance workouts," she says. "It takes only about a month to start seeing a difference.

"Do two sets of each of the moves on these pages three days a week. When you can comfortably complete two sets, add 3 to 4 repetitions on each move, building up to three sets.

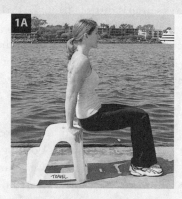

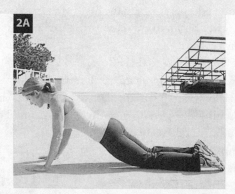

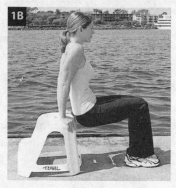

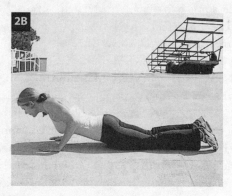

SHOULDER PUSH-UP

1A | You'll need a bench or a chair for this move. Place your hands about shoulder width apart on the lip of the seat and grasp it firmly. Straighten your arms without locking your elbows. Supporting yourself with your arms, slide your butt off the chair.

1B | Slowly lower your body by letting your shoulders come up toward your ears. Then raise yourself using the muscles in your shoulders and upper back. Do two sets of 8 to12 repetitions.

TRICEPS PUSH-UP

2A | Begin on your hands and knees with your hands shoulder width apart and far enough forward that the line from your shoulders to your knees is straight. Keeping your knees and toes on the ground, straighten your arms without locking your elbows.

2B | Bend your elbows to lower your body to the ground. Return to the starting position by straightening your arms. As you push up, tighten your triceps and keep your abdominal muscles taut to support your back. Try not to bend at the waist. Do two sets of 8 to 12 push-ups.

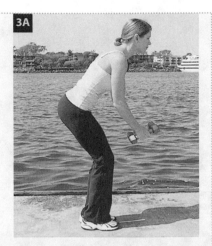

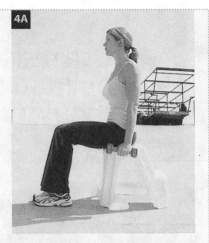

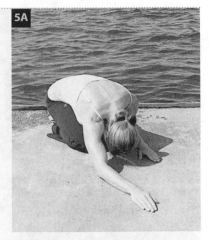

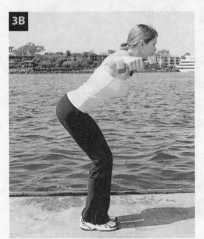

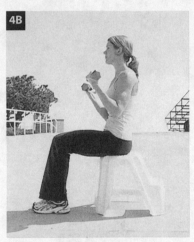

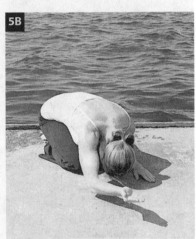

REVERSE FLY

3A | Hold a 3- to 5-pound dumbbell in each hand in front of you with your palms facing one another. Stand with your feet shoulder width apart and your knees slightly bent. Lean forward from your hips, keeping your back flat and your abdominals taut.

3B | Raise both arms out to the side until the weights are nearly level with your shoulders. Hold for one count, then return to the starting position. Keep your shoulders down and relaxed throughout. Do two sets of 8 to 12 repetitions.

BICEPS CURL

4A | Hold a 5-pound weight in each hand and sit on a chair with your feet flat on the floor, back straight, and shoulders relaxed. Hold the weights with your palms facing your sides.

4B | Bending at the elbows, curl both weights up toward your shoulders while turning your palms toward your chest. Hold for one count and lower to the starting position. Do two sets of 8 to 12 repetitions.

REACH, ROLL, AND LIFT

5A | Start on your knees with your butt on your heels and your left forearm on the ground at your side. Extend your right arm in front of you, keeping your palm facedown and your forearm on the ground.

5B | Without lifting your butt off your heels, raise your right arm as far as you can, rotating it so the palm faces up. Hold for 3 to 5 breaths, then lower to starting position. Repeat with left arm. Do two sets of 8 to 12 repetitions, alternating arms.

body work

Use resistance bands to build strong, shapely shoulders.

WORKOUT CREATED BY PETRA KOLBER   PHOTOGRAPHY BY DAVID MARTINEZ

WHAT YOU GET
Strong, shapely shoulders in time for summer.

WHAT YOU DO
An overhead press, external rotations, and a front-to-side raise; you'll perform these with resistance bands. Resistance bands vary in thickness: For all three exercises, choose one that presents a challenge but doesn't make you shake.

ALL IT TAKES
• Ten minutes, three days a week.
• In one month, you'll see better definition in your shoulders.
• In two or three months, you'll have gained more power for swimming, tennis, or golf.

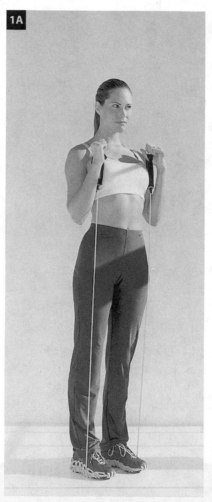

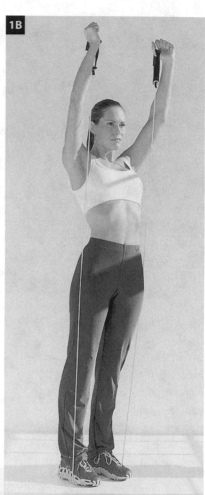

overhead press

1A | Stand on the band with your feet hip-distance apart. Pull the handles up until they rest gently on your shoulders. Your elbows should be at your sides, and your thumbs should be facing you.

1B | Using your shoulder muscles, exhale as you slowly press your arms straight up, taking care not to lean back or lock your elbows. Hold for one count, then lower to the starting position. Repeat 8 to 12 times. Add a second set in one month.

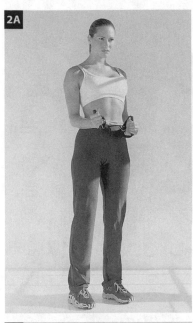

external rotations

2A | Wrap the resistance band around your waist and cross the handles in front of you. Your hands should be level with your hips, elbows at your sides.

2B | Holding your left hand in place, rotate your right shoulder until your right hand extends straight out from your side. Keep your elbow tucked in. Repeat 8 to 12 times; switch. Add a second set in one month.

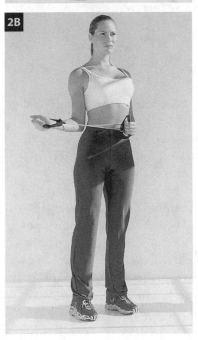

You can strengthen your entire body using the bands. And they fit easily into a suitcase for workouts on the road.

—trainer PETRA KOLBER

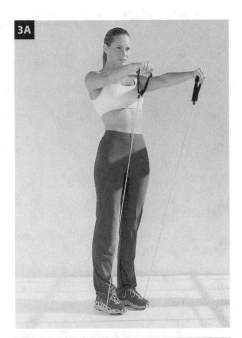

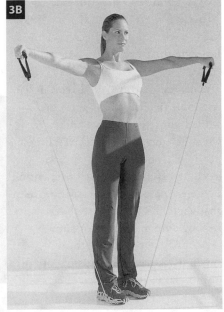

front-to-side raise

3A | Stand on the band with your feet hip-distance apart. Lift your arms up in front of you until they're at shoulder height. Keep your wrists straight and hold for one count.

3B | Now rotate your shoulders, opening your arms out to form a T with your body. Hold, then lower your arms to your sides. Repeat 8 to 12 times. Add a second set in one month.

CoreStrength Workout

for smoother abs and an injury-proof body

Smooth, firm abs aren't just for looks anymore.
Experts are finding that a strong midsection is
key to feeling centered—and staying well.

BY ELIZABETH B. KRIEGER

Every time I work out, I go through the same inner dialogue. I've finished my 45-minute sweatfest, plodded through a few basic strength-training exercises on either the machines or the free weights, and I'm ready to make a beeline for the locker room. Then I glance down at the floor mats, where I see people assiduously doing their abdominal and back work. "I should do those, too," I think. "Ugh, I hate floor work." Or, "No! I'm tired." Or, "I'm late for dinner."

Still, my torso area could certainly use some firming up, so once in a while I plop myself down and dash off a set of crunches and, if I'm feeling particularly dedicated, a few back stretches. But most of the time, I don't. I congratulate myself on having at least made it to the gym, toss my sweaty towel in the hamper, and hit the shower.

According to the latest thinking of many sports medicine experts, I'm missing out on a critical part of any workout, if not the very heart of it. By lopping off the part that really focuses on my "core" muscles—the large muscle groups of my abs, back, hips, and pelvis—I've just eliminated one of the best ways not only to look better in a bathing suit, but to keep injury-prone areas of my body healthy.

Sure, you've heard that sit-ups can help your back, but that's just the beginning of what core strengthening can accomplish. These days, leading injury specialists recommend core exercises to prevent and overcome all sorts of troubles, from shoulder pain to ankle strains. Just forget one-size-fits-all crunches as a panacea; with a few moves that work these muscles, you can maintain a healthy body no matter what your pursuit may be.

The concept is catching on: Classes such as yoga and Pilates are in heavy rotation at health clubs everywhere, due in part to the regimens' focus on the core. And the exercise gurus at Reebok and at Crunch Fitness have introduced new workouts based solely on core conditioning.

"The center of the body is where your strength and ability to move comes from," says Joel Press, assistant professor of physical medicine and rehabilitation at

> The center of the body is where your strength comes from. Ignore your center and you're setting yourself up for problems all over.

Northwestern University Medical School in Chicago. "It's simple, really. Experts are realizing that if you ignore your center, you're pretty much setting yourself up for problems all over."

I don't immediately think of my belly as having any effect on my feet, but Press sets me straight. He likens the body to an assembly line, and any weak link along the line means the end product will suffer. Imagine an assembly line for toasters in which the guy attaching electrical cords is having a bad day. The toasters may look fine, but they're going to give someone a nasty shock. Same with the body—all of your parts must work together. If one area isn't doing its job, you're going to end up in pain. "It's a carefully balanced system—a system of links in a chain of events," he says.

Think of walking: As you take a step, muscles in your hips, pelvis, abs, and back contract as the joints roll with the motion. This helps dissipate the force that each footfall places on these joints, and it provides energy and momentum for your next stride. If, say, the muscles in your hips are weak, you may begin to exaggerate the natural roll of your feet, putting pressure on your arches to do the work of those muscles—to soften the impact and absorb some of that force. That can lead to knee problems, foot fatigue, arch pain, and other injuries.

It works much the same way whether you're jogging, golfing, or playing tennis. "Your core is the anchor for those movements," says Press. "Without a strong anchor to support the effort of rotation, the strain on your limbs is greatly increased."

But strengthen the anchor and those movements get easier. It's not just your sporting life that improves, says Walter Thompson, professor of kinesiology and health at Georgia State University. "These often-neglected muscles stabilize you as you move, keeping everything—especially your hips and pelvis—in its proper place and in balance," he says. This area is the starting point for many activities: Digging in the garden, carrying groceries, pushing open a heavy door, lunging to grasp a precariously perched wineglass, hoisting a box to a top shelf—the list goes on and on.

"Your gait will improve, your breathing—everything is connected to your core and will benefit," says Gray Cook, orthopedic clinical specialist with the American Physical Therapy Association, and one of the

are you hard core?

Before you jump into a core-strength workout, assess how strong your center already is. These two tests—adapted from the Reebok Core Training program by Annette Lang, a Reebok master trainer—can help you gauge your level of strength and stability.

Test 1 | Find a spot at home where you can see a clock with a second hand. Standing with your feet together, arms at your side, slowly raise one knee up to waist height and balance. Count how many seconds you can hold this position without putting your foot down or wobbling.

Test 2 | Lie on a carpeted floor on your back. Prop yourself up on your elbows so that your forearms are flat on the floor at your sides. Raise your midsection so that you're supported only by your forearms and heels. Your body should be straight. Count how long you can hold this position without shaking.

0–15 seconds each: You need some core strength. Start with the workout on pages 118 and 119, but don't worry if you can't complete all the repetitions. Go slowly and stop if you feel unsteady.

16–45 seconds each: Not bad, but your midsection could still use some attention. You should be able to do one set each of the moves on pages 118 and 119. If that seems too easy, try holding the positions longer or doing up to 15 repetitions per set.

Over 45 seconds: Congratulate yourself on a good start. You're probably already doing regular ab exercises (or you're just lucky). If you want to do this workout, start with two sets of each move.

Another way to challenge yourself is to try one of the huge rubber balls you see in gyms. For proper technique, get an instructional video or hire a personal trainer. Or consider investing in the CORE board from Reebok ($190 with video; call 800-688-8623 to order). This is an oval platform balanced on a fulcrumlike pedestal, and it's key to the CORE class workouts you can find in gyms around the country. Most core moves can be done on these devices; their natural instability makes the workout more demanding.

developers of the Reebok Core Training system. There's your future to consider as well, says Richard Stein, adjunct professor of applied exercise physiology at Teachers College at Columbia University. "Looking good and feeling good is nice," he says, "but really the most important thing is whether you're able to do all the things that you want, and whether you'll be able to do all of them for the next 20 years. The muscles of your core are 'long-run' muscles."

Unfortunately, crunches alone don't cut it. Sure,

they're better than nothing to keep your abs up to snuff, says Annie O'Connor, clinical manager of the Center for Spine and Sports at the Rehabilitation Institute of Chicago. But several groups of muscles make up your core, and trying to work them all by doing just crunches is like expecting your arms to get strong from doing leg presses.

O'Connor stresses that the exercises you do should mimic the movements and functions you do in real life. "Look at a sit-up," she says. "That little curling

six steps to core strength

PHOTOGRAPHY BY JOHN HUET

These moves, designed by Reebok University master trainer and *Health* contributing editor Petra Kolber, put you on the path to a strong and toned center.

All it takes is about five to seven minutes, two to three times a week. After a few weeks, you'll start to feel stronger—from the inside out.

THE PLANK

1 | Lie facedown on the ground with your legs extended behind you, toes curled under. Support yourself on your forearms—elbows directly under your shoulders. Now raise your midsection. Hold the pose for 30 seconds. The plank strengthens your entire back and abdominal region.

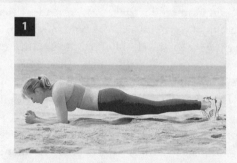

V-SIT

2 | Sit on the ground with your knees bent and feet flat. Maintain the small natural curve in your lower back. Lean back slightly so your thighs and trunk form a V-shape. Cross your hands over your chest (or, if that's too difficult, place your hands on the ground behind you). Raise one foot at a time, making sure to keep your abdominals firm. Do 8 to 12 repetitions on each leg. Staying balanced throughout this move works your abs, obliques (the big muscles that wrap around the side of your torso), and back muscles.

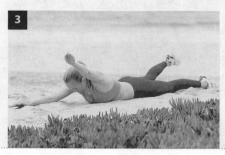

BACK EXTENSOR

3 | Lie facedown with your arms and legs extended. Lift your left arm a few inches off the ground and allow your head to follow. At the same time, raise your right leg. (With time you'll be able to get your arm and leg higher.) Hold for three to five breaths, then do the opposite arm and leg. Do 8 to 12 repetitions on each side. This move strengthens the muscles in your lower and upper back.

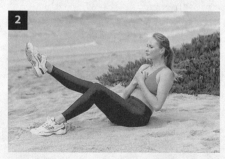

motion. When in your real life do you do that? Not very often." That's why the workout below includes six different moves. So-called "functional" ab and core exercises challenge these muscles in ways that you actually use them, incorporating stability and balance challenges at the same time.

It may sound like a lot, but remember, there's an aesthetic payoff as well. I've never seen a Pilates instructor or yoga teacher with a less than taut torso. All this work on your core helps you stand up straighter, a surefire way to look 2 inches taller and 10 pounds lighter. Combine core work with regular aerobic exercise and you're bound to have a tighter, trimmer middle, no two ways about it.

For me, it's clear that as much as I gripe about wanting to cut my workouts short, the very worst thing would be to have an injury cut them out of my life entirely. So save a place on the floor mats for me. ✷

Elizabeth B. Krieger is a freelance writer in San Francisco.

SPINAL ROTATION

4A | Start on your hands and knees. Place your right hand on the back of your neck, fingertips pointing down your spine and elbow pointing ahead. Creep your hand down your neck as far as feels comfortable.

4B | Keeping your hips steady and in line with your knees, curl under and point your right elbow to your left knee. Hold for three to five breaths. Bring your right elbow up and back, so that it's pointing toward the sky. Hold for three to five breaths. Do 8 to 12 repetitions with the right arm. Repeat on the opposite side. This move works the muscles along the spine and at the top of your butt.

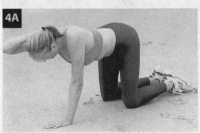

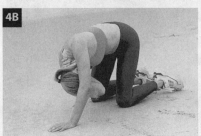

TRANSVERSE TWIST

5A | Lie on your back with your arms straight out from your shoulders, knees bent, and feet flat on the ground. Tuck your heels up close to your rear.

5B | Keeping both shoulders on the ground, slowly lower your knees to the ground on the right. Then bring your legs back to the starting position and continue over to the left side. That counts as one repetition; do 8 to 12. This strengthens your obliques, your abs, and the muscles along your spine.

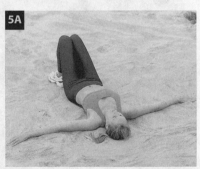

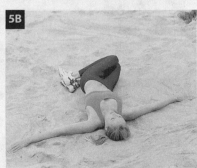

OBLIQUE TWIST

6A | Lie on your back with your knees bent and feet flat. Extend your arms on each side, palms up and elbows bent at a 90-degree angle.

6B | Bring your right elbow and shoulder off the ground toward your left knee. At the same time, raise your left knee toward your chest. Keep your lower back flat by pressing your belly button toward the floor. Do 8 to 12 repetitions per side. Your obliques and abs will benefit.

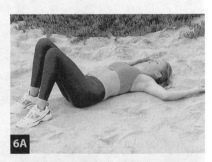

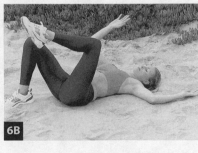

body work

Take three steps to a tighter tush.

WORKOUT CREATED BY PETRA KOLBER   PHOTOGRAPHY BY DAVID MARTINEZ

WHAT YOU GET
An effortless stride and
a tighter tush.

WHAT YOU DO
A single-leg bridge, a squat,
and a lunge.

ALL IT TAKES
• Ten minutes, three days a week
• In one month, your favorite
jeans will fit better.
• In two months, you'll bound
up stairs with ease.

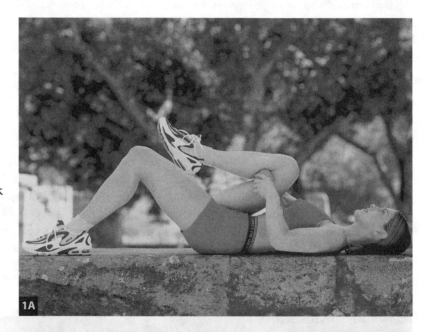

single-leg bridge

1A | Lie on your back and bend
your left knee, keeping your left
foot flat on the ground. Clasp your
hands behind your right knee and
pull your leg close to your chest.

1B | Contracting the muscles in your
rear, lift your pelvis several inches off
the ground, while keeping your right
leg pulled into your chest. Hold for
three counts, then lower. Do 8 to 12
repetitions, then switch legs; add a
set when you can easily do 12.

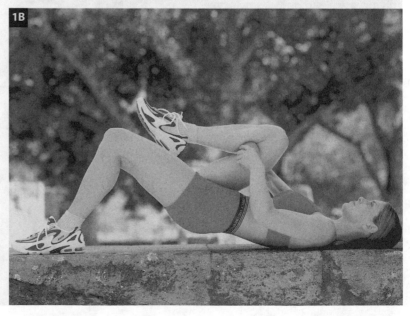

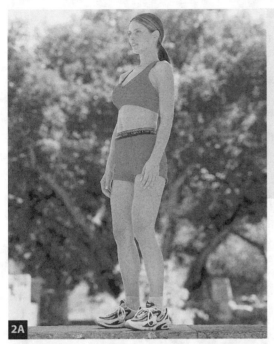

squat

2A | Stand with your feet hip-distance apart, toes pointing forward and arms at your sides.

2B | While bringing your arms out in front of you, slowly bend at the knees, as if taking a seat in a chair. Your knees should not extend past your toes. Hold for two counts and rise up. Do 8 to 12 squats; add a set when you can easily do 12.

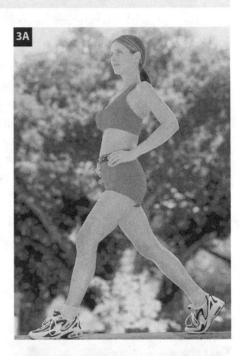

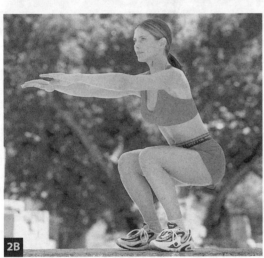

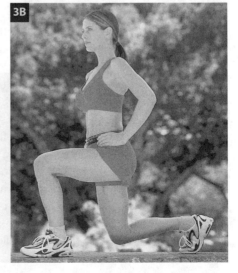

lunge

3A | Standing with your feet hip-distance apart and hands on your hips, step back with your right leg, keeping your right heel off the ground.

3B | Slowly lower your trunk, keeping your weight on your left leg but making sure your knee doesn't travel past your toes. Hold for three counts and rise up. Do 8 to 12 repetitions, then switch legs; add a set when you can easily do 12.

body work

Tone your hips to move with ease.

WORKOUT CREATED BY PETRA KOLBER

PHOTOGRAPHY BY DAVID MARTINEZ

WHAT YOU GET
Strong, toned hips; better balance; and more power in your step.

WHY THIS WORKOUT WORKS
These three exercises play on lateral (side-to-side) training, an often-overlooked component of fitness. Most physical activities involve forward or backward motion, so by adding lateral moves to your exercise program, you help balance muscle strength.

ALL IT TAKES
• Ten minutes, three days a week.
• In six weeks, anything involving side movements will feel effortless.

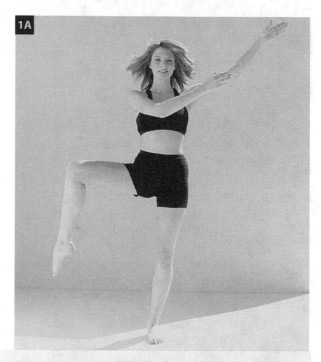

1A

lift and cross

1A | Stand on your left leg, knee slightly bent. Lift your right leg out and up to the side until your thigh is parallel to the floor and your toes are pointing at the ground. Lift your arms diagonally up to the left so your right arm crosses your body.

1B | Keeping your hips level with the floor and your chest lifted, slowly bring your right leg down and across the midline of your body, leading with your heel. At the same time, swing your arms down in an arc and then up so that your left arm crosses your body. Repeat 8 to 12 times; switch legs. Add a second set when you can easily do 12 and build to three sets.

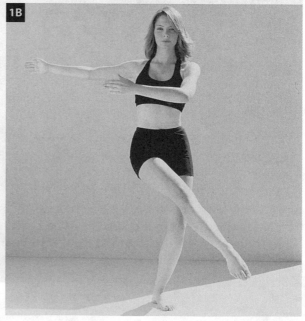

1B

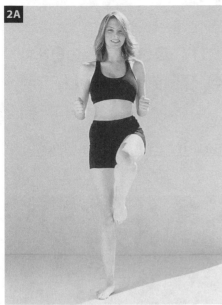

external rotations

2A | Stand on your right leg and lift your left knee until your thigh is parallel to the ground.

2B | Lunge out to the side with your left leg, keeping your right leg straight (knee soft). Make sure your left knee is directly over (not past) your toes. Keep abdominals tight and your chest lifted. Hold for 2 counts and push back up to the knee lift position. Repeat 8 to 12 times; switch legs. Repeat on the opposite leg. Add a second set when you can easily do 12 and build to three sets.

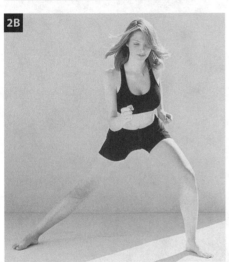

> Side-to-side training is a great addition to any workout. Whether you're lunging to return a tennis serve or tickle a toddler, you'll be able to move with ease.
>
> —trainer PETRA KOLBER

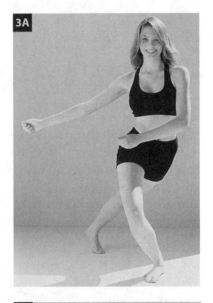

lateral leap

3A | Stand on your right leg, knee slightly bent and directly over your toes. Place your left leg diagonally behind you with the ball of your foot resting lightly on the floor.

3B | With abdominal muscles tight and chest lifted, push off with your right knee and leap to the left side. As you land on your left foot, bend your left knee and bring your right leg diagonally behind you, with the ball of your foot touching the floor. Do 8 to 12 repetitions. Add a second set when you can easily do 12 and build to three sets.

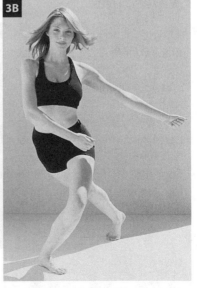

body work

Aim for strong, shapely thighs to power your lower body.

WORKOUT CREATED BY PETRA KOLBER

PHOTOGRAPHY BY DAVID MARTINEZ

WHAT YOU GET
Shapely, powerful thighs that provide power to your lower body.

WHY THIS WORKOUT WORKS
Instead of isolating one muscle, as most exercises do, these moves call on the two major players in the upper leg: the hamstrings and quadriceps.

ALL IT TAKES
• Ten minutes, three days a week.
• In two months, you'll have strong, firm thighs that will help you move efficiently, whether plowing through powder on snowshoes or racing to keep up with your toddler.

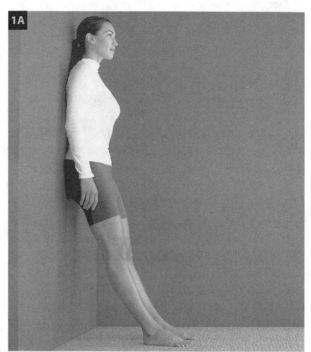

wall squat

1A | Standing with your back flat against a wall, place your feet hip-width apart, about 18 inches in front of you. Keep your abdominal muscles tight and your shoulders relaxed.

1B | With your weight centered over your heels, bend your knees and slide your back down the wall until your thighs are almost parallel to the floor. (Knees should be in line with your toes). Hold for 3 counts, then push up to the starting position. Do 8 to 12 repetitions; add another set when you can easily do 12. Build to three sets.

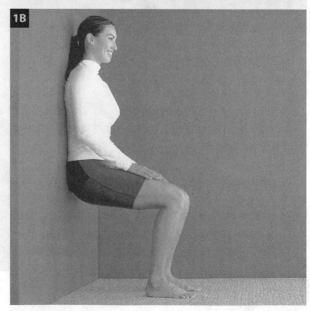

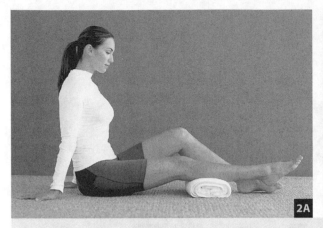

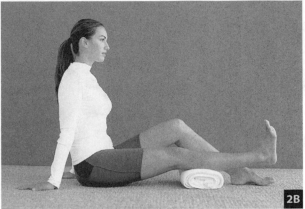

quadriceps lift

2A | Sitting on the floor, extend your right leg and place a rolled towel under your upper calf. Bend your left leg and place your left foot on the floor. Rest your hands behind you, fingers pointing away from your body.

2B | Contract your right thigh until your foot is flexed. Count to 3, then lower your foot. Do 8 to 12 repetitions on each leg to complete one set. Add a second set when you can easily do 12 and build to three sets.

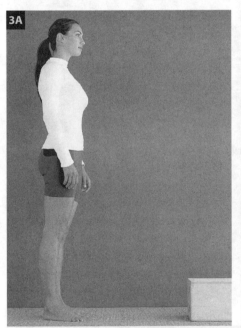

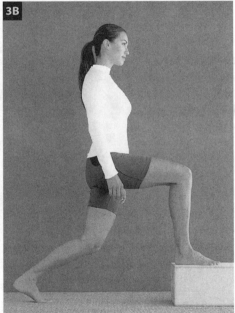

In one month, your legs will feel more powerful; in two months, they'll look as capable as they feel.

—trainer PETRA KOLBER

forward lunge

3A | With your feet hip-width apart, stand 2 feet in front of a step that's 8 to 10 inches high. Abs and chest are lifted, arms hanging loose by your sides.

3B | Step forward and place your right foot on the step. Bend both knees until your right thigh is parallel to the floor. (Keep right knee in line with right toes.) Hold for 3 counts; return to starting position. Repeat with your left leg (one move on each leg counts as 1 repetition). Do 8 to 12 repetitions. Add a second set when you can easily do 12; build to three sets.

body work

Build trim, limber calves.

WORKOUT CREATED BY PETRA KOLBER

PHOTOGRAPHY BY DAVID MARTINEZ

WHAT YOU GET
Sculpted legs and healthy feet.
Strong, limber calves that can
reduce your risk of injury.

WHAT YOU DO
A standing calf raise, a calf stretch,
a seated calf raise, and an inverted
calf raise.

ALL IT TAKES
• Fifteen minutes, three days a week.
• In one month, your calves will begin to look
stronger and more shapely.
• By next spring, you'll be primed for
prancing in your new capris.

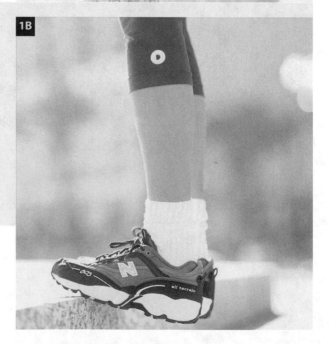

standing calf raise

1A | Stand on the balls of your feet on the edge of a
step using a wall or pole to balance yourself. Slowly
rise onto your toes as high as is comfortable and hold
for two counts.

1B | Gently lower your heels below the curb. Using
your calf muscles, rise back onto your toes. Do 8 to 12
repetitions. In one month, add a second set.

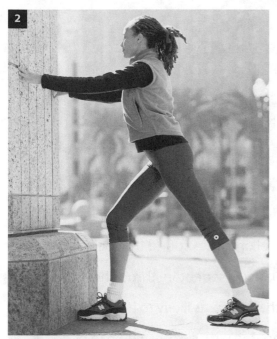

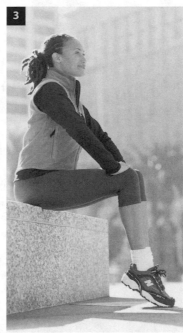

seated calf raise

3 | Sitting on a bench or chair, place your hands on your knees, keeping your shoulders back. Slowly lift your heels while pressing down with your hands for resistance. Hold for five counts, then relax. Do 8 to 10 repetitions. In one month, add a second set.

calf stretch

2 | Before you walk, do a 5-minute aerobic warm-up followed by this stretch to prevent injuries. Place your hands against a wall. Bend your right leg and extend your left leg back until you feel a gentle stretch while keeping your heel on the ground. Hold for 20 counts on each leg; repeat.

We often neglect training our calves. They're key to the powerful stride.

—trainer PETRA KOLBER

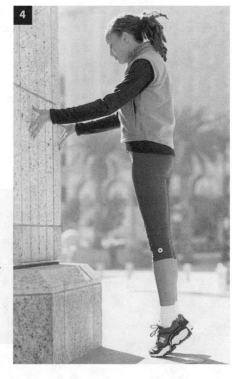

inverted calf raise

4 | Stand facing a wall and support yourself with both hands at a comfortable level. Your feet should be shoulder width apart with your toes pointed inward. Flexing the muscles in your calves, slowly rise onto your toes. Hold for five counts, then lower. Do 8 to 12 repetitions. In one month, add a second set.

Q+A
Why your body can get hooked on yoga classes

Is it possible to get addicted to yoga? If I miss a class, I end up feeling tighter than before I started.

We know just what you mean: A few days after a weekly yoga class, your hamstrings can feel as taut as a stretched rubber band. Why? Yoga loosens tense muscles, helping you to relax. Sometimes, though, if you stretch too vigorously, you create microscopic tears in the muscle fibers. These aren't serious and take only a few days to heal. But during that time your muscles protect themselves from further overextension by tightening up.

If, while this is happening, you continue to do yoga, the gentle stretching will coax your muscles into loosening again. Stop the cycle, and you'll feel stiff.

What's more, yoga puts you in touch with your body. That means you're more apt to notice even subtle sensations of tightness that you may not have focused on in the past.

There's a simple solution. When you're doing yoga, don't push your muscles too far; stretching should never hurt. And try to take a few minutes each day to practice some poses on your own. Your muscles will be looser, and you'll carry more of that delicious post-yoga relaxation into your everyday life.

EXERCISE TO OUTSMART ALZHEIMER'S

Want to retire with a sound mind and a fit body? Get off the couch. Researchers at Case Western Reserve University interviewed more than 500 older people about their lifelong participation in dozens of activities, from gardening to bowling to walking. They found that people who had been relatively sedentary throughout their lives were more than twice as likely to have Alzheimer's disease compared with people who had been active. This doesn't prove a cause-and-effect relationship between exercise and the disease, but it fits with other studies that have found a lower instance of Alzheimer's among people who have led active lives. And doesn't your tomato patch need weeding?

Go for the burn—not the heartburn.
Eat lunch, then hit the weights, and you may feel the burn in your heart. Lifters who eat before a session are three times as likely to suffer heartburn as other athletes, a recent study found. Wait an hour or two after fueling up prior to pumping iron.

Bicycle helmets save grown-ups too.
They're not just for kids and bike racers. New research offers more proof that they can save you from a serious head injury.

WHEN IT COMES TO EXERCISE, EVEN A LITTLE BIT HELPS

Talk about a fitness regimen you can manage. Researchers at Harvard University's Medical School and School of Public Health found in a study of nearly 40,000 women that those who exercise moderately (even as little as one hour of brisk walking per week) have about half the risk of developing heart disease as nonexercisers. This is welcome news for many, because heart disease is the leading cause of death among women in the United States. "Walk just an hour a week, and you can cut your risk of heart disease in half," says the study's director, I-Min Lee, M.D., Ph.D. "That's a very doable goal for someone who hasn't exercised before."

HEALTH BUZZ

THUMBS UP

cats
Score one for the fur ball. Researchers say that keeping a kitty in the house may actually protect kids from getting asthma.

drug companies
Sure, their motives are sketchy. Yet there's little doubt their move to lower prices on AIDS drugs will save countless lives.

THUMBS DOWN

fatty foods
It's bad for your heart, your waistline, and, now, your brain. In a study, rats fed high-fat chow had impaired learning and memory.

vitamin E supplements
As scientists debate whether the vitamin can fight disease, new research indicates it has no antioxidant effect. Stay tuned.

Exercise with the Stars

How did Julia Roberts get in shape for Erin Brockovich? How did Oprah manage to run a marathon? How can Angela Bassett look so fit all the time? Hours of lung-busting exercise, that's how. Here's the skinny on their sacrifices and rewards. Just remember: It's a star's job to look fabulous.

SUPERSTAR	WORKOUT	HOURS A WEEK	INDULGENCE
Angela Bassett	jogging, weight lifting	14	regular facials
Madonna	ashtanga yoga	14	toffee pudding
Julia Roberts	step aerobics, yoga, jogging, strength training, horseback riding	at least 7	biscuits and gravy
Sela Ward	stair-climbing	3	Krispy Kreme doughnuts
Oprah Winfrey	jogging	9	potato chips

YOGA

fitness without sweat

Combine the wisdom of the ages with modern-day science, and you get a newer, safer form of yoga that won't get you in a twist.

BY MARTICA K. HEANER

PHOTOGRAPHY BY DAVID ROTH

Perhaps the most appealing thing about yoga is that, compared with most other types of exercise, it seems so easy. Instead of a hard-body instructor demanding 50 more push-ups to the beat of a hip-hop hit, a catlike yoga teacher purrs at you to exhale as soothing chants transport you to a higher place. No wonder many yoga neophytes, empowered by exercise that doesn't involve such painful-sounding words as "fat-burning," attempt to contort their bodies as if they've been downward-dogging and head-standing for years.

Despite its gentler appearance, yoga isn't a one-size-fits-all activity. "Because yoga is a meditative, stretching-based workout, it's promoted as great for everybody from the complete beginner to the seriously fit—but it's not without risks," says Shay McKelvey, an exercise physiologist for the American Council on Exercise. "No matter how fit you are, you could strain joints in some positions or be pushed too far by an overzealous instructor."

As more people get their *om* on (the number of yoga classes offered at health clubs has increased by 26 percent in the past five years, according to IDEA, the association for health and fitness professionals), reports of yoga-related pains have increased as well. All styles, from Iyengar to Ashtanga, share standard poses that can stress the body: The swinging sun salutation series flexes the spine accordion style, which can strain the lower back. The cross-legged lotus pose can aggravate even healthy knees, while inverted postures such as the shoulder stand and headstand plough can put too much pressure on the neck.

Still, yoga's advantages shouldn't be discounted. Research suggests that regular practice improves blood pressure, muscular endurance, lung capacity, strength, balance, and, of course, flexibility. It works wonders for the mind too: Yoga may improve one's mood and decrease anxiety.

Something so good in so many ways doesn't need to be so hard on your body, says Washington, D.C.-based instructor Dawn MacLear, a yogi who has practiced for 23 years. In 1988, she experienced debilitating chronic neck pain. Thinking that yoga was helping the problem, she continued to suffer through her daily yoga poses. "Even though I had studied exercise physiology and kinesiology and knew that joints can be strained when put into certain positions, I never integrated the knowledge into my practice because I considered yoga to be sacred," says MacLear. "One day, I realized that the cause of my pain was the shoulder stand. I stopped doing it and the pain stopped." That revelation sparked Evolved Yoga, her user-friendly style that combines the benefits of centuries-old postures with today's knowledge of the human body.

"Most yoga teachers do not study exercise science," she says. "Instead, they concentrate on beliefs that have

join the evolution

The main tenet of Evolved Yoga is to create a safe, satisfying series of moves. To that end, postures like the spine-straining head and shoulder stands are out, as is the cross-legged lotus, because, as yoga teacher Dawn MacLear says, "Knees are hinge joints, meant only to bend and straighten, not twist." She also avoids moves that bend the body forward since most people already have a considerable desk-jockey slouch. Instead, MacLear favors positions that gently open the chest, loosen the back, lengthen the spine, and improve balance. In MacLear's method, as with all types of yoga, breathing helps you focus; as you move through the exercises on the following pages, inhale through the nose as you prepare for the posture, then exhale through the nose as you move into it. Continue to breathe deeply as you hold the position; remain in each one for 45 seconds to 3 minutes. Contact Evolved Yoga at 866-857-5858 or visit www.evolvedyoga.com.

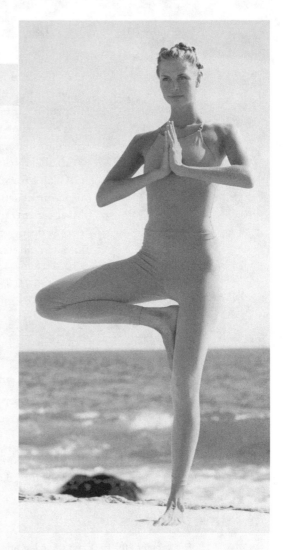

modified tree pose

WHAT IT DOES: Strengthens lower leg muscles; improves balance and poise.

HOW TO DO IT: Standing tall, raise your right leg, bend knee, and place your foot on the left inner thigh or calf. Focusing on one spot in front of you for balance, rotate the right knee, opening at the hip, and press your palms together in front of your chest. Switch sides and repeat.

HOW IT'S DIFFERENT: The traditional tree pose calls for the outside of the raised foot's ankle to be placed in front of the standing leg. The modified version puts significantly less stress on the bent knee joint, allowing you to focus on balance and posture.

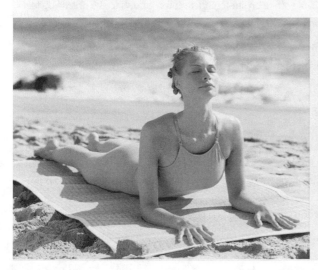

modified cobra

WHAT IT DOES: Stretches the lower spine.

HOW TO DO IT: Lying on your stomach, with legs together and the tops of your feet touching the ground, raise your shoulders up and rest on your forearms. Look forward or slightly up as you keep your shoulders relaxed and rib cage lifted.

HOW IT'S DIFFERENT: The typical cobra, in which the body weight rests on the hands, forces the back into an extreme arch and can hurt the wrists. By shifting the weight to the forearms, this pose still extends the spine but doesn't overdo it.

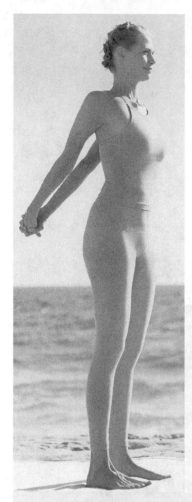

been passed down from yogi to yogi. But the past few decades of research have taught us how best to train the body. Applying this knowledge to yoga can improve it immensely." MacLear has done that by modifying many positions so that everyone—regardless of fitness level—can participate without getting hurt. She eliminates moves banished by mainstream fitness pros for safety reasons.

MacLear's one- to two-hour sessions have been a staple at Gold's Gyms in the D.C. area for years, and she regularly spreads the Evolved Yoga philosophy to fitness instructors at conferences. However, the most gratifying thing for MacLear isn't presiding over a class. "One of the most beautiful things is seeing people doing yoga off in a corner by themselves," she says. "That's when you know it really feels good." As good—and as easy—as it looks. ✳

Martica K. Heaner wrote Cross-Training for Dummies *(Hungry Minds, 2000).*

chest expansion

WHAT IT DOES: Stretches the shoulders and upper arms.

HOW TO DO IT: Stand with your feet hip-width apart and clasp your hands, palms together, behind you. Open your chest by pressing your shoulder blades together and down. If it's difficult to clasp your hands behind your back, open your arms to the side and press your palms back.

HOW IT'S DIFFERENT: Most instructors incorporate a forward bend into this position; eliminating it reduces stress on the spine and lets you focus on the upper body.

modified child's pose

WHAT IT DOES: Stretches the back and shoulders and helps improve circulation.

HOW TO DO IT: On your hands and knees, extend your arms in front of you as you lower your shoulders and drop your forehead to the ground. Concentrate on stretching from the elbows to the ribs. If you feel any strain in your knees, raise your hips higher; for comfort, kneel on a padded mat or a folded towel.

HOW IT'S DIFFERENT: In the typical child's pose, you sit back on your ankles, which places your knees in a weight-bearing, possibly stressful position. When your hips are raised, the knees are more stable.

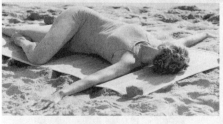

lying spinal twist

WHAT IT DOES: Loosens tight back and torso muscles.

HOW TO DO IT: Lie on your back in a T, with legs together and arms straight out at your shoulders. Cross your right knee over the left side of your body, keeping your hips on top of each other. If it's comfortable, look over your right shoulder. Switch sides and repeat. (If you have a pre-existing back condition, don't force the top knee to the floor.)

HOW IT'S DIFFERENT: This version lengthens the spinal muscles by twisting rather than by rounding the back.

the
absolute truth

Somewhere out there, amid all the 'killer abs'
hype and silliness, are things that really can flatten
your tummy. Here are the facts.

BY LEN KRAVITZ, PH.D.

PHOTGRAPHY BY MISHA GRAVENOR

If late-night infomercials are any indication,
ab anxiety ranks right up there with death and
taxes. Maybe that's why there are so many
myths about how to tone your midsection:
Desperate times call for desperate measures. But
beneath all the get-fit-quick schemes and goofy
ab-gadgets are truths that can help you to a
firmer tummy. We've culled the research and
called the experts on our mission to debunk
abominable abdominal myths, finding out not
only what doesn't work—but also what does.

Myth: Three hundred crunches are better than 30.
Truth: Who *hasn't* tried the more-is-better approach
when it comes to ab work? Problem is, lots of repetitions are not the best way to a firmer abdomen. "The
standard recipe for training any body part—whether
it's arms or abs—is to do one to three sets of no more
than 15 repetitions," advises Los Angeles chiropractor
and fitness instructor Eric Swartz. Any more sets
than that, and you're training the abdominals for
endurance, which is important only if you're a line-
backer who gets hit in the gut for a living.

Myth: The crunch is the most effective ab exercise.
Truth: Fact is, exercises that put you facedown in a
push-up position, or even standing, can give your

entire core—abs, back, and other torso muscles—a very
challenging workout. During crunches or sit-ups,
it's easy to focus on raising your chin and shoulders
rather than isolating and tensing the abdominal muscles. Core exercises remove that temptation: Lying
prone or standing forces your muscles to support
your back and improve your stability (see "True
Moves" on pages 134 and 135 for essential how-tos).

Myth: You should exercise your abs every day.
Truth: To make muscles stronger, you must first work
your abs until you can no longer maintain proper
form, then give them a rest. It's actually during
recovery that muscle fibers adapt and strengthen. As
with any muscle group, you'll get the best results from
training your abs two to three days a week, with a rest
day in between. "Remember, your abdominals
deserve a break along with the rest of your muscles,"
says personal trainer Tracy York, star of *Shaping Up
With Weights for Dummies* and *Breakthru Pilates* videos.

Myth: You should flatten your back before you start
to perform a crunch.
Truth: This standard advice from many trainers and
aerobics instructors is a bit off, says Lisa Singer,
president of Fitness Finders, a placement agency for
instructors and personal trainers. "Your back flattens
when you curl up anyway," she says. Instead, focus on
hollowing your midsection by pulling in your belly

button. This will engage your deepest abdominal muscle, the *transversus abdominis,* the muscle you need to target for a flatter abdomen.

Myth: You can whittle away your waist if you twist vigorously enough.
Truth: Repeatedly twisting from side to side won't do anything for your waist, but it could strain your back, Swartz says. The muscles deep in your back—not your abs—bear the burden when you're twisting.

Myth: For the ultimate ab training, take a 30-minute abs-only class.
Truth: Ten minutes is all you need to get a complete ab workout, York says. In fact, you could complete a total-body toning workout in the same amount of time it takes to finish one of the abs-only classes offered at many gyms. "But as long as you aren't

overtraining, taking one of these classes to vary your ab routine every now and then can't hurt," Singer adds. And it may help: Research shows that you can benefit from switching the order, speed, and kind of exercises in your fitness routine.

Myth: To exercise your abs the most effectively, you need to do different exercises that focus on the upper and lower ab muscles separately.
Truth: Some people believe most common ab exercises, like the crunch, target only the upper abdominals (near the ribs). Other exercises, such as the reverse curl—where you raise your hips instead of your shoulders—supposedly work only the lower abdominals (ones that are beneath the belly button). But new research from San Diego State University shows that these moves actually contract both upper and lower abs. "When a muscle contracts, all of it contracts—not

True Moves
three ab exercises that really work

STANDING STABILIZER
This exercise forces your core muscles to keep your body balanced as your center of gravity shifts.

1A | Stand with feet parallel, hip-width apart. Place hands on hips. Inhale as you raise right knee in front; stop at hip level. Pull belly button in and hold. Use a wall or chair for stability if necessary.

1B | Holding abs tight, extend leg straight and make a quarter-circle with toe to bring leg out to side. Lower; repeat 10 times. Switch legs. Do two to three sets.

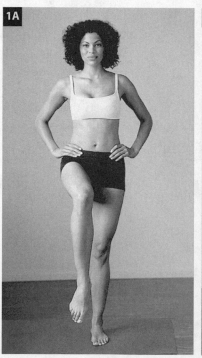
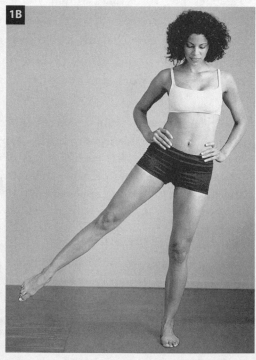

just parts of it," York explains. But moves that require you to lift your lower body, such as the reverse rotation and the foot push (see "True Moves" below), are tougher because legs are heavier than the head and shoulders, and therefore require more effort to lift.

Myth: If you still have ab flab, you aren't using proper technique.
Truth: "If you can't see your abs, you have to get rid of the fat that smothers them," York says. The best way: Burn more calories through aerobic exercise (aim for at least 30 minutes of brisk walking or another moderately intense activity every day) and cut out excess calories. Abdominal exercises will strengthen and tone your muscles but won't burn off the fat surrounding them. York adds, "if you're genetically programmed to store more fat in your abdomen than in other parts of your body, it might be harder to lose."

Myth: Your abs get a good workout only when you're doing exercises that target them.
Truth: Actually, your abs and other core muscles are working hard even when you least expect it—when you're walking, running, doing step aerobics, or playing your favorite sport. "You can improve your core control when you exercise by contracting your abs whenever you do any kind of movement, from walking to jumping," says physical therapist Suzanne Countryman.

Not only will your efforts result in a firmer midsection, but also it could save you from some aches and pains. "By maintaining an ab contraction, you'll suffer less wear and tear on your back, neck, and knees," Countryman says. ✴

Len Kravitz, Ph.D., is the coordinator of exercise science at the University of New Mexico.

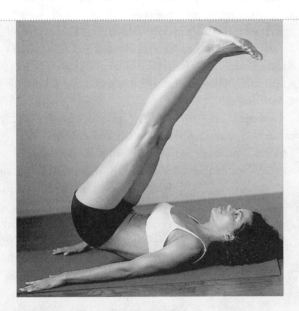

FOOT PUSH
2 | Because legs and hips are heavier and harder to lift than your upper body, this move is more challenging than a crunch.
• Lie on back, hands at sides, holding legs in the air straight out from hips.
• Exhale and contract abs by pulling belly button toward spine, while pushing feet to the ceiling. Hips will tilt forward slightly, and legs will lift up a few inches. Hold; then inhale as you lower and repeat 15 times. Do one to two more sets of 15.

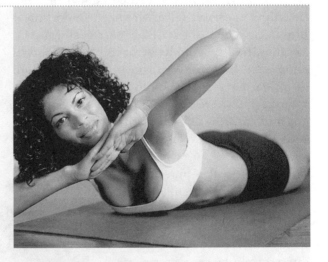

REVERSE ROTATION
3 | A variation on the elbow-to-knee crunch, this move works the obliques (the muscles that cover your ribs and sides) and back muscles.
• Lie on stomach with elbows out to the sides and chin resting on both hands.
• Keeping abs tight, exhale as you raise chest a few inches off the floor and rotate chest to the right; hold. Rotate back to center and then to the left; hold. Inhale as you lower; repeat 10 times on each side. Then do one to two more sets of 10.

gardening:
the perfect exercise

Want to prevent osteoporosis and beautify your environment? Get to work in your own backyard.

BY LOUISE RAFKIN

As someone who is addicted to pruning, enamored of raking, but reluctant to set even a single toe inside a gym, I've often wished the hours I spend in my yard could legitimately be tallied as exercise. I'm already proud of my blooming rosebushes and clusters of summer peaches, but it would be great to be able to gloat about, say, building stronger bones while I tend to my garden. Ha! I'd say to my friends rapidly running nowhere on those treadmills. So you've got buff muscles on a strong frame? I've got the muscles, the bones, and the peonies, too.

Researchers at the University of Arkansas must have been eavesdropping on my fantasy. According to their groundbreaking (so to speak) study of mature women, there's a direct correlation between yard work and healthy bone density. Among 3,310 women aged 50 and older, those who were gardeners had denser bones than those who regularly engaged in seemingly more "active" pursuits, such as jogging, swimming,

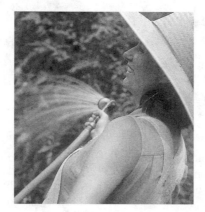

walking, and aerobics. In fact, these researchers found that gardening was as good as weight training at preventing osteoporosis, the brittle-bone disease that steals strength and independence from hundreds of thousands of older women each year.

These results are great news, as far as I'm concerned: Facing the choice between repetitions and rhododendrons, I'd happily choose the latter. But I can't help wondering: Can gardening be as good for my bones as working out?

Osteoporosis—which means "porous bones"—is caused by genetic, dietary, and hormonal factors. Especially of concern to women after menopause, when falling estrogen levels slow the process of bone building, the condition can leave you vulnerable to fractures. As experts have told us for years, weight-bearing exercise—in which stress is put on the bones, spurring bone-building cells to get busy—is one of the best ways to prevent osteoporosis.

Yard work, it turns out, puts a lot more pressure on bones than might be apparent at first glance. "While some people see yard work as a dainty activity," says Lori Turner, the

Because gardeners don't see their work as drudgery, they are more apt to continue tending their plots well into their later years—while their bodies steadily reap the benefits.

dietitian who led the study, "it actually includes a lot of weight-bearing motion: digging holes, pulling weeds, pushing a wheelbarrow."

To which I might add: pushing a shovel into the soil, stomping on the blade, pulling up the loose dirt, and tossing it aside. And doing all of the above over and over and over again. Because gardeners don't see their work as drudgery, says Turner, they are more apt to continue tending their plots well into their later years—while their bodies steadily reap the benefits.

By the time I've finished chatting with Turner about her study, I feel almost superior to those aficionados of gyms and machines: all this and sweet peas, too.

But while it's news to me that my private passion is bone beneficial, I have never considered working in the garden to be a "dainty" activity. Dainty is not what I feel when I am pushing the lawn mower over thick patches of grass or standing knee-deep in manure, spade in hand. Dainty is not what I feel when I am schlepping great drifts of downed leaves from rake to garbage bag. And dainty is certainly not what I feel when, after three or four vigorous hours of autumn cleanup, I retire to a hot bath with an aching back and a scrub brush to work the dirt out of my rough, calloused hands.

What I do feel while gardening is a sense of both calm and achievement. I feel present with the earth (and the snails, and the worms, and all the rest of the critters that share my plot of land). Working year-round in my garden makes me more acutely aware of the changing of the seasons. I revel in the blossoming of spring, when the emergence of the dormant bulbs and the flowering of the fruit trees makes my work light—mostly a matter of watering and weeding and admiring. But I also appreciate the return of the chilly, quiet winter months with their more demanding chores of pruning and hauling and clearing of old growth.

Perhaps most of all, I love the sense that I'm in partnership with the weather and the powers that be (not to mention the bees themselves). When a new season approaches, there is always some uncertainty about what's to come. The light rainfall in 2000, for instance, brought forth a bumper crop of daisies and a

exercise that pays off—in spades!

OKAY, so gardening is good for your bones—but how does it measure up to the Lycra-bearing types of exercise for burning calories? Surprisingly well: 45 minutes of vigorous yard work equals 30 minutes of aerobics. The chart below tells you how many calories a 140-pound person burns in 30 minutes while doing some common gardening tasks. If you're tempted to grab a power tool as an easy way out, don't. Crunch the numbers, and you'll see there's a big difference between motorized and manual labor.

Mowing (riding mower)	79	Digging, spading, tilling	159
Mowing (push with motor)	149	Weeding	143
Mowing (push only)	191	Planting seeds	127
Trimming shrubs (power)	111	Planting trees	143
Trimming shrubs (manual)	143	Laying sod	159
Raking	127	Watering	48
Bagging leaves	127	Hauling branches	159

SOURCE: BARBARA E. AINSWORTH, UNIVERSITY OF SOUTH CAROLINA SCHOOL OF PUBLIC HEALTH

wayward sunflower that, uninvited, popped up its cheery head near the back fence. I eventually beheaded that sunflower and brought it into my kitchen. Flowers brighten my windowsills and those of my friends. The fruits of my labor—peaches, lemons, and apples—travel home with visitors. I'm not ashamed to admit that it's always a treat to harvest the oohs and aahs of the folks who leave carting bags of my bounty.

Even tossing aside these somewhat touchy-feely benefits of tilling and tending for a minute, I'm certainly not averse to burning calories, and Turner tells me that some of this work consumes quite a lot of them (see the chart above). I can pretty much guarantee that if I spend a half hour poking around my yard—potting plants, turning compost, and trimming trees—I'll burn around 140 calories.

For bone building, Turner recommends gardening two to three times per week, depending on the strenuousness of the chores you're doing. "I'm a great believer in women's independence," she says, "and having healthy bones ensures autonomy well into our senior years." It is her belief that a beautiful, groomed garden is a perfect symbol of this independence.

I'm apt to agree. And after fully digesting Turner's research, I'd like to add that my particular garden now symbolizes my independence from the gym. ✳

THE BEST
personal trainer:
your computer

Can using your computer as a personal trainer keep your workouts on track? Our writer shares her lessons in logging on.

BY NANCY ROSS-FLANIGAN

Just as 1999 donned its tiara and dangling earrings, preparing to morph into the glamorous Y2K, my husband started talking transformation too. "Starting tomorrow, we're going to walk every day, rain or shine," Ray announced that New Year's Eve. It was welcome news to me. I'd already started my own walking and weight-training program, but going it alone was tough on dreary Michigan days.

Through winter's raw winds and well into spring, we stuck with our routine, striding along our blacktop road after dinner and hiking through local parks on weekends. When one of us felt lazy, the other coaxed, cajoled, and shamed the slacker off the futon and onto the footpath. Our bodies—and our whole beings—felt lighter. Bad moods melted instead of festering, and even on the most stressful days, we laughed at little ironies.

Then one day Ray said he wouldn't be walking with me anymore, at least not for a while. He claimed his legs were bothering him, but I suspected backlash against the extra-long hikes I'd dragged him on during our recent trip to the Tetons.

While my friends all lived too far away to fill in as replacement exercise partners, there was one constant companion who might be willing—the same one who takes me shopping, organizes my appointments, and balances my checkbook. Of course! I could recruit my computer to help me keep fit too. Giddy as a hopeful single placing a personal ad, I fantasized about finding my ideal online trainer. It wouldn't force me into a rigid routine but would understand my need for variety. It wouldn't make unreasonable demands on my time or be unforgiving if I didn't check in for a day or two. Like the closest of confidants, my cyberbuddy would help me know myself better—revealing the realities of my habits and foibles. I'd browsed enough to know that there were Web sites offering diet-and-fitness tracking programs, exercise tips, and support groups—most at no charge. I figured one could surely provide the structure and motivation I needed.

Since walking was my main aerobic activity, JustWalk (www.justwalk.com) seemed a good place to start logging my daily treks. After spending only a few minutes with the site, I could tell that it would offer even more. I was able to set monthly goals for distance, time spent exercising, or calories expended, and every time I logged on I could see how close I was to meeting them. After each walk, I could record just about anything I'd ever want to—distance, duration, time of day, minimum and maximum heart rates, type of terrain, and even the shoes I was wearing. Then I could call up colorful graphs to show total monthly distance, time versus distance, calories versus distance, or the number of miles I'd put on my favorite pair of walking shoes. When I felt competitive, I could compare my walks to those of the site's top five striders. If I craved camaraderie, I could join an online walking club to trade tips and mutual support.

Despite its name, JustWalk isn't just about walking. I was also able to record my bike rides and yoga sessions in the same way, and my strength training in enough detail to keep track of sets, repetitions, pounds for each lift, and even changes in the bulk of my biceps. Easy and quick, the site seemed to have everything I wanted—except a way to keep tabs on my diet.

So I then turned my attention to OnHealth (www.onhealth.com), which claimed its "Diet and Fitness Journal" would generate plenty more charts and reports for me. In return for entering daily exercise and diet details, I'd get end-of-the-day summaries of calories consumed and expended. I could see how my diet stacked up against Food Pyramid guidelines and play "what-if" to gauge what would happen over time if I exercised more or ate less. Sounded fun.

In addition to wearing my pedometer everywhere, I started logging every mouthful. The site made tracking exercise easy but didn't offer as many options or useful stats as JustWalk did. At OnHealth, I simply set a weekly goal—the number of calories I wanted to burn—and followed my progress on a chart.

When I first tried logging diet data, the only workout I got was an exercise in frustration—it took me all week to enter one day's meals. But when I checked back a few months later, an updated version of the journal had made the task easier. I could create a frequent food list so I didn't have to search the whole database for soy milk every time I poured some on my oatmeal. In fact, I could save groups of foods I usually eat together. As promised, OnHealth served up plenty of stats once I entered my meals and workouts. My favorite was the "Daily Nutrition Status" chart that I could check throughout the day to see if I'd hit my fat limit or needed a little more calcium.

OnHealth was an entertaining playmate, but when my mouse began to wander a few weeks later, CBS HealthWatch (www.healthwatch.medscape.com—click on "tools") made my heart race.

On the exercise side, I could choose from among 36 activities, entering duration, distance (or number of sets), and heart rate. I was rewarded with little dumbbells on a calendar each time I worked out, and I could also generate a table that showed all the dates I'd exercised and what I'd done. Still, I wished for a slicker way to monitor my progress by automatically comparing times, distances, rates, and reps. In my explorations, I had found that only at JustWalk.

Food was more satisfying than exercise—isn't it always? Using my current and goal weights, HealthWatch created daily recommendations for calories, protein, carbs, fat, and so on. When I entered each day's foods—a snap, even with my own recipes and favorite brands—the calculator tallied my totals and compared them with the recommendations.

I was getting a better handle on healthy eating habits than ever before—and having fun doing it. For years I'd been trying to follow diet recommendations I'd read about, but until now I'd had no idea whether I was really getting them right. Now I had proof that when I think I'm eating well, I am.

The ideal online trainer in my fantasies would understand my need for variety, be forgiving if I didn't check in for a day or two, and, like the closest of confidants, reveal the realities of my habits and foibles.

After a few months, though, my fling with online trainers began to lose its spark. If they'd been my only fitness-partner options, I might have stuck it out, or at least kept up the flirtation. But wouldn't you know—just as I tired of my cyber-companions, my real-life one came back.

One summer evening after dinner, Ray leaned back in his chair and looked across the lake behind our house.

"Starting tomorrow," he said, "let's ride our bicycles around the lake every morning." And so we have. Sometimes I keep track of how far we've gone. But often I just enjoy the scenery, knowing that I've been to the cyber side and found the grass no greener. ✳

Nancy Ross-Flanigan is a contributing Health *editor.*

Staying on Track with Regular Workouts

Changes in your life can shift fitness to low gear. Here's how to keep your workouts revved up.

BY KERRI WESTENBERG

About a year ago, I packed up my apartment in the Southeast and hit the road to join my fiancé in Los Angeles, 2,000 miles away. Before I left, my days were consumed with hauling around boxes of books, making endless trips to the Salvation Army, and performing other energy-consuming tasks. Up until that time, I had been a five-days-a-week gym-goer, but when I was packing, the last thing I wanted to do was put on a sports bra. So I didn't. And I didn't worry. After all, I was moving to California, the land of year-round sunshine and running paths, where everyone tops off a good workout with a healthful fruit smoothie.

Well, once I got there I downed plenty of smoothies, but I sure didn't find time—what with job hunting and organizing my new apartment—to start exercising again. Before I knew it, I had gained 12 pounds.

My story is common. Almost every woman has, at some point, had her workout routine disrupted because of a life transition, be it a move like mine, marriage, divorce, job change, deciding to stay home with the kids—you name it.

To make exercise really accommodate the changes in your life, the kind of workout you do has to change too.

"When things change in our lives, exercise can get squeezed out," says Richard Cotton, an exercise physiologist and a spokesman for the American Council on Exercise. Ironically, it's during these life-changing times that we need a good workout the most. "Change causes stress," says Cotton, "and exercise is one of the best methods of stress management going." But when things get a little crazy in your life, how on

Morning workouts are the ones you're least likely to skip because that time slot isn't affected by the surprise events and errands that crop up as the day goes on.

earth do you find the time and the motivation to stick with your regular workout routine? I began looking for answers to that question when my landlord told me he planned to sell the apartment my fiancé and I had recently settled into. Faced with yet another move (and I had only recently been able to drop that extra 12 pounds), I knew I needed a game plan.

Schedule Exercise in Red Pen

"You absolutely must set aside workout time, even though you have other things competing for your attention," says exercise psychologist Jack Raglin, Ph.D., a professor at Indiana University. Raglin says it's essential to write down a time for exercise in your day planner. He also recommends morning workouts as the ones you're least likely to skip because that time slot won't be affected by the surprise events and errands that crop up as the day goes on. If afternoon workouts are just a better fit for you, surround your-self with "reminders," such as keeping your gym bag next to your desk or posting a "When are you going to exercise today?" sign on your fridge. These kinds of tricks may sound silly, says Raglin, but they really work.

Do a Little Exercise Multitasking

My sister Kelli Harris decided to go back to college while juggling a full-time job and being a mom to her 12-year-old son, Saul. Her first semester back in school, Kelli cut back on her regular workouts and soon had difficulty sleeping. So she got wise during her second semester and devised a plan that would allow her to work out and be with Saul at the same time. Now, three times a week, Kelli runs while Saul rides a scooter or bike next to her. "That way, I don't feel as though I'm taking time away from him, and we both have fun," she says. Similarly, my friend Laura Samuel Meyn used to work out regularly, but that routine went out the window once she got married. "After a day at the office, I just wanted to spend time

with [my new husband] Till." After spending months parked on a couch watching *The Sopranos,* the duo recently decided to do something more active with their time together—they took up tennis. "We are both conscious of having gotten out of shape, so now we take lessons together one night a week and usually play a game on the weekend," she says.

Do Something Completely Different

Sometimes, to make exercise really accommodate the changes in your life, the kind of workout you do has to change too. For example, if you're a new mother who used to be a gym rat, but now you just don't have time to get to a gym, buy weights and lift at home while the baby sleeps (or buy a jogging stroller and take the baby on runs with you). If you used to take an aerobics class, but your new job leaves you feeling too exhausted at the end of the day to enjoy such a tough workout, switch to something gentler, like yoga or tai chi. Another idea: Allow a new town or office to be the catalyst for a new kind of workout. For example, my friend Julie Lyke's new route to her office near Washington, D.C., sweeps her past the Potomac River. Observing the rowers on the river day after day, Lyke was inspired to try it and has since become an active participant in the sport. "It was a challenging sport to learn, but once I got the hang of it, it was fun and a great workout," she says.

It's during life-changing times that we need a good workout most. Change causes stress, and exercise is one of the best methods of stress management.

Finally, if you just can't get yourself going in the midst of whatever's happening in your life, just bite the bullet and hire a personal trainer—if only for a few weeks—to get yourself back on track. I took that route. Recently, I told my trainer about my weight gain during my last move and my fear that something similar would happen this time. She raised an eyebrow, smiled, and said, "That's not going to happen again." ✳

Kerri Westenberg is a writer based in Santa Monica, California.

THE SPARK:
10-MINUTE WORKOUTS FOR WEIGHT LOSS AND WELLNESS

ARE YOU MISSING OUT on exercise benefits because your life is overbooked? Physiologist Glenn A. Gaesser has a plan for you. The noted researcher—coauthor of *The Spark* (Simon & Schuster, 2001)—has found that splitting workouts into 10-minute bursts can help you lose weight and stay healthy. *Health* spoke with him about his new program.

Q: How did you happen upon this idea?

A: I helped develop the American College of Sports Medicine's fitness guidelines. We recommended people work out up to an hour most days of the week and do strength-training and flexibility exercises. Afterward, I realized this was unrealistic for the average American. Exercise needs to be accessible to sedentary people.

Q: So what does the program entail?

A: Each 10-minute bout of exercise is called a spark. In my study, I had women perform 7 to 10 aerobic sparks (mainly brisk walking), 2 to 4 strength-training sparks (using 8-pound dumbbells), and 2 to 4 flexibility sparks a week. They averaged about 15 sparks weekly for the duration of the study. I also asked them to include more fiber-rich foods in their diet and drink more water.

Q: How well does this work?

A: After three weeks, on average the participants improved their aerobic fitness by 10 to 15 percent; in other words, they gained the endurance of a woman 10 to 15 years their junior. The women's strength improved by as much as 100 percent, the equivalent of what you'd see in a person 15 to 20 years younger. Their flexibility increased and their cholesterol and triglycerides declined significantly.

Q: What about weight loss?

A: The average loss during the study was about a pound a week. But my guess is that for long-term weight control—and that's what counts—a woman could drop as much as 10 pounds. It's incredibly difficult to lose much more than that and keep it off.

Q: So can I stop slaving away at the gym?

A: If you're exercising regularly, that's great—keep it up! But if, like a lot of people, you find it tough to make it to the gym, my program will work for you.

chapter 4

anti-aging
secrets

a busy woman's guide to healthy looks

the face of health

These five women have it: confidence, inner beauty, and a vitality that turns heads. Here's how they make it happen.

BY LYNNE CUSACK

PHOTOGRAPHY BY JENNY ACHESON

The so-called standards of beauty seem to grow more unattainable every day—as in impossibly thin and wrinkle-free. At the same time, there are women who know better, who care for themselves without obsession or checklists, who don't panic over stretch marks or a few extra pounds. These women are comfortable in their own skins, and that comfort inevitably translates into confidence, which is the foundation for good looks.

We set out to celebrate these women with our Face of Health contest, asking readers to nominate someone they felt epitomizes the great looks that come with being healthy, happy, confident, and connected. More than 800 readers wrote in to tell us about yourselves or someone you know—in one winner's case, a husband nominated his wife—and what it means to be truly beautiful. Virtually everyone said a positive outlook is the single most important aspect of feeling beautiful. Some reported a defining moment when they chose to go against the pull of negativity, but most came by their attitudes gradually or naturally. Whatever the source, though, it's clear that developing a confident, healthy respect for your body and spirit is truly the secret to looking your best.

"I've learned to find joy in everything, even the negative."

Lisa Relling
30, mom
West Vancouver, British Columbia, Canada
Married for 1 year
Children: Max, 6, and Lola, 8 months

"Now that I am 30," wrote Lisa Relling in her entry, "I define beauty as an energy and a feeling, rather than a look or a size." That wasn't always the case. Her head-on-straight outlook began about six years ago with the birth of her son, Max. Her pregnancy cast her in a new light: Instead of comparing herself to others, she began to marvel, "Look what my body can do!" Before that, she says, "I wanted to look 'perfect' and fit in. Now I see I wasn't meant to fit in. I don't think any of us are. We're meant to stand out."

Her attitude was put to the test when she went through a divorce when Max was a year old. "On my own with a child to raise, I was really stressed out and knew it wasn't doing me or Max any good." Relling decided to take a positive view. "I've learned to try and find joy in everything, even the bad. It's made me who I am."

Although Relling's not hung up on size, she finds it fairly easy to keep hers a healthy one. "I'm not neurotic,

Looking Good: Lisa's Lessons

• Lisa says a visit with a dermatologist was a great investment. She learned how to cut through a sea of creams and lotions and use products geared to her sensitive skin.
• A favorite beauty shortcut: Mixing foundation with moisturizer to even out her complexion.
• Lisa says she loves the ease of her wash-and-go cut and likes the bonus that her style "isn't like everyone else's."
• "Even my son will tell you, 'Mommy feels naked without her lipstick,'" she says.

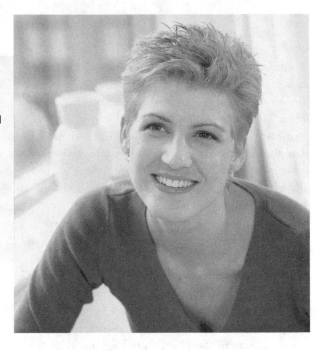

and I don't deprive myself," she says. "I eat foods in the amount my body tells me to. I think that's what healthy living is all about: listening to your body."

Her exercise routine revolves around her family. A power walk with Lola riding in a carrier is Relling's exercise of choice, while inline skating with Max lets her spend time alone with her son. "It may be a cliché," she says, "but exercise gives you a natural high."

"Beauty is a feeling."
Karen Smith

51, training consultant
Branford, Connecticut
Married for 4 years
Children: Dawn, 32; foster son, Spencer, 10 months

If you're lucky, the next time you walk into a room full of strangers, you'll find yourself alongside someone like Karen Smith. She's one of those people who has a gift for putting you at ease and making you feel special. She gives you plenty of signs that she's not just listening, she's interested.

What fuels her is reaching out to people in need. Besides being a foster parent, she helps immigrant

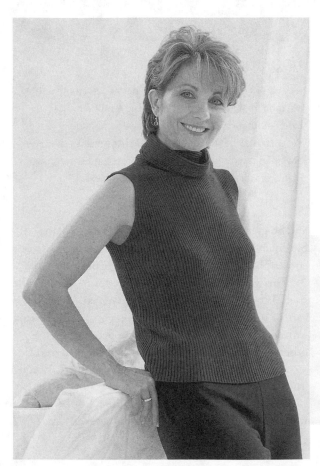

Looking Good: Karen's Counsel

• "My hair never does the same thing twice," Karen says. So she favors hairstyles that take advantage of her natural wave and body. "Why fight it?"
• Ease is critical to her busy lifestyle. Karen likes to freshen up with Oil of Olay Daily Cleansing wipes, which she carries along wherever she goes.
• "I never used to use a lip liner, but lip lines tend to fade as you get older, and liner helps define them."

families acclimate to her community. In 1992, Smith, who's of Croatian descent, traveled to Bosnia during the war to help open up a medical mission for children. "The sheer joy I get out of helping others is immeasurable," says Smith. "You can't feel happier than that." She believes that nothing affects a woman's looks more than her outlook. "Inner beauty is a feeling and a state of mind. It illuminates the darkest moments as well as the worst of bad hair days."

Smith came by her sunny disposition in her early 20s when she became a single parent. "I had a daughter I had to be happy for. In my way of thinking, you can be positive or take a less-than-positive approach," she says. "Facing things—both good and bad—with an upbeat attitude starts your day on the right foot."

It probably keeps her going too. A part-time training consultant for Southern New England Telephone Company, she attends college at night (maintaining a 4.0 grade point average). A doting foster mother to 10-month-old Spencer, Smith is also grandmother of R.J., 5, and Michael, 3.

Working out and eating right are important parts of Smith's way of life. She and her husband, Richard, walk and swim near their home on the Long Island Sound and cook healthy meals together. And while she admits that her shape may not be identical to what it was in high school, she's proud that she weighs the same today as she did 33 years ago. Her instant destressing solution may be partly responsible: When feeling tense, she runs up and down the three flights of stairs in her house. "The nervous energy dissipates quickly," she says, "and I feel better instantly."

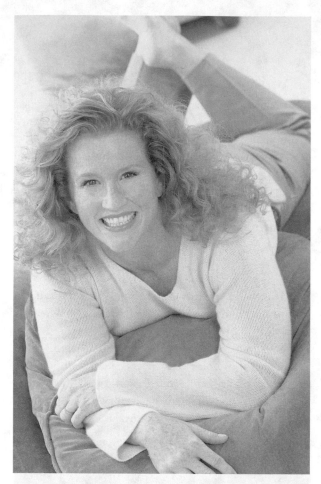

Looking Good: Susan's Secrets

- Susan says her long red hair is a part of her identity. "It's a symbol that I've beat cancer. Having temporarily lost it to chemotherapy, I wear it with a newfound pride."
- Susan is diligent about protecting her sensitive skin. She always uses a moisturizer with sunscreen, and she drinks plenty of water, which brightens her complexion.

"I don't waste a minute."
Susan Shulman

33, volunteer
Mill Valley, California
Married for 8 years
Child: Max, 6

"My wife is radiance personified," wrote Barry Shulman. In a couple of succinct paragraphs, he told the story of how she had been diagnosed with aggressive breast cancer just before their son Max's first birthday and how she now has more vigor than ever. Susan Shulman had no clue Barry had sent off an entry to our contest, but she was thrilled when he broke the news.

"This whole year has been a celebration for me," she says. "When you hit the five-year mark as a breast-cancer survivor, your survival rates go up. There's an untold story of how all sorts of people come out the other side of cancer better than when they entered. It's so ironic that I of all people would now be considered 'the face of health'!"

Since her diagnosis, Shulman's life has gone from full to fulfilled. "When you have the eye-opening experience of being told you may have only a few years to live …" she says, unable to finish the sentence. "Well, I don't waste a minute."

That makes her certain about what's important. "I believe that health is about finding a balance in life between what you really like to do and what you have to accomplish," she says.

Finding that balance is especially easy, since saying that she likes to exercise is like saying that Faith Hill likes to sing. Shulman, who has done several marathons and triathlons, devotes as much time as possible to working out and is now preparing to become certified as a personal trainer.

Shulman rises at 5 a.m. most days for her workout. She swims three times a week, does a Spinning class about four times a week, lifts weights twice a week, and does Pilates three to four times a week.

Reaching out to other women boosts that radiance her husband wrote about. She volunteers in a program that offers emotional support and information to women newly diagnosed with breast cancer and those undergoing related surgery.

For Shulman, beauty is about a lot more than what shows up in a picture. Her ultimate fulfillment: "When I can accomplish what I set out to do. I am the happiest when I'm doing my best at being a mom, a partner, a friend, and an athlete."

"I believe there isn't anything I can't do."

Frances Jucutan

35, project manager and MBA student
Concord, California
Single

There's a reason Frances Jucutan's friends have been known to call her "Saint Frances." She was raised in a traditional Filipino household, where doing for others was expected of daughters. Jucutan fulfilled this role, accommodating just about everyone but herself.

Then something changed. Around 30, Jucutan realized she had to stop living by a phantom list of "shoulds" and consider her own needs.

This self-acceptance gave her the confidence to do things she wouldn't have before. She ended a long-term relationship that promised security but not much more. She got past a paralyzing guilt and moved away from her family. And she set off into the unfamiliar waters of a career outside her comfort zone. "I needed to challenge myself," she says. "Now I really believe there isn't anything I can't do."

As if to prove it, she's handling a heavy-duty schedule as a full-time project manager for hospital group Kaiser Permanente and is a part-time MBA student at the University of California at Davis. And she keeps up her exercise routine with the mantra, "Make it convenient, and you don't make excuses." Walking the trails in the East Bay area near her home is her preferred workout. Or if Jucutan can't fit in walking, tennis, or yoga, it's not too late. "I'll use my home weights or pop in my Tae-Bo tapes," she says.

Jucutan says life is great, and she knows what to do to keep it that way. Now that she's traded wariness about the future for optimism, this woman has no intention of turning back.

Looking Good: Frances' Finds

- Since Frances began getting monthly deep-cleansing facials six months ago, breakouts are very rare.
- She found that adding layers to her short hair saved precious time in the morning.
- Recent discovery: Brow Zings from Benefit. This soft, pigmented wax is brushed on to define unruly brows.

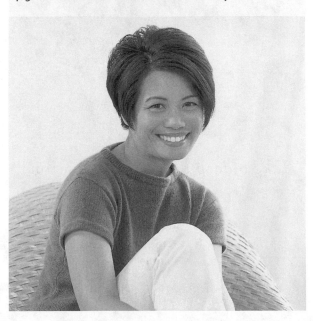

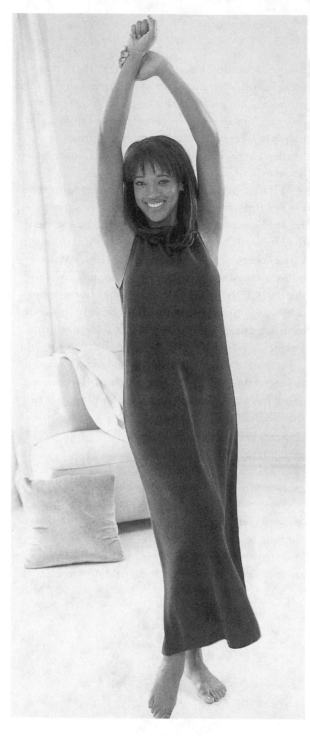

"Take a deep breath and move on."

Inga Savage

33, sales-support specialist
McLean, Virginia
Single

Looking Good: Inga's Advice

• Inga never had acne growing up but started having flare-ups in her late 20s. Her dermatologist recommended a line of cleansers, toners, and lotions that contain glycolic acid, which exfoliates the skin. Since then, she says, "My complexion feels renewed, and my pores seem so much smaller."

• Whenever Inga went without eye makeup, people would ask if she were tired. Then she discovered that wearing mascara on her upper lashes makes her look more awake.

There's something about Inga Savage. You hear it in her voice. You get the sense that she knows something good is going to happen.

If it does, don't assume it was just chance. Savage is a woman who engineers her own contentment. A sales professional for NetDecide, a computer software company, Savage admits it hasn't always been this way. "It took dealing with some disappointments for me to realize that I'm responsible for my own happiness," she says. Savage has learned to put things in perspective from some of life's typical obstacles: relationships that didn't work out and difficult job challenges. "At recent points in my life, I could have chosen either to get trapped in one place or take a deep breath and move on," says Savage. "I chose to keep moving."

She recently took moving literally, relocating to an area where she could delve into a smorgasbord of new pursuits—and the old one of exercising. Her gym is right across the street from her home, making it easy to start the day with a session instead of an excuse. Resistance training is a three-times-a-week habit, and she hits the stair climber or stationary bike daily. In good weather, she walks, inline skates, or cycles outside.

After work, anything can happen. On the roster these days: stress-relieving yoga, salsa lessons, and a course in jewelry making that brings out her creative side and has a mental payoff as well: "It's very relaxing," she says.

"I believe you're never too old to learn something new. The more things you experiment with, the more likely you are to find your niche. I go to bed tired," she says, "but I'm definitely happy." ✳

Lynne Cusack is a New Jersey–based freelance writer.

ANTIOXIDANTS:
the best defense against wrinkles

Antioxidants are naturally occurring substances that neutralize free radicals—molecules that are missing electrons and that try to steal them from healthy cells to make themselves complete. "When a gang of free radicals teams up on a healthy cell, that cell becomes damaged and much more prone to degenerative diseases, such as heart disease or cancer," says Jim Baral, a dermatologist in New York City. An antioxidant, then, is a hero that swoops in to interact with the free radicals and stop this sequence of events.

Many dermatologists attribute wrinkles to free-radical overload. "Studies show that antioxidants, such as vitamins C and E or topical polyphenols, can help decrease signs of aging," says Baral.

Some power-packed products: Revlon's Vitamin C Absolutes line, Sothys's Noctuelle, and Merle Norman Luxiva Preventage.

It's normal for the body to carry around small amounts of free radicals. But stress, pollution, or too much sun can cause an overload. The best defense? Load up on antioxidants by eating foods that are rich in vitamins C or E—like citrus fruits, leafy greens, and nuts.

THE LOWDOWN ON COENZYME Q10

First off, Q10 has more names than a member of the British royal family. You've seen it on labels as ubiquinone, Q10, coQ10, and coenzyme Q10, but it's all the same thing. "Q10 is a fat-soluble vitamin that our bodies produce to help protect cells from free radicals," says Richard Glogau, a San Francisco–based dermatologist. The levels of Q10 in our bodies decrease with time, so doctors recommend it as a supplement to prevent heart disease and other ailments associated with aging. Now, it's being touted as an anti-wrinkle agent.

But can Q10 really make you look younger? Some doctors think that the same free radicals responsible for heart problems also cause wrinkles. So applying Q10 topically should, theoretically, work. Studies done by several major cosmetics companies report impressive results, but the jury is still out. "There's no independent medical proof that Q10 in a skin cream can stop wrinkles," says Glogau. But for the chance of younger looking skin, many dermatologists say it's worth a try.

Sex really *does* keep you young

Keep your sex life robust, and the only place you'll be finding wrinkles is in your sheets. Clinical neuropsychologist David Weeks, of the Royal Edinburgh Hospital, questioned 3,500 people judged to look young for their age. Having sex three times a week seemed to take 7 to 12 years off their looks. But before you get too excited, know that having even more sex won't compound the benefits. And casual sex, because it increases stress, seems to speed up the aging process.

Cosmetic Dentistry

what you need to know

Your teeth are one of the first things people notice about you but may be last on your list of things to fix. It's never been easier to get the smile of your dreams.

BY LYNNE CUSACK

A pink sign on the desk in the dimly lit reception area reads "concierge." The scent of a lavender candle and the sound of a babbling fountain waft through the room. The woman behind the counter wants to know if I would care to try an herbal neck wrap as she graciously presents me with a platter of fresh fruit and sparkling water. I find myself beginning to unwind. Not 10 minutes earlier, I'd been knee-deep in midday Manhattan gridlock, running late for my dentist appointment.

Yes, my dentist appointment. You'd think I was at a luxurious beauty center awaiting my masseuse, but I was actually in the lobby of the Rozenberg Dental Day Spa, waiting to have my teeth bleached. And that's only one of a number of things I could have had done at this plush establishment. If I'd wanted to, I could have had my teeth straightened, a chipped tooth repaired, or a silver filling replaced with a light-colored one. In less than an hour, I could even have had my gums trimmed.

Dental spas are the latest spin in the burgeoning world of cosmetic dentistry. These days, a swarm of baby boomers (and their younger siblings) want youthful smiles as much as they want toned bodies, and more dentists are getting into the act to accommodate them. It ain't cheap: Most cosmetic dental procedures are not covered by insurance and run anywhere from $300 on up. But the payoff is great—and extends way beyond your teeth. As Dean Lodding, president of the American Academy of Cosmetic Dentistry (AACD), puts it, "The wonderful thing is that in less than an hour you can help boost someone's self-esteem as well as their appearance."

I'd benefited from cosmetic dentistry before. When I was a child, my well-meaning parents had put their trust in a not-too-savvy dentist, and I was left with crowded, crooked teeth. Over the years I'd heard many whispered remarks, like "Why doesn't she do something about those teeth?" or "Jeez, she'd look so good if it weren't for her teeth." The criticism was devastating. Eventually, old obstacles—fear, inertia, skimpy savings—fell away,

> **These days, baby boomers** (and their younger siblings) want youthful smiles as much as they want toned bodies.

and as I neared my 40th birthday, I decided to straighten my teeth. The effects on my smile—*and* my self-esteem—were miraculous.

Now, two years later, I'm ready for more. This time I've decided to really pamper myself. No medical office for me; I'm here at the Rozenberg spa, relaxing under the influence of that herbal neck wrap, waiting for my dentist to erase the souvenirs of too much wine and roses (my favorite rose tea, that is). I'm actually giddy at the prospect of improving my smile again.

Interested in perking up your own pearly whites? Whatever you feel is marring your smile, one of these procedures might help.

"My front tooth has an irregular edge. Can it be fixed?"

Quite easily with bonding, one of the simplest and most effective cosmetic procedures. Basically, the dentist applies an enamel-like resin to your tooth, contours it to suit your smile, hardens it with intense light, then polishes it. "Bonding is quick and usually requires no anesthesia," says Mike Malone, a cosmetic dentist in Lafayette, Louisiana. In addition to evening out irregular edges, it's great for repairing cracks, chips, and small gaps. Expect to pay about $300 to $800 for each tooth—and to have it last for three to eight years.

One caveat: "Bonding tends to attract stains because it's a porous material," says Lana Rozenberg, a cosmetic dentist and owner of the Rozenberg Dental Day Spa. If you smoke or drink a lot of stain-causing beverages like tea, coffee, or cola, your bonded tooth may yellow over time.

"I've tested quite a few tooth-whitening pastes, but my teeth don't look that much brighter. Any suggestions?"

It's no surprise these pastes don't offer dramatic results. Their whitening ingredients are mild in strength, and a quick brushing doesn't allow for much contact time.

If you want to up your smile's wattage, talk to your dentist about professional bleaching. Most dentists

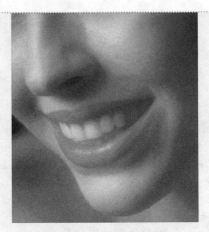

how to find a good cosmetic dentist

Don't just go by the certificate on the wall. "Scientific skills are important, but so is the dentist's artistic ability," says Renee Tarnutzer, a spokesperson for the American Academy of Cosmetic Dentistry. It's wise, therefore, to ask your dentist how often he or she has performed a particular procedure and to speak with patients who've undergone a similar treatment.

It also doesn't hurt to request a series of before-and-after photos so you can see for yourself whether you like the results. Even more important, find out whether your dentist participates in continuing education courses to stay abreast of the latest cosmetic techniques. (The AACD maintains a free referral service of member dentists who have taken the academy's courses. Call 800-543-9220 or visit www.aacd.com.)

offer two choices: Either they'll do it for you, or they'll make you a kit to use at home. Interestingly, the results are about the same. Those not inclined to be their own taskmaster may opt for the costlier in-office treatment. In that case, the dentist can use a stronger whitening solution (because he'll be sure to protect your gums properly) and jump-start the effects with a laser or intense light. In-office bleaching takes from one to two visits. Fees start at $600 and can go as high as $1,200.

If you go the at-home route, the dentist will make custom trays for your upper and lower teeth and provide you with bleaching agents. You'll fill the trays with this paste and wear them every night for two weeks or during the day for up to two hours.

A beautiful smile gives you more than just a pretty face. It boosts your confidence and helps you reach out to the world at large.

The cost is $300 to $600. Depending on your habits, your teeth will stay bright for one to three years. Please note: Bleaching is out of the question if you've got any underlying gum disease or decay or cracks in teeth. "You don't want to pour bleach into an infection," says Barry Morse, a family and cosmetic dentist in Montvale, New Jersey.

"I'm 45. Is it too late for braces?"

Not at all. According to the American Association of Orthodontists, one in five orthodontic patients is an adult. "Teeth will move at any age, if the gums and bones are healthy," says Terrie Yoshikane, an orthodontist near San Diego. The transformation can be impressive, as are potential health benefits. "Crowded or crooked teeth make it difficult to keep teeth clean and may increase the risk of decay or gum problems," explains Yoshikane. "A bad bite may cause chewing problems or even wear down the enamel."

Many adults are tempted to go straight because braces are so much more user-friendly these days. The metal bracket that's bonded to the tooth is much smaller than the one you would have had when you were 12. The wires are softer and more flexible, so they exert less pressure on your teeth. And there are several new types of braces that will appeal to your vanity.

Many people opt for clear or tooth-colored porcelain braces, which are hardly visible. Lingual braces are actually placed out of sight behind the teeth (though they're more expensive than traditional braces and harder to work on). And last year a smile-friendly alternative to braces, called aligners, came on the market. Aligners are customized, clear removable trays, each of which is worn for about two weeks. Though you're supposed to wear them all the time (except when eating or brushing), you can pop them out for job interviews,

parties, and other occasions when you don't want any distractions or potential embarrassment. Aligners are not suitable for every orthodontic problem, though, so check with your orthodontist to see if they're right for you.

How much of a drag is wearing braces—however enlightened their form? It depends on the extent of the fix. You may only need to straighten the top or bottom teeth, and you could need them for as little as six months or as long as three years. Expect to pay $5,000 or more for a comprehensive treatment.

"Are braces my only option for crooked teeth?"

No. If you really can't stand the idea of wearing braces, and if you have a lot of money, very few procedures rival the effect of veneers, says Larry Rosenthal, a New York City cosmetic dentist. Veneers are thin, tooth-shaped porcelain shells that are applied to the front surface of existing teeth. Then they are shaped and aligned with the neighboring teeth (or veneers) to create a straight line. In the process, they also cover stains and even out teeth that are unattractively shaped.

Of course, it's not quite as simple as it sounds. Veneers require a truly discriminating eye on the part of the dentist, who has to make calls on the size, shape, color, and angle of the veneers. First, he must remove a minimal amount of enamel from each tooth to allow for the thickness of the veneer. Then he takes an impression of your teeth and sends it to the lab. The completed veneers are checked for fit and color, then cured in place with intense light. Finally, the dentist fine-tunes their shape and polishes them to a natural, attractive finish. Veneers cost from $800 to $2,500 per tooth and with proper care should last 10 years or more.

"For years, I've closed my mouth for photos because I'm so self-conscious about a 'gummy' smile. Can this be fixed?"

Yes, in one of three ways. The least invasive procedure is a gum lift. Using a laser or scalpel, the dentist removes tiny bits of gum to expose more tooth. The procedure costs about $800 to $1,300. Depending on the structure of your mouth, you might be a candidate for crown lengthening, in which the dentist also removes a bit of the bone underlying the gums. That costs $450 to $600 per tooth.

For people with the opposite problem—too much tooth and too *little* gum—gum grafting is an option. In some cases, the dentist literally pulls down the gum tissue at the problem site. In other instances, tissue may be taken from another site and grafted onto the area. Depending on the complexity of the problem, grafting will run you between $500 and $1,500.

"Every time I grin I feel like the only thing people see is my mouthful of silver fillings."

If you grew up in the 1950s and '60s you didn't have the benefit of fluoride that kids do today—which means there's a good chance you've had a cavity or two packed with a silver filling. Smile wide, and you'll expose those shiny, dark reminders of too many sweets and less than perfect oral hygiene.

Today, garden-variety cavities can be filled with a tooth-colored composite that's nearly undetectable as an impostor. Even old fillings, assuming they're not too deep and you haven't suffered additional decay hidden beneath them, can be replaced with this natural-looking alternative. Composite fillings cost about $300 per tooth and last indefinitely.

Depending on the tooth's location and its amount of decay, other options can still beat silver in the looks department. If there's not enough tooth structure left to hold a filling, for example, the next step is a porcelain inlay or onlay. An inlay fits entirely within the confines of the inner walls of the tooth; an onlay fits over the biting points of the tooth. A simple composite inlay or onlay costs from $800 to $1,500 per tooth.

Finally, a dentist may recommend a crown to restore the shape and size of a tooth that has fractured. Depending on materials used (a crown can be made of porcelain, alone or fused to another material, or gold) and the location and condition of the tooth involved, crowns can cost between $900 and $2,000 apiece. They'll last about 10 to 15 years. ✳

Lynne Cusack is a writer in Township of Washington, New Jersey.

Q+A
the pros and cons of do-it-yourself teeth bleaching

Are the tooth-bleaching kits I've seen at the store worth a try?

If you're hoping for a megawatt grin like Julia Roberts, probably not. But if you have the cash flow of a graduate student and the patience of a kindergarten teacher, you may want to check these kits out.

Each over-the-counter kit is $10 to $50, versus $250 to $1,000 for dentist kits, says Cary Ganz, D.D.S., a cosmetic dentist in New York. "But they're also made with weaker bleaching solutions, so it can take six months to see any change, and it will be slight—just one or two shades brighter, as opposed to four to eight shades with a dentist-prescribed kit."

Because the do-it-yourself drugstore products aren't supervised by a dentist, you may not know if you have tooth decay, a problem that makes teeth ultrasensitive to chemicals used to whiten teeth. Also note that the one-size-fits-all trays in drugstore kits (as opposed to custom-made trays dentists use) increase the risk that chemicals can leak out and irritate your gums.

If you want to try a kit from the toothpaste aisle, see your dentist first to make sure you'll get the results you're looking for.

THE SMART WAY TO SAVE YOUR SKIN FROM SUN DAMAGE

Do you feel invincible after slathering on sunscreen with a sky-high sun protection factor (SPF)? If so, you may want to hear about the latest research before you go soak up some rays.

Robert Bissonnette, a dermatologist at the University of Montreal, tested six lotions with an SPF of 21 or higher that claim to block exposure to ultraviolet A (UVA) and ultraviolet B (UVB) rays. Twelve volunteers had a few sunblocks rubbed on sections of their backs and then got zapped by a heat lamp. Later, Bissonnette examined their skin to see how much the lotions limited ultraviolet damage.

It turns out that SPF is an incomplete measure of safety. Bissonnette found that two of the lotions with the highest SPFs—45 and 50—provided the least protection against UVA rays, which can cause wrinkles, damage the skin's immune system, and lead to cancer. That doesn't mean that a high SPF isn't important—it is a good measure of sunburn protection (caused by still-dangerous UVB rays). But don't take UVA protection for granted.

For optimal protection, Bissonnette suggests picking a lotion with a high SPF and Parsol 1789, a substance that's known to block UVA rays. Only two of the products he tested in his study contained Parsol: PreSun 30 and one not available in the U.S. But you should be able to find more lotions that fit the bill.

Of course, these fine points don't change the bottom line about protecting your skin. "Wearing a hat, avoiding the midday sun, and seeking out shade are all more important than the brand of sunscreen you buy," says Bissonnette.

HEALTH BUZZ

THUMBS UP

honey
How sweet it is: A new study indicates the golden nectar boosts power and endurance as much as fancy sport gels do.

aspirin
More good news about the painkiller. Now experts say gals who take it regularly may cut their odds of getting ovarian cancer.

THUMBS DOWN

dozing on the side
Sleep on this: Researchers say that people who always snooze on one side are far more likely to get kidney stones than are others.

protein bars
Are you sure what you're getting? Consumer groups say many bars are falsely labeled to understate their carb content.

Q+A
if sunscreen makes you break out, try this

Every time I wear sunscreen to the beach, my skin breaks out. Can I wear my SPF 15 foundation instead?

Yes, says Flor Mayoral, a dermatologist in Miami. "But in direct sunlight, foundation will mix with sweat and slide off your face," she says. "For prolonged exposure, reapply your foundation every hour or so—a little more often than with normal sunscreen."

Don't feel like being so diligent but do have acne-prone skin? Then you should look for sun-shielding lotions that say "non-comedogenic" on the label. Try Clinique Sun-Care Body Spray 30 SPF SunBlock or Neutrogena's Oil-Free Sunblock. Another idea: Sunscreens in gel form have a high alcohol content that will dry out oily skin.

WAVE GOOD-BYE TO CHAPPED "WINTER" HANDS

Like slushy streets and icy windshields, chapped hands seem to be a seasonal hazard. Between dry heat indoors and harsh conditions outdoors, it's no surprise that your regular moisturizer can't seem to keep your hands soft and smooth for long. Here's how to help curb winter's wrath:

wash with care Detergent-laden soaps are drying to the skin, so try a milder version, such as Earth Therapeutics' Gardener's Anti-Bacterial Wash. Also, give your hands a gentle exfoliation twice a week to help scrub away those dry, dead cells—it will make your hands feel smoother.

switch moisturizers Go for specially formulated hand creams, advises Debbie D'Aquino, vice president of product development for Clinique. Look for such ingredients as shea butter, petrolatum, and cholesterol that lock in the skin's natural moisture by pumping up its lipid barrier—the fatty substances that serve as the body's first defense against water loss. And use hand cream more than once a day. D'Aquino recommends keeping it in your purse and applying it at least three times. Try Clinique's Stop Signs Hand Repair, Lush's Helping Hands, or Source Océan's Hydro-Active Barrier Hand Cream. Also, drink lots of water and consider using a humidifier to add moisture to your environment.

go the extra mile Once a week, try giving yourself one of these moisturizing treatments: Soak hands in hot water with a few tablespoons of baking soda for half an hour, recommends Vera Kantor, owner of Verabella Skin Therapy salon in Beverly Hills. Next, dry hands and cover them with a heavy hand cream. Then put them in plastic bags inside old socks for 20 minutes. Paraffin wax treatments work on the same principle; try Conair's Paraffin and Manicure Spa kit. Another option: Spend the night in BlissLabs Glamour Gloves. The gel lining contains soothing agents like grape seed and jojoba oils.

Q+A
causes and cures for chapped lips

Even when it's warm outside, my lips are always chapped. Why does this happen, and how can I prevent it?

As temperatures rise, many people start licking their lips more, trying to keep them cool and moist. Ironically, they end up doing the opposite, which may be what's happening to you. If you're not a lip-licker, matte lipstick could be the culprit, or you may be allergic to an ingredient in your lip balm, toothpaste, or something else that touches your mouth. If you eat a lot of fruit, you might even be reacting to acid in the juice.

To keep your lips smooth and flake-free, dermatologist Debra Jaliman, M.D., a clinical instructor at the Mount Sinai School of Medicine in New York, suggests using a lip balm that has sunscreen and petrolatum, the key ingredient in Vaseline (a great substitute if your lips are sensitive to regular balms). Avoid cinnamon-flavored balms; they smell yummy, but they're just too harsh on lips. When you're shopping for a new lipstick, choose a sheer, glossy color. And if you think you might be fruit-sensitive, keep it away from your lips by cutting it into small pieces and eating it with a fork.

Learning to See

Most of us are happy if we can fumble through the chart on the wall at the DMV. But true vision is about much, much more—and if you work at it, you can attain it.

BY ANN JAPENGA

PHOTOGRAPHY BY JIM FRANCO

Laura Sewall is trying to answer my questions. She really is. But perhaps we should have met in a bare room. As it is, we're sitting by a hotel pool on the edge of the desert in Palm Springs, California, surrounded by a jagged horseshoe of rocky hills. Sewall, here for a conference, is seduced by hundreds of beckoning images. In the breeze a green palm frond catches the sun flashing gold, and Sewall's attention darts away from the interview. Then she glimpses a nearby ridgeline where corrugated mountains collide with blue sky, and she spins off again in visual delight.

I can't really blame her for being preoccupied. She's in love, and the object of her affection—the visible world—won't leave her alone.

"I must be weird to think this is exciting—the color red, light on water, a sparkle in a piece of mica," says Sewall, a 45-year-old professor at Prescott College in Arizona. "But there's so much to see out there. It makes it fun to be alive."

You probably think of enhanced sight as the province of artists, astronomers, and wildlife trackers. But, as Sewall says in her book, *Sight and Sensibility: The Ecopsychology of Perception* (Putnam, 1999), visual rapture is available to everyone. Just put down the magazine, look away from your e-mail and TV, and revel in the vibrant and juicy (two of her favorite words) world. "Just look, and look again," Sewall urges.

Sewall has a wide, white-toothed smile and a woodsy glow—picture Joni Mitchell as an Outward Bound instructor. Her Ph.D. is in the neurophysiology of vision, so she can dumbfound you with her grasp of neural networks and how the brain is wired to comprehend visual stimuli. At Prescott, she teaches in the new field of ecopsychology, which explores how our physical and psychological well-being is tied to our relationship with nature. Sewall cites one study that suggests our senses have diminished as we have become more removed from dependence on and interaction in natural environments. Most people, according to Sewall, can no longer see the subtleties in color because it isn't important for us living in cities and suburbs to be able to differentiate shades of green. But she says this is reversible, and awakening the sense of sight is her mission.

Most people can no longer see the subtleties in color because it isn't important for day-to-day living.

But what we see helps us understand the world: What we see *is* our world.

Sewall is one of a new wave of researchers and writers who urge us to push the bounds of vision. James Elkins, Ph.D., an art professor at the Art Institute of Chicago, discusses the subtleties of viewing grass and postage stamps in *How to Use Your Eyes* (Routledge, 2000). In *The Eye Care Revolution* (Kensington, 1999), Robert Abel Jr., M.D., clinical professor of ophthalmology at Thomas Jefferson University in Philadelphia, argues—like Sewall—that vision is more than the ability to read the fine print on a food label.

Yet we've been looking at flat surfaces for so long—computer and TV screens, newspapers, and books—that we no longer perceive the magnificence all around us. "In the visual science model we all grew up with, eyes are passive receivers," Sewall says. We have accepted the mechanical model of vision; we think of our eyes merely as machines—little cameras—and grow irritated when they falter, as they do for most people at midlife. We want them fixed, pronto. So popular are mechanical fixes that laser eye surgery has been called the procedure of the millennium, with the other standard mechanical fixes—contacts, bifocals, and more—close behind.

depth perception Once you discover that your eyes aren't just small cameras and you tap into your awareness of the visual world, you will be bombarded by qualities in images you've never noticed before: the explosion of color and texture at the center of a flower, the razor tips of a palm frond.

visual delight Enhanced sight isn't just the province of artists, astronomers, and wildlife trackers. Anyone, really, can learn to discern and appreciate the vibrancy of colors, the variation of textures in seemingly flat images, the sharp edges where objects collide with their surroundings.

But Sewall says sight is too important to dismiss in such a utilitarian fashion. After all, what we see is our ultimate source for understanding the world. About 70 percent of all the sensory information we take in is visual. What we see *is* our world.

Laura Sewall's own journey to enhanced vision began in the mid-'70s, when she was living on a small island off the coast of Washington state. Having become nearsighted as a teenager, Sewall hated wearing glasses. On frequent sea-kayaking trips in the Puget Sound, the ocean spray would coat her lenses, and she would struggle to navigate through a salt-scummed world. About this time, Sewall discovered the work of William H. Bates, M.D., an ophthalmologist in the 1920s who advocated eye exercises to relax strained eye muscles and correct vision problems. Although his theories have been discredited by many ophthalmologists, his 1943 book, *Better Eyesight Without Glasses,* was a best-seller, and some people reported modest improvement in their vision if they did the Bates exercises regularly.

Sewall turned out to be one of them. She left Washington and moved to Los Angeles to work with Janet Goodrich, a disciple of the Bates method. Every day Sewall met with Goodrich. She practiced looking at a distant object and then a close one in an exercise called "near-far swings." Some days Sewall wore a halolike device that dangled a piece of colored tape in her field of vision—an exercise meant to awaken the less-dominant eye. After less than two months, Sewall no longer needed glasses.

But her ability to clearly see road signs wasn't the only thing that had changed. Behind glasses, she had the sort of fearful personality she says is typical of people with near-sightedness. Clear vision begat a bolder Laura. "It was so empowering to be able to drive without glasses and to feel unafraid," she says. "It just transformed me."

Sewall had shifted not only her focus but her whole way of perceiving. Visual perception embraces dimensions the 20/20 chart doesn't measure; these include the capacity to gauge depth, color, patterns, peripheral vision, aesthetics, and the ability to glean meaning from what you see. For Sewall, these unmeasurables suddenly zoomed beyond any chart.

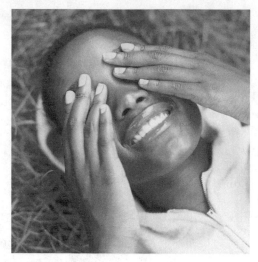

"Palming" is a way of teaching your eyes to see the world in a different way. Try it two to three times a day.

Rhode Island. Now her vision was filled with diagrams with of such things as retinas, neurons, and the lateral geniculate nucleus (where the brain mixes and matches visual signals). Among her scientist friends, it was heresy to suggest that the visual system in adults could be intentionally altered—could, in fact, soar to extreme heights. When Sewall raised the possibility in classes, she was met with vague answers and uneasy glances. But she continued to investigate and found some studies that suggest structural changes to the visual cortex do indeed occur in adults. "Scientists don't even have a way to track the true potential of vision," she says. "Exceptional performance is not something they measure."

Though supersight lies outside the purview of routine eye exams, some doctors say it may indeed be possible to enhance perception (as opposed to acuity) through rigorous training. "There is something to be said for becoming more aware," says Philadelphia ophthalmologist John Jeffers, M.D., a spokesman for the American Academy of Ophthalmology. "It's as if you're saying to the eyes, 'Yo, wake up.'"

deeper reflection Your eyes aren't simply passive receptors. You can train them to look beyond the obvious and take in layers of imagery: the play of light on a glass decanter, a clustering of leaves below the shimmery surface of a lake, the slow dance of clouds and sun across a placid pond.

"I began to glimpse sharp, razorlike edges and neon colors," Sewall writes in her book. "Fabulous shapes and vibrant colors signaled to me, edges were sharp all the time, and whole stories revealed themselves to me on street corners. I was developing a true vision, one that continues to inform and orient my life."

If this could happen to her, Sewall thought, it could happen to others. She now believed people had the power to supercharge their sight. Nothing in the glasses-wearing culture had prepared her for this revelation, one that launched her career.

Hooked on sight, Sewall enrolled in a Ph.D. program in vision at Brown University in Providence,

If it were up to Sewall, this would be big news in every paper across the land: The visual equipment in your brain can perform miracles, if you learn how to use it. Your eyes are not mechanical cameras; the world is not a flat screen after all.

Finally, I just have to stop talking with Laura Sewall about enhanced vision and try it for myself. So I put down the reporters' notebook and take a look around.

The visual equipment in your brain can perform miracles,
if you learn how to use it.

sensory seduction True vision is almost a total-body experience: It requires intense focus and complete awareness.

There, resting on a palm frond, is a plain old dove. I know doves. They flutter about my yard every morning and scatter when I step outside to shake a rug. They're small creatures with beady black eyes and are as common as pill bugs. But have I ever really seen one?

I watch this particular dove for a few moments, bringing my full intention to the task as if this were my most important job of the day. "As in any intimate relationship, what we bring to the exchange determines the quality of the experience," Sewall quietly explains.

If you had asked me before about the color of a common dove, I would have said it was a drab khaki. Now I can see that the dove's feathers are really a cool cream color—velvety perfection that would make a modernist designer weep.

My body tenses as the dove grips the branch for balance. It's almost—and this is how real seeing works—as if I am becoming the dove. When the dove takes off, I stop short of flying away myself, but I do feel a sympathetic surge in the muscles between my shoulders.

Go deeper: Your field of vision encompasses more than what's right in front of you. Focus on objects that are varying distances from your eyes to help improve depth perception.

It's only a quick experiment, but already I can see there's something to Sewall's message: Vision is not just for spectators—it's the ultimate action sport. ✳

Ann Japenga is a Health *contributing editor.*

seeing 101

Learning to use your eyes in new ways can bring layers of pleasure to your daily life. The following exercises, suggested by Laura Sewall, Ph.D., author and professor of ecopsychology at Prescott College in Arizona, can give glimpses of a dazzling world if you make an effort to see deeply.

Try "palming." Sit or lie down in a quiet place and gently cup your palms over your eyes. Wait until all the flashes and squiggles have vanished and you see total blackness. (If you are aware of activity under your closed lids, your eyes are still working.) For maximum effect, do this exercise two to three times a day for 15 minutes each. But if you try it even once, colors and edges will likely be more defined when you open your eyes.

Strengthen your intention. Select a color, a shape, an object—or even something abstract like beauty—and attend to that cue for an hour. Afterward, you should continue to notice the cue even though you're not looking for it. If, for instance, you focus on the color red, Sewall says, "red starts showing up all over the place. The one-hour exercise teaches us how much more we see when we're actively prepared to see something."

Paint the world. Most people spend a good part of their days with their eyes focused on what they habitually see. To loosen up the small muscles in your eyes, pretend you have a paintbrush on the end of your nose. When you look at an object, trace its contours with your nose and let your eyes follow. Sewall calls this "painting the world." Your eyes will get a workout, and you'll take in more visual information than you would if your eyes were static.

Reaquaint yourself with depth. Most of the surfaces people look at every day are flat—computers, televisions, newspapers, road signs. The eyes and brain almost forget how to factor depth into a scene. Get into the habit of intentionally looking into the far distance, middle distance, and the spaces in between that you rarely pay attention to. Says Sewall, "When your eyes move in and out of various depths, there's always something else revealed."

FOREVER young

the new plastic surgery

Many dermatologists are venturing into what used to be strictly plastic-surgeon territory, performing cosmetic techniques—and often researching and improving on them.

But is a youthful face worth the risks?

BY LISA MARGONELLI

I n Los Angeles, you get used to a certain made-for-TV air about people, but this woman is different. With her empathetic eyes, fine solid nose, and sturdy eyebrows, the judge looks nothing like the glamorous actors on *Ally McBeal* or *The Practice.* She appears no-nonsense, by-the-book, "real."

Except for her tattooed lips. "You can't put on lipstick on the bench," she explains to dermatologist Ronald Moy, M.D., in his office on the fifth floor of the University of California at Los Angeles (UCLA) Medical Plaza. Getting permanent makeup was one of the first things her female colleagues advised her to do when she joined their ranks. Now, though, she thinks she needs something more dramatic: maybe a face-lift. Wearing a black robe all day draws an inordinate amount of attention to her face—or more precisely, to her

wrinkles, her pores, her age spots. "I'm not interested in being on the cover of *Vogue,*" she insists. She just wants to look "fresher."

Like a good consumer, the judge has done her research and has settled on Ron Moy as the best doctor in Los Angeles, maybe anywhere, for the job. A dermatologist rather than a plastic surgeon, Moy has helped pioneer techniques that achieve many of the effects of the traditional face-lift, but with much less cutting, tugging, and stitching. The result is more natural looking than the scary *Sunset Boulevard* stereotype. The recovery time is much shorter and the cost far lower, making these procedures more appealing and attainable for the average professional person than ever before. According to the American Society of Plastic Surgeons, its members performed

Many of these "**plastic surgery lite**" procedures are so new and so untested that no one knows how they compare with traditional plastic surgery—or what complications may ensue.

approximately 2 million cosmetic procedures last year, up 198 percent from 1992. Although no one group monitors the number of what we'll call "plastic surgery lite" procedures, rough estimates suggest that dermatologists did 6 million, including Botox injections, laser treatments, and liposuction.

On any given day, Moy might "tweak" the face of a lab tech, a surfing instructor, or a department-store saleswoman. Then there's his Hollywood clientele (don't even try to book an appointment before the Emmys). Until recently, Moy also edited one of the leading dermatological journals in the country, explaining the dos and don'ts of virtually every cosmetic procedure developed in the last 10 years. In this appearance-obsessed, media-driven culture, all this means that Moy isn't just a big-deal dermatologist (or megaderm, as they're known in the beauty business)—he's one of the people helping redefine how 21st-century American women think women their age should look.

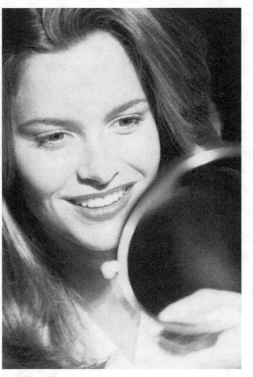

The judge thinks she should look something like Susan Sarandon—not screen-goddess stunning, necessarily, but youthful and glowing. Moy, on the other hand, thinks she looks just fine. "You don't need a face-lift," he says mildly. Her only problems, if she wants to call them that, are a few crow's-feet, a little slackness around the eyes, and some lines around her mouth. Years of sun exposure have damaged the collagen layer under her skin. Collagen is the skin's support structure; when it thins and loses elasticity, the skin buckles and wrinkles form. Moy suggests using a CO_2 (carbon dioxide) laser to zap the offending areas. The laser's heat stimulates the collagen to start growing again. This will make the judge's skin become tighter and her furrows less noticeable—without a single nip or tuck.

Moy's voice is soft, his words carefully considered. At a boyish 43, he has the reassuring charm of a self-professed nerd. His low-key demeanor is comforting; the judge's eyebrows, which have been locked in a scowl, start to unknit. Then Moy throws his sales pitch into reverse. He shows the judge a photo of a woman covered with oozing crusts: Lasered skin needs at least seven days to heal, he explains. Other snapshots show patients who are very wrinkly before the treatment and only slightly less wrinkly afterward. In other words, Moy says, don't expect any miracles. The judge rattles off questions with the authority of someone who's spent her entire professional life searching for answers and weighing consequences, but, plainly, she's ready to sign on for whatever he thinks would work best.

Some big questions, however, remain unasked. Most fundamentally: What are the societal consequences of air-brushing a woman's history from her face—of erasing signs of laughter, anger, bright summer days, and normal aging—as if they were flaws? Surely someone as intelligent and successful as this dispenser of justice shouldn't have to care what anyone thinks of her lip color and crow's-feet.

Moy certainly doesn't seem bothered by her aging signs, but the judge is. And the work of Moy and his fellow megaderms is one catalyst for her desire to look younger. By figuring out how to make cosmetic surgery quicker, cheaper, and less traumatic, dermatologists have transformed the field. Cosmetic surgery has become more like normal skin care—just one step removed from slathering your face with an alpha hydroxy acid cream at night. The new accessibility of procedures such as laser resurfacing makes them not just an option but a necessity, like good grooming. If you can look younger and prettier, why on earth would you choose not to?

Once upon a time, dermatologists devoted most of their practice to treating conditions such as acne and psoriasis with lotions and creams. Anything that required cutting into the skin, even the removal of an unsightly mole, was considered plastic surgery.

But the field started to change in the 1970s and '80s, thanks to a convergence of coincidences. New drugs were making the old standby complaints all but obsolete. The restructuring of the medical industry was making traditional doctoring—with its standard $10 co-payments—unprofitable. Technologies such as lasers and fillers, like collagen, came on the market. Cosmetic procedures, which patients paid for out of pocket, became far more lucrative.

By the time Moy, a Southern California native, began his residency at UCLA in 1981, a few daring dermatologists had begun to tread on the plastic surgeons' turf. Moy discovered that he loved surgery and that he was good at it.

Once they started cutting, the early dermatological surgeons didn't stop. They began to do face-lifts and eye-lifts, using the skin's healing powers to their advantage and teaching each other their tricks. But the dermatological surgeons didn't just replicate old techniques; they figured out how to improve on traditional plastic surgery.

Take, for instance, the face-lift. In a full-scale face-lift operation, the surgeon makes a long incision around the face: behind the ears, into the scalp, and below the chin. Then he or she delicately separates the skin from the flesh below it and the flesh from its underlying support structure of muscle and bone, pretty much the way a cook skins and debones a chicken breast. As the surgeon gently tugs the flesh toward the forehead or neck, deep furrows, such as the naso-labial folds—those cheeky, matronly trenches that run from the sides of the nose to the mouth—become less noticeable. This is major surgery, requiring four or more hours in the operating room, general anesthesia, a month of recovery time, and a fat bank account (none of the cost, which can be upwards of $20,000, is covered by insurance).

Compare that to a kind of mini-face-lift, known as an S-lift, favored by dermatologic surgeons like Moy. Instead of cutting and lifting the entire face, Moy just removes a small scroll-shaped piece of skin from in front of the ear. Then, working under the skin as though he's rearranging apples beneath a piecrust, he takes a few stitches and tugs the underlying layer of fascia and muscle upward to smooth out furrows. Moy performs the operation in about two hours, under local anesthetic. The patient recovers in about a week, though it takes longer for bruises and swelling to subside. The cost is around $5,000.

Of course, the results aren't as dramatic as those created by a traditional face-lift: The S-lift delivers almost exactly what you see when you look in the mirror and pull the skin back near your temples. But then, most people don't have the money or the time to spring for the full-scale operation. Many are frightened of the risks. What's more, a face-lift is most appropriate for someone with major sagging and bagging. An S-lift is a tweak, the kind of work you have done when gravity is just beginning to make your cheeks droop.

To many prospective patients, derma-surgeons offer not just beauty and youth, but healing. A good doctor and a few thousand dollars can erase emotional scars from the past—and reshape the future.

The dermatologic surgeons have been quick to adapt every new piece of technology to achieve the effects of plastic surgery with less muss and fuss.

With his skill and training in surgery, Ronald Moy has led the pack in these adaptations. He became co-chief of dermatologic surgery at UCLA at age 35 and editor in chief of the journal *Dermatologic Surgery* by 38. Almost constitutionally devoted to research, he has pushed other doctors to innovate, to conduct more research into aging skin, and to understand why the new techniques work or fail.

Although Moy is widely respected, there's plenty of controversy about the direction that dermatology has taken—and not just among plastic surgeons, who naturally resent this intrusion into their territory. Lawrence Field, M.D., of the University of California at San Francisco, was one of the first dermatologists to perform face-lifts. Since the '70s, he has reconstructed about 35,000 flaps. (That's how dermasurgeons rate themselves: flaps of skin they've cut open and sewn down.) But after years of advocating an aggressive approach to surgery, Field has reconsidered. "The great thrust today is money," he says. "Too many people are doing things for which they're not really trained. As a specialty, we need to go more slowly."

Field has a point: Economics is one of the biggest factors behind the dermatology community's recent interest in cosmetic surgery. Under pressure from insurance companies, primary-care physicians no longer make automatic referrals for such "trivial" problems as rashes and pimples. They treat them using the same drugs that dermatologists prescribe. So, forced to generate new sources of income, more dermatologists have taken up the laser, the chemical peel, the scalpel. But unlike board-certified plastic surgeons, who spend years learning their specialties, many dermatologists have not done residencies in surgery. Like their own patients, they may assume that "lunchtime procedures" are so simple and safe that special skills aren't necessary. "Moy is a very careful young man," Field says. "A lot of people aren't that careful."

In Moy's office, the excitement of innovation is almost palpable. The studies being conducted there, the newness of the equipment, and the enthusiasm of the staff and patients give the bland dermatology office an energy that must resemble NASA in its mission-to-the-moon heyday.

Moy sets the pace. "Next to him I feel like a slouch," says Victor Neel, director of dermatologic surgery at Mass General Hospital/Harvard University Medical School. Neel has a Ph.D. in genetics and an M.D.,

and has done residencies in both pediatrics and dermatology. He's drawn to doctors who push the envelope—and Moy pushes harder than anyone else. "He's constantly thinking of the next thing," Neel says.

In his quest to develop objective measures and new techniques, Moy has done a lot of clinical trials. Some are rather ungainly: In one study, for instance, laser-resurfacing patients had half their faces covered with a dressing, while the other half was occasionally uncovered and sprayed with oxygen for several days. In another, liposuction patients stayed at the nearby Hilton, waking every two hours so a technician could check the levels of anesthesia in their blood. Moy has many subjects. And some of these guinea pigs keep coming back.

One is Kim Luna, who has had four experimental procedures at Moy's hands. Yet the 48-year-old doesn't fit the stereotype of some neurotic, overstretched plastic-surgery victim. Luna is attractive and vivacious but has left one mark on her cheek untouched: a large mole with, as she says, "hairs growing out of it." Why would someone who's had so much work done decide not to remove a hair-sprouting mole? "This mole is part of me," she explains, "but my wrinkles are new."

When the last of her three kids left home, Luna says she had a funny reaction. "I didn't feel any older than when I had them. What happened?" Her poochy tummy bugged her, and so did the sad wrinkles around her eyes. In 1997, she signed up for a liposuction study conducted by Moy.

To tighten Luna's tummy, Moy used ultrasonic waves in addition to the standard liposuction, hoping to make the process easier and prevent bleeding. Luna remembers that the only disturbing part of the procedure was that when she stood up, water "leaked like a faucet" from the holes in her skin. She was so pleased with the results, though, that she had her thighs done. Since then, however, Moy has abandoned the ultrasonic technique; the potential complications, the doctor decided, outweighed the benefits.

In another of Luna's experimental procedures, implants were used to eliminate the deep folds running from her nose to the sides of her mouth. For a demonstration video, Moy inserted Soft Forms, spaghetti-size tubes of Gore-Tex, into Luna's furrows to lift and smooth them. Though the forms were stiff at first, they soon became more supple and natural looking. Luna says she was happy with them. Unfortunately, dermatologists and many patients were not. In some cases, the Gore-Tex fibers unraveled and pushed through patients' skin. Moy has since abandoned this technology, too—like almost all the techniques used on Luna.

But all that matters to her is that they were quick and relatively painless, and that Moy, a doctor she trusts completely, was in charge. She's not worried that almost every technique he employed is now obsolete. She'd get more cosmetic surgery if she could afford it. "My husband thinks I'm a little weird," she admits. But she adds, "I did it for myself."

Luna's story highlights the little-seen flip side of dermatology's cutting edge. Many of the innovations pioneered by hotshot megaderms like Moy are so new and untested that no one knows how well they really work—or what complications might ensue. Take the CO_2 laser. For patients whose only problem was mild wrinkling around the eyes and lips, doctors used to zap just those areas, leaving the rest of the face alone. But a few months after treatment, patients began returning with "hypopigmentation"—the treated skin had lost its pigment, leaving permanent "owl eyes" and pale blotches around the mouth. Now doctors have changed their techniques, using more gentle lasers, treating the entire face, and taking more precautions to prevent complications.

Moy ticks off a dozen procedures he no longer performs because the side effects proved too numerous or nasty. Yet he defends the process of innovation and believes any good surgeon, in any field of medicine, is constantly experimenting with new techniques and tools, trying to perfect his art. What's more, with constant introduction of new machines, peels, and other products, it's important to study and test them rigorously before they're widely used.

Moy, says fellow megaderm Arnold Klein, is doing the public a huge service by removing the "hocus-pocus" from cosmetic surgery. Still, you get the feeling Moy has some qualms. In the midst of the culture he's helped to create, he finds himself saying "no" a lot, especially to techniques that aren't safe and to technology that's moving too fast. And he has become almost notorious for saying "no" to his patients. He talked his own mother out of a face-lift. "No liposuction," he tells a woman in her 50s. "Buy an Ab Roller."

"That procedure may be worth your time," he tells another woman, "but probably not your money."

"I need a miracle," says another patient. "No," Moy says firmly, "no, you don't." He even ends his session with the judge by refusing to schedule a laser-resurfacing appointment. "Think about it a bit," he tells her as he leaves the room.

As the judge could tell you, the irony is that Moy's "no" is so compelling it has the unintended effect of making his patients want the procedures more.

Moy told 46-year-old mother Janet Jackson three times that he would not give her a neck-lift. Finally, moved by her persistence, he gathered his staff to see what they thought.

Jackson had an abdomen you could bounce a quarter on and the face of someone in her early 30s. Moy was afraid that whatever was wrong with her neck was just in her head, which is a big problem in the cosmetic-surgery biz. Unrealistic expectations can lead to unhappy clients—and lawsuits. However, his staff saw it differently: They said yes, Jackson seemed level-headed; yes, she knew what she was getting into.

And they pointed out that if Moy didn't do her lift, she would just find another surgeon—almost certainly one with less experience than Moy.

So Jackson came to Moy's office and waited to be prepped for the procedure. A traditional neck-lift, like a traditional face-lift, is a big-deal operation. The technique Moy favors, called a suture suspension, involves local anesthesia, minimal amounts of cutting, and a two-week recovery. Moy sat down next to Jackson and began to draw dotted lines on her neck.

"You think I'm a frivolous, airheaded woman," she told him at one point. On closer inspection, however, her neck was different from the rest of her body; weak and flubbery, it started at her chin and fell gracelessly to her collarbone. It seemed her neck's problem was not fat, Moy said, but a sagging platysma muscle. To correct the drooping, he planned to run a cord through the flesh and muscles, gathering them slightly as if he were a tailor easing a lapel into a jacket, and anchoring the suture to the bones near her ears. As the neck heals, it will grow taut. When Moy was finished marking her up, the dotted lines extended from ear to ear and from the back of her jaw to her chin. She looked like a kid's construction project.

Jackson was thrilled to be in the operating room at last. She cracked jokes with the nurse. "I'm not a vain woman," she said. "If I were, I wouldn't have 32A breasts." As the nurse finished injecting the anesthesia, Jackson relaxed into the pillow. "This is a good day," she sighed. "This is the end of all this."

Jackson's reasons for wanting this surgery were far from frivolous after all. For years, she had been married to an abusive man. She endured all manner of torment, finally leaving after her husband broke her neck. Once she recovered, she quit her job, picked up her children, and moved to California to begin a new life. "I'm one of the 5 percent that don't go back," Jackson says proudly. But her sagging neck continued to haunt her, a constant reminder of the broken bones, the horrible past. "I had to get this fixed," she says.

Jackson's story explains better than anything else the success of the new dermatologists. They offer not just beauty and youth, but healing. Many of Moy's patients use the word "empowering" to describe their experience. All you need is a good doctor and a few thousand dollars, and you can change what once seemed irrevocable: not just the future, but the past. You can erase the acne scars that made adolescence so miserable or recapture enough of your youth to imagine finding love again after a divorce. You can gain confidence to switch careers at an age when many women feel devalued and stuck or clear up your surface imperfections so that people will focus instead on your brilliant ideas. According to one study, 59 percent of women getting plastic surgery on their faces said it was to improve their self-esteem. "We can make people feel better about themselves with surgery," Moy says.

This is the upside of the dermatology revolution. No woman, whether a judge or a secretary, should have to care about her lip color or crow's-feet, but if she does care, she can fix the problem fast. "We dye our hair, we use a microwave, we don't get up to change the TV channel," Jackson says. The newfangled cosmetic surgery fits right in.

Perhaps it's not surprising, then, that so many women are willing to take the plunge—even with procedures that are relatively new and untested, like Moy's suture suspension. Jackson says she understood the potential complications. She understood she might not see the dramatic result she desires. The cord could break; she could be forced to have another operation.

None of that mattered. Jackson was confident that she had made the right decision. "With the risks I've taken in my life," she says, "this is nothing. This is not a risk." ✳

> Moy has gained an almost notorious reputation for saying "no" to patients. "No liposuction," he tells one woman who has come to him for the procedure. "Buy an Ab Roller."

Lisa Margonelli, based in San Francisco, is a contributing writer for Jane *magazine.*

nonsurgical face-lifts

Could partaking of sugar, caffeine, and wine make you more attractive? Cosmetics companies think so—if they go on your skin, not in your mouth. The latest skin care products are chock-full of these goodies that promise real benefits. Here's the news.

The Goods on Grapes: Polyphenols are the wonder workers here. Derived from grape skin, polyphenols were recently discovered to be powerful free-radical scavengers. They neutralize the body's unstable oxygen molecules—the silent force behind wrinkles. And they won't irritate the skin like vitamins C and E can. But polyphenols' biggest claim is that they don't break down as quickly as vitamins C and E, so they stay effective longer in creams. Try Lancôme's Vinéfit SPF 15 Complete Energizing Moisturizer.

The Skinny on Sugar: Middle Eastern women have used sugar as a depilatory for centuries, but the beauty world is reinventing it as an exfoliant. The grainy texture removes rough skin but, unlike traditional exfoliants such as salt, won't dry it out. Try Osmotics's Sugar Scrub and Estée Lauder's Idealist Skin ReFinisher.

The Juice on Java: Caffeine's diuretic properties fit the bill for eye and skin creams. By drawing out fluids, caffeine temporarily reduces puffiness, for a more toned appearance. Get your fix from facial moisturizers such as L'Oréal's Plénitude Revitalift Slim or Origins' Have a Nice Day Super-Charged Moisture Lotion SPF 15.

EARLOBE AID
for women who love big earrings

Break out those jewelry boxes, because big earrings are back and as much fun as ever. "Whether you're in a suit or shorts, an eye-catching pair of earrings can add color to any ensemble," says Shaune Bazner, jewelry designer for Mei Fa.

But one thing is for sure: Whether you opt for wiry hoops, dangling chains, or beaded extravaganzas, super-sized accessories can wreak serious wear and tear on your earlobes. So, choose wisely.

First, look at your lobes. Women with elongated holes that are close to the bottom of the ear should go with small, lightweight styles. The safest options are sets with a sticklike post held securely in place by a metal back that's surrounded by a clear plastic disk. These can give you much-needed stability; if an earring gets caught on your collar, it can easily tear through your flesh.

For those with holes smack-dab in the center of the lobe, a sticklike post is still best for heavier styles. A hooklike one is okay for lightweight earrings, but pay attention to where they dangle. Loose knits and turtlenecks can catch those free-flowing numbers.

Finally, be sensible. If your lobes start to ache after an hour, the earrings are too heavy, so switch to a lighter pair.

A WOMAN'S *sexiest scent*

Woman's most alluring essence may not come from the Givenchy counter. Researchers at the University of Texas at Austin asked men to rate the smell of a month's worth of T-shirts worn by women they'd never met. The test group consistently rated the shirts worn during the women's most fertile stages as sexier and more pleasant smelling. The women in question had not worn perfume, nor had they used unscented products, so as not to lead the men's noses astray.

So the next time you're in search of an enticing fragrance midcycle, consider going au naturel.

Strengthen Your Nails

You may have heard that a lack of calcium is the culprit of weak nails or that eating gelatin is the fix. But Boni Elewski, a professor of dermatology at the University of Alabama at Birmingham, says it ain't so. "Nails split because they're dry; diet has little influence."

The best solution is to condition nails with lotions and oils often. Give nails intense therapy by soaking them in warm olive oil for 10 minutes. Topical nail strengtheners are also a no-no (especially ones with formaldehyde) because they coat the nail and prevent conditioners from penetrating.

That said, there are two oral fixes that might help. Soy protein can strengthen nails, so you should load up on soy milk and tofu. Or try biotin, a member of the B-complex vitamin family. In supplement form you'll need 80 milligrams a day; or you can get it from egg yolks and yeast.

Q+A

help for dry scalp

Can a shampoo containing hydroxy acids help my dry scalp?

If you're only a little flaky, these products are effective. "Hydroxy acids are mild exfoliants that may help remove excess scaling and flaking from your dry scalp and ease slight itching," says David J. Leffell, M.D., author of *Total Skin* (Hyperion, 2000) and professor of dermatology and surgery at the Yale School of Medicine. Some to try: Goldwell Definition shampoo with alpha hydroxy acids, Merz's Aqua Glycolic Shampoo & Body Cleanser, and Therapy Systems' Glycolic Cleansing Gel.

Major itching, though, is a cry for moisture. Treat your scalp to an over-the-counter dandruff shampoo, such as Nizoral. If that doesn't work, see your doctor. You may have seborrheic dermatitis, an inflammation of the scalp that can be cleared up with a prescription hydrocortisone lotion.

Products aren't your only defense against flake-outs. Keep showers short and low on steam (hot water dries out your scalp); skip daily, oil-stripping shampoos; and go easy with the hot blow-dryer.

the risk of acrylic nails

I've heard acrylic nails can cause all sorts of health problems. How can I protect myself?

The safest option, is to grow your own. But if you'd like to try them, be aware that "many people are allergic to the glue used to apply acrylic nails," explains Jeanine Downie, M.D., a dermatologist at Image Dermatology in Montclair, New Jersey. If you're one of the unlucky ones, try silk wraps. They require less glue than acrylic tips and may help you avoid the redness, flakiness, and puffiness that come with an allergic reaction.

If you're not allergic and want to stick with acrylic, this simple safeguard may help: Make sure the nail is placed properly. "When the weight or misplacement of the acrylic tip causes your original nail to lift up, it leaves an opening for fungus or yeast to enter and multiply," Downie says. That can translate to pain and a yellowish-brownish discoloration—as well as set you up for a bacterial infection. Another option at salons or at home: Original Organic Nails, a nail system that uses nontoxic glue and decreases the risk of nail lifting.

the real-woman's guide to all-day pampering

Just because you're overscheduled doesn't mean you have to look it. Take the stress out of a jam-packed day with these seriously easy, superfast spa treatments.

BY LEAH ROSCH

PHOTOGRAPHY BY AMY NEUNSINGER

Pampering, for the majority of us, is a Martha Stewart concept in a *Survivor* world. And its cruelest irony is that the more you need pampering, the less likely you'll be able to fit such an indulgence in—let alone afford it. Or so you may think.

We've found that the pluses of pampering don't come only from all-day spa packages or 30-minute deep-conditioning hair treatments. By fitting quick treatments into "found" moments—the two minutes you're on hold, five seconds after lunch, one minute before bed—you can get that just-back-from-a-country-weekend look and the relaxed feeling that comes with it, even in the middle of a time-crunched day.

We canvassed experts at some top spas across the country for their most innovative, and least time-consuming, sybaritic secrets. Then we worked their tips into a typical overflowing schedule. None of them takes more than 15 minutes, so you can look renewed, feel relaxed, and still get most everything crossed off that to-do list. Who knew feeling at ease could be so easy?

6:00 a.m.

RISE-AND-SHINE STRETCH. Set an energizing tone for your entire day with a deep-breathing routine. Deborah Evans, general manager of Red Mountain spa in Ivins, Utah, offers this invigorating plié stretch to start you off on the right foot. Match the following instructions with the photos at right.

1. Stand with feet shoulder-width apart, toes slightly pointed out. Cross your arms in front of your body and bend your knees in a half plié.

2. Take a deep breath through your nose and gently raise your arms overhead, straightening your legs as you bring your arms up (this should be one fluid movement).

3. Exhale slowly, while lowering your arms. "The deep breathing increases the level of energizing oxygen in the blood," says Evans, "and the lengthening movement loosens your shoulders, helping to

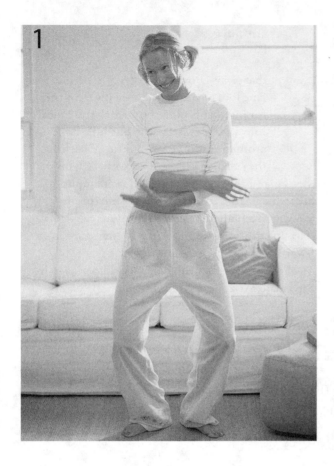

1

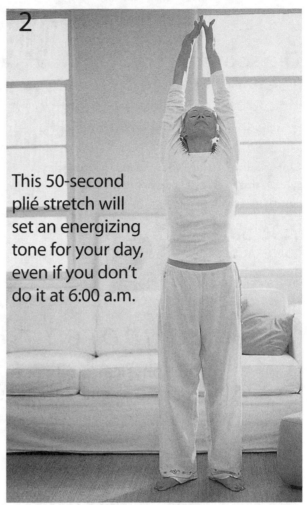

2

This 50-second plié stretch will set an energizing tone for your day, even if you don't do it at 6:00 a.m.

alleviate tension." Repeat five times. **Total investment:** 50 seconds.

6:30 a.m.

MORNING FACIAL MESSAGE. How bad can a day be when it starts with a caress? Treat your skin to the soothing power of touch when applying moisturizer, suggests Deborah Bakhtiari, institute training coordinator at the Clarins Spa in Houston. A big proponent of a little patting, Bakhtiari cautions that vigorous facial rubbing can tug on collagen and elastin fibers, which over the years can lead to a loss of elasticity and firmness. Her gentler approach: Apply moisturizer to hands and lightly press them to your cheeks, working from the middle to the sides. Then, using your fingertips, massage the temples, working upward to the middle of the forehead; walk fingertips down the bridge of your nose to the area above your lips. Apply the same gentle pressing motion to the chin area, up the jawline to your ears. Finish by lightly squeezing your ears, from the top to the lobe. Clarins' Aromatic Plant Day Cream, suitable for all skin types, features a blend of violet extract, geranium, and palma rosa essential oils.

3

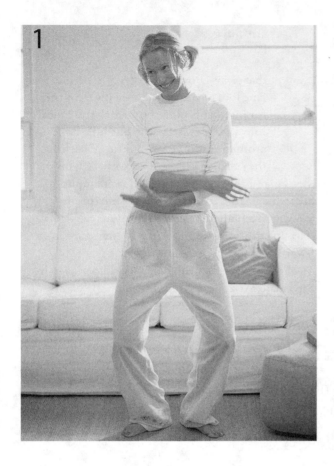

The soothing scent of lavender and rosemary is relaxing but keeps you focused. In your car, it could even spare you a few frown lines and speeding tickets.

Or try Laura Mercier's Tinted Moisturizer with SPF 20; this multitasker saves precious time when you're in a rush. **Total investment:** 1 minute.

7:36 a.m.

ROAD-RAGE ERASER. You'll get to work at the same time whether you fire off a few choice obscenities at that cigar-chomping, 45-mph-in-the-fast-lane lout or not. Avoid even the temptation for highway hostility by turning your Saturn into a spa on wheels with one little device: an aromatic diffuser for your car. Check out the Aeron dashboard diffuser, $17, on www.amaranthine.com, or the ceramic amphora, $10, which hangs from the rearview mirror, on www.buyaromatherapy.com. They quiet nerves by releasing a calming scent—and may even spare you a few frown lines and speeding tickets.

John DeFontes, spa director at the Phoenician in Scottsdale, Arizona, suggests the following plant and

add more grace to your life

From physical practices to mental ones, there are many approaches to grace. These suggestions can get you started.

BY NINA SCHULYER

1. Get in touch with your body. Holding your body correctly is key to physical grace. One way to learn how is by using the Feldenkrais method, which teaches people better ways of using their bodies. One basic Feldenkrais lesson you can try: Lie on the floor on your side, with one shoulder facing up. Slowly move the shoulder forward and back, up and down, in a circle. By repeating this movement, you'll begin to sense how your shoulder blade glides over your ribs. To learn more about Feldenkrais or to take an online lesson, visit www.feldenkrais.com.

2. Straighten your back. To improve your posture, spend a few minutes before a full-length mirror. Is your spine crooked or sagging? Shift your body so that it looks straighter and taller. To maintain this posture during the day, imagine you're wearing a $10,000 necklace and hold your chest out proudly.

3. Sit upright. Long days hunched at a desk can lead to repetitive strain injuries and a permanent slouch. With your feet flat on the floor, notice how you sit. Do you feel more weight on your right or left buttock? Does your body feel cramped and contracted? Now see how you feel when you put equal weight on both buttocks. Experiment by adjusting your chair and computer height, or by placing a thin pillow at the small of your back.

4. Stretch. Tight muscles often lead to poor posture. One good stretch for your lower back: Lie on your back with knees bent and feet on the floor. With both hands, pull one knee to your chest, then the other. Hold your legs against your chest for a few seconds, then release, putting one foot, then the other, on the floor. Repeat several times. Yoga is another good way to relieve muscle tension. For yoga postures that target your spine, go to www.yogasite.com.

5. Volunteer. The Greeks understood that grace is inseparable from charity. If you'd like to give back, but aren't sure where or how, check out

flower essences: Geranium promotes peacefulness; a combination of lavender and rosemary relaxes while keeping you focused; citrusy bergamot has a refreshing and balancing effect. You can also try spearmint or sandalwood—both offer a spicy fragrance with relaxing properties. Total investment: 3 seconds (for plug-in or positioning).

10:15 a.m.

CONFERENCE-CALL ENERGIZER. Treat your hands to a simple acupressure massage while closing that big deal on speakerphone. Place a pair of Chinese therapy balls in one hand and then rotate them clockwise to

stimulate acupressure points, suggests Dale Rutkin, a senior massage therapist at Carapan Urban Spa, a day spa in New York City. The motion alternately contracts and relaxes the muscles of your fingers and forearm, helping relieve fatigue and improve circulation. A pair of hollow-steel cloisonné balls is available for $6 from ZLB International at www.uran.net/zlb. Total investment: 2 minutes per hand.

1:00 p.m.

POST-LUNCH PICK-ME-UP. Start the afternoon with morninglike freshness by misting your face with a toner that has an essential-oil base, says Lynne

www.communityservice.org (the site also lists virtual volunteering options that you can do from home).

6. *Rub out stress.* Massage is ideal for loosening stressed-out muscles. Take a few minutes every day to smooth on some lotion and knead out areas where stress tends to settle, such as your neck and upper shoulders. Better yet, have your mate or a professional masseuse do it for you. To find a certified massage therapist in your area, try the Massage Therapy Web Central at www.qwl.com.

7. *Savor.* Do little things throughout the day to slow your mental clock and to help you appreciate the moment.
• When you eat, take smaller bites and truly taste the flavors of the food.
• Instead of running those errands, stroll them. Pay more attention to the buildings and the people around you.
• Resist the urge to multitask: Read, talk on the phone, or cook dinner—but not all three at once.

8. *Breathe deeply.* Taking slower, deeper breaths can help to reduce stress, headaches, hot flashes, and even your blood pressure, while also heightening your stamina and exercise performance. For suggestions on improving your breathing, check out www.authentic-breathing.com.

9. *Free your mind.* If you're new to meditation, try these suggestions from Tibetan monk Sogyal Rimpoche, author of *The Tibetan Book of Living and Dying* (Harper San Francisco, 1994).
• Find a quiet place, such as a guest room or a corner of the garden.
• Sit with your legs crossed and your back straight.
• Gaze straight ahead at a 45-degree angle.
• Try not to think about anything except breathing. If your mind drifts, gently nudge it back—maybe by focusing on a single object.
• After four or five minutes, take a break of perhaps a minute, then meditate again for up to half an hour.

10. *Go outdoors.* Studies show that just looking at photos of nature can have a beneficial effect on spiritual and physical health. Go for a hike, feed birds in the park, or watch the kids play at the beach. To find places to hike in your area, visit www.gorp.com.

11. *Get strong.* Doing weight-bearing exercises, lifting barbells, walking, climbing stairs, and working out on machines strengthens bones and muscles, making it easier for you to sit straight and stand tall. Exercises that target your back and midsection—your body's core—are especially useful.

Nina Schulyer is a writer, painter, and teacher in San Francisco. She is working on her first novel.

Vertrees, director of the Lake Austin Resort and Spa in Texas. "It revives your complexion and refreshes your senses—all without disturbing your makeup." Her homemade spritz recipe: a light, hydrating rose-water-based toner made of 3 drops rose-water oil to 8 ounces distilled water. When poured into a cobalt-blue glass mister bottle to shield oil from sunlight, it can keep for six months. Also check out Sonya Dakar's Aromasol Toning Mist, available in four skin-type formulas, or Enessa Aromatherapy's Hydra Mist. **Total investment:** 5 seconds for 2 spritzes.

2:25 p.m.
TENSION HANDOFF. Has all that pounding away on the keyboard made your hands feel more tired than an insomniac's eyelids? Then run cold water over your wrists and hands. "This stops the excess flow of blood to your fingers," says Carapan's Dale Rutkin, "and instantly relaxes them." Afterward, pat hands dry and massage them with a thick and luxurious cream. The fast-absorbing Shea Butter Hand Cream from Elizabeth Arden's Spa 7/52 line is a boon at the office because it's practically greaseless. **Total investment:** 3 minutes.

3:11 p.m.
MIDAFTERNOON DEFOGGER. Inhale an energizing scent for a quick, caffeine-free refresher, suggests Laura Hittleman, beauty director at Canyon Ranch in the Berkshires. Lace a tissue with a few drops of a fatigue-fighting essential oil, such as rosemary or peppermint, and wave it under your nose. Or try Aveda's Blue Oil Balancing Concentrate, which combines stimulating peppermint and menthol oils in a portable .24-ounce vial capped with a roller ball; dab under each nostril and take a deep breath. **Total investment:** 2 seconds per sniff.

4:33 p.m.
WAKE-UP CALL FOR TIRED EYES. If you've been up all night with a sick child or staring at a computer screen since Monday, your eyes will show—and

got a minute?
secret beauty shortcuts

6:00	rise-and-shine stretch	50 seconds
6:30	morning facial massage	1 minute
7:36	road-rage eraser	3 seconds
10:15	conference-call energizer	4 minutes
1:00	post-lunch pick-me-up	5 seconds
2:25	tension handoff	3 minutes
3:11	midafternoon defogger	2 seconds
4:33	wake-up call for tired eyes	5 minutes
5:50	yoga lift	5 minutes
6:38	news-break brushup	5 minutes
7:45	cooling feet treat	5 minutes
9:36	head calmer	15 minutes
10:19	evening glow	15 minutes
10:30	sleep relief	1 minute

feel—the strain. Lara Wright, co-owner of Green Valley Laboratory at the Green Valley Spa in St. George, Utah, offers this cool antidote: Fill a snack-size plastic bag about three-quarters full with uncooked rice and chill in the freezer for two minutes. Place the bag over your eyes, then lean back and relax. "It's the gentle pressure and cooling texture that relieves eyestrain," says Wright. Some other favorite eye soothers: zucchini soaked in chamomile or ginseng tea, or the 3 Cool Eyes packet from Stone Spa in New York City. **Total investment:** 5 minutes.

> There's nothing quite as blissful as a scalp massage. The benefits are more than just relaxing: It encourages circulation and cell renewal.

5:50 p.m.
YOGA LIFT. Unkink your body and mind from a crazy day with this pose, recommended by massage therapist Cheryl McKereghan. You can do it even if you're

yoga-impaired (and it's fun for kids to get in the act too): Lie on the floor with your legs raised against a wall and your arms in a comfortable position; exhale through your nose five times in short, sharp breaths and repeat a total of 10 times. "This position drains the blood that can pool in your lower legs and ankles after being on your feet all day, and the breathing clears your head, while filling your lungs with fresh air," says McKereghan. For added effect, try lighting a calming aromatherapy candle, such as Lancôme's AromaTonic Energizing Mood Candle, with the tangy scents of lime and ginger. **Total investment:** 5 minutes.

6:38 p.m.

NEWS-BREAK BRUSHUP. If your power-red polish has left your nails yellow, get them back in the pink with a soothing lemon-and-milk bath. While watching the nightly news, soak your nails in fresh-squeezed lemon juice (the citric acid serves as a bleaching agent), then moisturize cuticles in a bowl of warm milk for four minutes. Rinse in cool water and pat dry. **Total investment:** 5 minutes.

7:45 p.m.

COOLING FEET TREAT. Particularly welcome after a power walk, this refresher from Cat Petru, a massage therapist at California's Sonoma Mission Inn & Spa, soothes tired, swollen feet. Place ice cubes and water in a zippered sandwich bag. For a few minutes, alternately run each bare foot over the icy-cool bag. Finish by misting feet with a blend of tea tree and eucalyptus oils, known for their invigorating and naturally deodorizing properties—use 3 drops each to 8 ounces of distilled water mixed in a mister bottle. Or try Refreshing Foot Spray from the Body Shop. **Total investment:** 5 minutes.

9:36 p.m.

HEAD CALMER. When getting ahead just gives you a headache, there's nothing quite as blissful as a scalp massage. And the benefits are more than merely relaxing. "Massaging your scalp with a blend of essential oils encourages circulation and cell renewal," says Barbara Close, founder of Naturopathica, a holistic spa in

Looking for a good night's sleep?
A few drops of lavender oil on a hankie near your pillow could be just the thing.

East Hampton, New York. Use a premixed massage oil like French Lavender Soothing Massage and Body Oil from Naturopathica. Or try this homemade recipe from Close: Fill a glass bottle with 1/8 cup extra-virgin olive oil or avocado oil; add 2 drops tea tree oil and 5 drops rosemary oil; cover and shake well. Fill the bottle with an additional 1/8 cup olive or avocado oil, cover and shake again. Massage oils through hair; leave on for 10 minutes. Shampoo and rinse thoroughly. When stored in a cool, dark place, the mixture will keep for six months. **Total investment:** 15 minutes.

10:19 p.m.

EVENING GLOW. Before bed, smooth your skin by exfoliating with a sea-salt paste accented with a blend of calming oils. Measure 1/2 cup coarse sea (or kosher) salt into a glass bowl; mix with a few tablespoons of olive oil and 3 drops of lavender oil. Stand in the shower and slather it over your entire body from the neck down, rubbing in a circular motion; make sure to include heels and the bottom of your feet. Shower off in warm (not hot) water. Pat dry and finish with a light body moisturizer, such as Avon's BeComing Aroma-hue Replenishing Body Balm in Spirit. Try it twice a month. **Total investment:** 15 minutes.

10:30 p.m.

SLEEP RELIEF. Quiet your mind by dabbing several drops of naturally sedating lavender oil on a white cotton handkerchief and placing it on your pillow. Or try Sleep Time On-the-Spot Gel from Origins, which contains sleep-inducing chamomile and neroli; dab it on your temples, the center of your forehead, the back of your neck, and just below your navel—the body's four sleep-related points, according to Ayurvedic practices. Turn out the light and dream sweetly. **Total investment:** 1 minute. ✻

Leah Rosch is a writer in New York who reports on health and fitness.

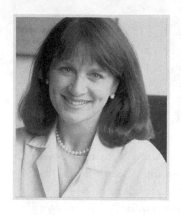

Good Question
about Beauty
by Nancy Snyderman

Help for Rosacea

This winter my cheeks get redder than usual. And the redness doesn't always disappear when I go inside. What's going on?

You may be suffering from rosacea, a relatively common skin condition that affects 13 million Americans, mostly women. Men tend to be afflicted with the more severe cases, but that's probably because they wait until their noses are about to fall off before seeing a doctor!

It's important to see your doctor early on because even though there's no cure for rosacea, you can keep it from getting worse. The first symptom is the one you've got: flushing on the cheeks that doesn't go away. Over the years the redness may spread to the rest of your face, and you could develop burst capillaries (which can show up as red lines) and little red bumps. Left untreated, those bumps can really do a number on your nose, giving it that bulbous look that W. C. Fields made famous.

Fortunately, there are steps you can take so you don't end up that bad off. No one is sure what causes rosacea, although some researchers think bacteria plays a role. But the key to managing the problem is clear: Limit your exposure to extreme temperatures, sun, and stress. Some people even claim that alcohol, spicy foods, hot drinks, and caffeine can cause flare-ups. Use only the gentlest cleansers on your face and be sure to slather on sunscreen every day.

Antibiotics can also help in some cases, either in cream or pill form. But be aware that certain antibiotics, such as tetracycline, can make you more sensitive to the sun, so you end up exacerbating the very problem you're trying to solve. If your skin is really marked up, laser therapy works wonders. In one or two treatments, small lines and bumps are zapped to oblivion.

Hair Dye Linked to Rare Form of Cancer

I've started dyeing my hair recently and would like to continue doing so, but I've heard that chemicals in hair dye can cause cancer. Is that true?

This worry has been circulating for years, partly because of research some time ago linking hair dye to lymphoma and leukemia. But that was only one study, and it hasn't been borne out as experts have checked further. Now, however, researchers at the University of Southern California (USC) have discovered a connection with a different cancer.

They compared 897 women who had bladder cancer to an equal number of women who were disease free. After looking at a number of lifestyle factors, they found that women who'd used permanent hair dye once a month for a year or more had twice the risk of bladder cancer of those who'd kept their locks au naturel. Even worse, women who had worked in salons for 10 years or more and handled hair dye on a daily basis had five times the risk. The study wasn't designed to show how hair dye could cause cancer, but we know that a family of chemicals commonly found in dyes, called arylamines, has been found to be carcinogenic in laboratory animals.

But here's where you should stop and take a deep breath. Bladder cancer is quite rare. Each year about 15,000 women are diagnosed with it, compared to 183,000 who developed breast cancer in 2000. And it's very curable when caught early. If you see blood in your urine—a warning sign of bladder cancer—let your doctor know immediately. If you really want to play it safe, switch to a semipermanent or temporary dye, neither of which was linked to cancer in the USC study.

Cracked, Brittle Fingernails Could Warn of Thyroid Woes

I've had nice fingernails all my life, but lately they've been brittle and prone to cracking. What's wrong?

Calcium deficiency and nail fungus are two possible explanations. But it could be a sign that you've developed hypothyroidism, which means your thyroid gland is producing too little thyroid hormone. This is the single most underdiagnosed condition in women, even though it's very common: About 1 in 10 women over 65 has it, and the numbers start climbing after age 40. Luckily, hypothyroidism is easily treated with thyroid hormone supplements; most women get back to normal pretty quickly.

The real question is whether you're experiencing any other symptoms; brittle fingernails alone don't necessarily signal a thyroid problem, even if you've developed them only recently. Are you often tired, or have you put on weight? Some women get constipated or notice that their menstrual flow is heavier than usual. Many also end up depressed.

If you have more than one of these complaints, ask your doctor for two blood tests: The T4 test measures the thyroid hormone thyroxine, and a TSH test checks levels of thyroid-stimulating hormone, which controls activity of the thyroid gland.

The Best Treatments for Eczema

I've had eczema for years, and I hear there's a new steroid-free cream. Should I switch?

It's always good to go with the mildest drug possible, but depending on the nature of your eczema, you may be better off with your regular treatment.

Steroid creams can thin the skin and cause pigment changes and acne; when they're absorbed, they can also harm the adrenal glands. But they work wonders on the red, scaly rashes that plague eczema sufferers.

Protopic, the drug you're referring to, provides the same symptom relief without the side effects of steroids. However, it does have a downside of its own; long-term use can make you more sensitive to the adverse effects of the sun. Plus, its safety has been studied for only one year, and there are lingering,

though mild, concerns about its effect on the immune system. Right now the Food and Drug Administration (FDA) has approved Protopic only for people for whom steroids don't work or who shouldn't take the drugs because of the potential risks.

If your eczema follows the typical pattern, meaning it occurs sporadically, your steroid cream is probably just fine. My feeling is it's only a problem if you use it daily for long periods of time, which most people don't need to do. Many sufferers get relief from moisturizers before even resorting to prescription creams.

You may want to discuss Protopic with your doctor if you get eczema on your face, where cosmetic changes from steroids are particularly troubling. Steroids near the eyes can even lead to cataracts or glaucoma.

How to Spot Melanoma

As I've gotten older, my skin has developed all sorts of spots and blemishes. Which ones should I be worried about?

First, the ones you don't have to worry about: liver spots, which are brown blotches caused by UV damage to the skin's pigment-making cells; small, red bumps known as cherry angiomas; and wartlike or waxy growths called seborrheic keratoses.

The shorthand for telling if something is cancerous is if it exhibits any one of the ABCDs: Asymmetry, Border irregularity, Color variation, or a Diameter greater than 6 millimeters. Another sign is if a mole, blotch, or mark bleeds or grows rapidly. And don't just wait for something new to appear; often skin cancer shows up as a change in a skin feature you already have.

See your doctor if you're the least bit unsure of what you've got. When diagnosed early, basal- and squamous-cell skin cancers are nearly always curable. And it's vital to catch melanoma early. It spreads quickly and is often fatal, accounting for 80 percent of skin cancer deaths. If you're over 50, have a skin exam every other year, preferably by a dermatologist.

Nancy Snyderman, M.D., is a medical correspondent for ABC News and author of *Guide to Good Health for Women Over Forty* (Harvest Book, 1996).

VITAL STATS

43 million
People who regularly lifted free weights for exercise in 1999

38 million
People who walked or ran on a treadmill

2 : 1
Ratio of women to men who work out with personal trainers

3 of 4
U.S. adults who do not get enough exercise

70
Percentage of Americans who purchased fitness clothing in the last year for casual wear, not exercise

50
Percentage of people who don't clean their cuts

I
Ranking of "because it hurts or stings" as the reason they don't

49
Percentage of adults who take vitamin or mineral supplements daily

12
Percentage who use herbal supplements daily

18
Percentage who never take supplements

Unless otherwise noted, statistics apply to the United States.

TEST YOURSELF
How much do you know about osteoporosis?

IF YOU THINK that osteoporosis is just about bad posture and weak bones, think again. Time to see what you know—and don't know—about this disease that affects 8 million women nationwide.

1. Hip fractures are the most common injuries for women with osteoporosis.
   True or False?

2. Tallness is a risk factor for osteoporosis-related fractures.
   True or False?

3. A person with osteoporosis can fracture a bone even by sneezing.
   True or False?

4. Hip fractures are serious, but not deadly.
   True or False?

ANSWERS
1. False. Vertebral compression fractures, which happen when the weakened bones of the spine collapse, are more than twice as common as hip fractures. One in three women over the age of 50 will suffer a vertebral fracture that can cause acute or chronic pain, height loss, and stooped shoulders.

2. True. According to the American Association of Clinical Endocrinologists, the most significant risk factor for fracture is low bone-mineral density (if you've never broken anything) and prior fractures from everyday activities. Other factors include family history of osteoporosis, older age, weight loss or low body weight, cigarette smoking, working in situations with a high risk of falls, and yes, tallness.

3. True. When bones become thin and weak because of osteoporosis, everyday activities such as walking—even sneezing—can cause them to fracture.

4. False. Each year, 65,000 women die from complications from hip fractures.

chapter 5

wellness

self-help and medical care for common conditions

finding peace amidst tragedy

Meet four women who have held on to hope, humor, and gratitude in the face of personal tragedy.

BY JANE MEREDITH ADAMS

PHOTOGRAPHY BY MELISSA SPRINGER

Pregnant with twins and wretchedly nauseated, I sat on the crinkled white paper of the examining table and described my pitiful state to Dr. Chin, an acupuncturist who I desperately hoped would poke me into digestive well-being. I was getting to the part about how my vomiting was like the launch of the space shuttle when Dr. Chin interrupted. "I see many women for infertility," she said sternly. "You're lucky to be pregnant."

There's nothing like being *told* to be grateful to put me in a vile mood. It's like telling someone that she ought to be happy—you can suggest the reasons why someone might consider happiness as an option, but you can't force it. The same thing is true with gratitude: The individual who's bald from doses of chemotherapy gets to decide when and whether she feels grateful.

Which is why it is all the more remarkable that women faced with genuine challenges can find their way to gratitude. We talked to four women who have dealt with deep adversity—the death of a spouse, a debilitating brain injury, breast cancer, and a brother's suicide—and come through transformed, with a renewed sense of thankfulness.

For each of these women, it's taken time and the development of certain skills: the willingness to express a range of feelings about their losses, an ability to connect with people, some type of creative expression, and a spiritual understanding. Using these tools, they've found their way. They're strong women whose gratitude is hard-earned.

In fact, the hardships they faced may have nurtured their joy of life. People who have endured life's harshest experiences seem to express the most appreciation of simple pleasures, according to Robert A. Emmons, Ph.D., professor of psychology at the University of California at Davis.

"You'd think that people with pain and disability would be the least grateful, but it's just the opposite," Emmons says. In his research, those who were ill expressed higher levels of appreciation for the good things in their lives, while the healthy more often expressed discontent. "There's no shortcut to gratitude," he says. "You have to work through the adversity first."

As for me, even when I was feeling my worst, I was grateful to share the details with my college roommate, who was pregnant and woefully queasy herself. We'd even laugh sometimes. I was thankful for that. And then, at long last, I held two babies in my arms and knew I was lucky indeed.

turning grief into song

A year after her husband, Ernest, died of lymphoma in 1994, singer-songwriter Beth Nielsen Chapman began recording her CD *Sand and Water*. During the first song, she started crying uncontrollably. "I had hardly cried at all since his death," she recalls.

For 45-year-old Chapman, whose songs have been recorded by Faith Hill, Bonnie Raitt, and Bette Midler, among others, the tears were an important part of letting go. "I had to keep it together—or so I thought—for my son, who was just 13," she says. "The only time I could connect to my grief was when I was writing songs."

In the studio, she was able to finally express her feelings through music. The songs on *Sand and Water* may have been born of grief, but they're not depressing. There's a sense of peacefulness about Chapman. Listening to her, it's impossible not to wonder how she transforms suffering into songs that speak of love and connection.

Through her music, Chapman seems to embrace difficult events. "As a culture, we're afraid of death," she says. "But the moment my husband died, I was holding his hand, and this incredible feeling of reassurance came over me. I knew in my heart that everything was going to be OK."

Her songs express an acceptance of how life is transitory; love is what's enduring. In the CD's title track she writes, "I will see you in the light of a thousand suns/ I will hear you in the sound of the waves / I will know you when I come, as we all will come / Through the doors beyond the grave."

Chapman's CD called *Deeper Still* also plays on the themes of loss, grief, and moving forward. "I'm grateful every day," she says. "Even when you're not having a great day, I think you have an underlying gratefulness you acquire after you go through things like this." What saddens her most, she says, are people who have health and material well-being but are spiritually empty. She says, "They don't have the connection to the amazing wonderfulness of what's right here right now."

peace through perspective

Searching for the amazing and wonderful is what 39-year-old Lisa Cunningham tries to do daily, despite a disabling brain injury that makes everyday tasks a struggle. On a summer afternoon in 1977, Cunningham was struck by lightning in her parents' West Virginia home. "There was a bright flash, the brightest light I've ever seen," she says. "I was flying through the air. I thought, 'I'm going to die.'"

Lightning had bolted through an open window.

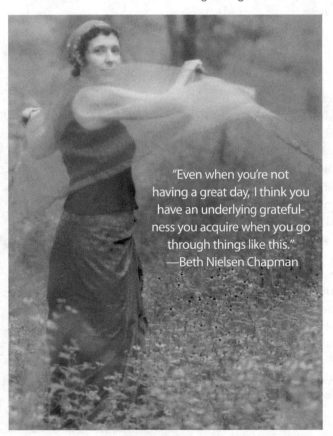

"Even when you're not having a great day, I think you have an underlying gratefulness you acquire when you go through things like this."
—Beth Nielsen Chapman

After about an hour, the tingling in her limbs stopped, and Cunningham thought that, miraculously, she was OK. And she was, for about 18 years. But then, in 1995, she began to have such severe dizzy spells that she couldn't walk across a room. A hissing sound filled her ears, and she found it impossible to drive or to even leave the house. Stationary objects seemed to move. Noise overwhelmed and confused her.

A neuropsychiatrist found that Cunningham had permanent brain damage probably

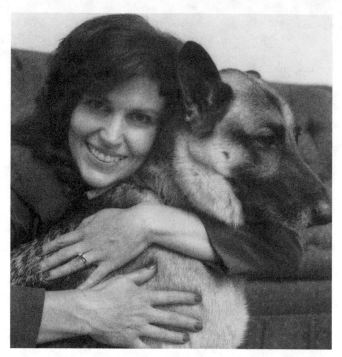

"I was able to say goodbye to the old life and look
for ways to make the new life as positive as possible."
—Lisa Cunningham

caused by the lightning and exacerbated by two con-
cussions and severe fevers she experienced in later
years. As depressing as the news was, it marked a turning point. "I was able to say goodbye to the old life and
look for ways to make the new life as positive as possible," she says.

Cunningham focused on another doctor's advice:
to find happiness wherever she could. One source of
strength has been her growing relationship with God,
she says. At first, she prayed for a complete recovery.
When that didn't happen, she thought of her mother's
adage: "God helps those who help themselves." She
began praying for direction to help herself.

Cunningham decided to start practicing yoga to
develop her balance, and slowly she began to improve.
After seven months, she says, "I could walk two miles
with a walking stick and go into small restaurants and
grocery stores." Some days, she is able to cook dinner
for her husband, Tim. Other days, she can't do more
than sit in the sun on the porch of her northern
Alabama home, babying her two German shepherds.
But she remains focused on the future. She's even
thinking about starting her own business. "A lot of
people don't realize how much inner strength we all
have," she says, "until we have to put it to use."

from hurt to healing

Feeling a little stronger, a little more alive, is what
San Francisco landscape architect Topher Delaney
hopes cancer patients experience in the healing gardens she designs for hospitals. "I'm trying to create
spaces where there is some joy, a little bit of energy,"
says the 53-year-old. "Hospitals can be scary, overwhelming places."

She should know. In 1989, after being told the
lump in her right breast was malignant, Delaney
wandered through the hospital looking for a place to
absorb the news. The small, dimly lit chapel reminded
her of a tomb. "I decided that if I got through this,
I would make gardens and places for people to go to
contemplate," she says.

While she's had a mastectomy and is now cancer-
free, her work has taken her into hospitals where others are not doing as well. Particularly saddening were
the children with cancer at the Norris Cancer Center
at San Diego Children's Hospital. Delaney rejected
the hospital's preference for an austere garden with
birch trees and granite. "I said, 'I want something that

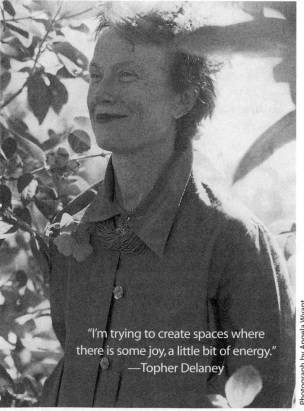

"I'm trying to create spaces where
there is some joy, a little bit of energy."
—Topher Delaney

Photograph by Angela Wyant

tells me I'm going to live.'" Her design is dynamic, its high stucco walls a brilliant orange and yellow. Kids run through a maze decorated with sea creatures, while a windmill sets mechanical birds in motion. In other settings, Delaney is more serious. For a leafy garden at Marin General Hospital in northern California, for instance, she chose medicinal plants that are the basis for cancer medications.

For now, Delaney is focusing on making residential gardens that function as sanctuaries. The work helps her live with her breast-cancer experience. "I make peace with my life through making gardens," she says.

the sacrament of suffering

Hospice counselor Kathleen Dowling Singh had spent decades developing inner peace by practicing meditation. But in 1998, a phone call put her inner calm to the test: Her brother Bobby, 43, had killed himself.

"There's always a certain measure of guilt in every experience of grief," says 54-year-old Singh, author of *The Grace in Dying* (Harper San Francisco, 2000). Still, Singh worked hard not to focus on "what if." Bobby had been unable to accept help, she says, and she thinks of his life as a testament to the importance of expressing grief. Their father died when Bobby was 9 years old, and instead of mourning, the boy shut down in his pain. After his death, she says, "I ended up feeling enormously grateful to be a woman. We give ourselves so much more permission to feel the range of all the things that are real in life."

Singh continues to draw strength from meditation. With practice, meditation peels off the false self, she says, just as a dying person stops worrying about appearance and security. Ultimately, death and illness can offer what she calls "the sacrament of defeat."

"In our slick lives that appear so safe," Singh says, "something of defeat, something of tragedy, can be a sacrament because it stops us and causes us to look deeper." ✻

Jane Meredith Adams is the author of a forthcoming book on faith called Beauty Tips: A Year in the Life of Junior Nun.

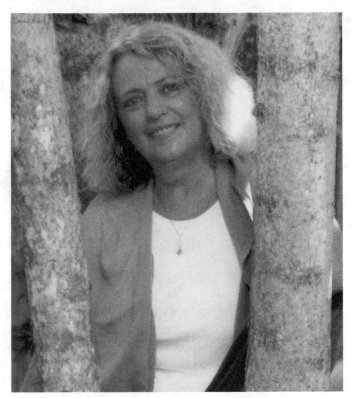

"In our lives that appear so safe and secure, something of defeat, something of tragedy, can be a sacrament because it stops us and causes us to look deeper."
—Kathleen Dowling Singh

amp up **your gratitude**

You can rewrite the story of your bad times, says Laura A. King, Ph.D., of the University of Missouri at Columbia.

In her studies, students were asked to write about the strengths they gained from the most traumatic event of their lives. "The students wrote about having a sibling who was raped, a son who was killed—horrible things," King says. Yet they were able to find a sense of meaning in their suffering. Some had become more compassionate, while others discovered the importance of forgiveness. Months later, the students who had rewritten their stories in a positive light had fewer doctor visits and reported greater life satisfaction.

To get on the road to gratitude, King suggests these steps. First, step back from your disappointment—rent a funny movie or chat with a dear friend. For three days in a row, write for 10 minutes about what you've learned from the negative experience. Finally, decide you want a happy ending and try to make the dream a reality. "We are our life stories," King says. "The way that story ends is really important."

10 STEPS TO BETTER
sleep

Most women over age 30 have some trouble sleeping.
If you're counting sheep in the wee hours, remember this:
The most powerful sleep aid is your own mind.
Here's how to make it work for you.

BY DOROTHY FOLTZ-GRAY

Before I switch off the light each evening, I turn to my husband to say not "good night" but "wish me luck." Until my early 40s, I fell asleep easily—and stayed asleep. I woke rested and eager to start my day. No more. Now, on most nights, I rouse between 2 and 3 a.m., wide awake, often for the next two hours. Sleep has turned from a comfort into a challenge.

Each night, I ask myself, "What will I report tomorrow morning?" Will it be an eight-hour knockout or interludes of slumber broken by the dog, the cat, my husband's snores, or my hot flashes and insistent bladder? I never know, and the uncertainty, the tease of possible sleep is sometimes more maddening than the resulting fatigue.

For at times, I do feel it's a tease I'm dealing with, a provocative bedmate who each night wins me completely, only to abandon

me in the wee hours. I lie there and try to remember the good times: Saturday naps, for instance, when all I have to do is curl on my side and I am fast asleep. But I am fooling myself. Whatever wooed me to sleep is long gone. Our relationship—at least the good part of it—is over. Soon, I'm feeling prickly, discarded, fretful.

If you're a woman in midlife, this scenario may sound familiar. According to the National Sleep Foundation, more than half of women ages 30 to 60 have trouble sleeping. Twice as many women as men suffer daytime sleepiness, and a quarter more have trouble snoozing at least several nights a week.

Lack of sleep can do more than make you irritable. It's long been known that chronic sleep loss can hobble memory, dull concentration, make it harder to learn new things, and perhaps even weaken the immune system. Driving while drowsy can be just as dangerous as driving drunk.

The latest research is even more alarming. Insufficient sleep, it seems, wreaks havoc on hormones and metabolic processes. A

Soaking in a hot bath does more than just relax you—it allows you to get more deep sleep. For extra indulgence, add some lavender aromatherapy oil.

study by Eve Van Cauter, a sleep specialist at the University of Chicago, found that for young, healthy adults, just a week of sleeping four hours a night gave rise to hormone profiles that looked like those of much older people. That doesn't mean the subjects were on the road to premature wrinkles. But they could be more vulnerable to age-related illnesses. For instance, the study found that the sleep-deprived volunteers' bodies used insulin in much the way they would if they were on the verge of diabetes. Other research has shown that sleeping less jacks up stress hormones and reduces the production of human growth hormone, a decline associated with muscle loss, weakened immunity, and increased fat.

Worrisome findings, to be sure. But there's good news too. In the past few years, sleep researchers have increasingly come to realize that people's sleep problems have a lot to do with their attitudes and beliefs about sleep. If you can change your expectations—and your coping strategies when reality falls short—better sleep will follow. True, your slumber may never again be the wonderful, uncomplicated affair it was in your 20s, but you can vastly improve the relationship with sleep that you've got now.

Sound Pollyannaish? Just think how stewing about sleep can become a self-fulfilling prophecy. We fret about whether we'll be able to get to sleep, which, in turn, just makes it harder to fall asleep. Lying awake, we agonize about being unable to function the next day, which keeps us awake longer. We start the next day grumpy because we figure we'll be foggy-brained all day.

As one of my friends puts it, "I wake up and I'm doomed. It's all so familiar to me now: the worry, the

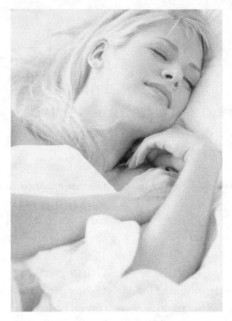

Can you sleep *too* much?

Sleepyheads beware: Researchers recently found that among a group of 1,400 people, those who got more than eight hours of nightly shut-eye had 9 percent more strokes than those who slept less. The scientists say that long, fitful slumber could be a sign of sleep apnea, a disorder linked to stroke.

stupid whirling of the brain that does no good except to keep you awake."

But researchers now have solid evidence that it's possible to break this vicious cycle. In spring 2001, Duke University scientists reported that teaching insomniacs to change their attitudes about sleep resulted in longer and better slumber. And in a 1999 study, Laval University researchers gave 78 poor sleepers either attitude-changing therapy, drugs, or a mix of both. After two years, only the people who'd learned to change their thinking about sleep consistently slept better.

It's a lot like managing a relationship with a difficult person. First, you need to understand your partner (your sleep habits) better. That means figuring out what makes him tick and how he may have changed since you first met. Then you can work on accepting the things about him that aren't likely to change—and tweaking those that are. Follow this path and you really can spend more time in dreamland. Here's how to get there.

Accept that some sleep changes are unavoidable.

In our 40s and 50s, as we pass through the hormonal storms of menopause, we sleep approximately 10 minutes less each night—and 30 minutes less on the weekends—than we did before menopause. We also wake more often during the night. By the time we reach our 70s, we sleep a half hour to an hour less than we did in our 20s, and the sleep is much more fragmented. Our body clocks also shift over the years, making us drowsy earlier in the evening and waking us sooner in the morning.

"It's like hair going gray," says Van Cauter. "Sleep

To smooth your path to slumber, **try a cup of valerian tea.**
This herb is widely used in Europe, and many studies have shown it works.
To tame its pungent odor, add some lemon juice or orange peel.
Drink it 45 minutes before bed.

quality deteriorates. But it's not a disease; it's a normal part of aging."

Realize you sleep more than you think you do.

According to Van Cauter, a person's appraisal of how much she's slept is dependent on how fragmented the sleep was, especially in the second half of the night. "A woman may get lots of sleep early in the night but have interruptions later," she says. So on mornings when you're sure you've done nothing but toss and turn, you may well have slept half the night—but only remember the later, more turbulent hours.

Don't panic if you're a midnight riser.

If your pattern is to fall asleep easily, then wake for several hours, it may help to know that during that first portion of the night, you're getting mostly deep sleep. That's the dreamless phase of slumber during which your body restores and repairs itself. While you lie motionless, your pituitary gland is churning out growth hormone, which is crucial for counteracting the toll that time takes on aging bodies. Your body is also synthesizing proteins that repair cellular damage, strengthen bones, and replenish immune cells. And if you're able to get back to sleep in a few hours, that second stage of slumber gives you several cycles of REM sleep, which is thought to bolster memory, learning, and mood.

Give sleep the attention it deserves.

Keeping track of your sleep habits can show you patterns you had been unaware of and help you make changes that will boost your chances of sleeping better. "Maybe it turns out that when you go to sleep earlier in the evening, your sleep quality is consistently better," says Van Cauter. Keep a notebook by your bed and write down anything you did during the day that might be relevant to your sleep, such as exercising or drinking coffee or wine. Also, note the time you turned off your light. In the morning, jot down when you woke up and how well you slept.

Put sleep first and others' needs second.

If a snoring partner is keeping you awake, you may need to sleep in another room. If you're always the one who tends to restless children or pets, it's time to talk to your partner about making some adjustments.

Need a good night's sleep?
get a new wardrobe

Whether you bed down in boxers and a T-shirt or something more Victoria's Secret is not just a matter of style. What you wear, says Barbara L. Heller, psychotherapist and author of *How to Sleep Soundly Tonight* (Storey Books, 2001), "can affect the quality of your slumber. And how well you sleep affects every aspect of your life, including your health, mood, and productivity."

When choosing what to wear between the sheets, go for comfort and warmth—especially for the feet. "Warm feet are a natural sedative," Heller says. "Slip on warm socks or PJs with feet, or stash a hot water bottle by your toes."

In the rest of your nighttime wardrobe, look for soft fabrics, such as cotton or flannel, which help you settle in cozily. Just avoid hot materials like fleece—especially if you've got a bedmate generating warmth.

Steer clear of embellishments such as buttons, sequins, or fancy appliqués that may poke and wake you during the night; also save form-fitting outfits for romancing rather than sleeping. Experiment with nightgowns of different lengths to find ones that won't tangle around legs. PJ gals should look for loose bottoms with drawstring waists rather than elastic. If you've got lines zigzagging across your body in the morning, it could mean your sleep clothes are constricting.

Shield your sleep from worry.

For too many women, the moment their heads hit their pillows is the first quiet moment of their day—which becomes the time to start fretting. To keep this sleep-robbing anxiety at bay, experts recommend that you schedule 30 minutes of worry time during the day, well before bedtime. Make a list of the things you're troubled about—big and small—and how you might cope with them.

Soothe yourself to sleep with comforting rituals.

If you pay bills just before going to bed, it's unlikely that you'll nod off easily. Instead, spend a little time each evening pampering yourself. Taking a few minutes to stretch or meditate before you turn in will help you wind down.

Don't reward yourself for not sleeping.

"Even when they complain about being unable to sleep, some women really like those hours of the night when they're awake," says Joyce Walsleben, director of the New York University Sleep Disorders Center. "That's when they have time to themselves." If you've inadvertently trained yourself to wake at night because you treasure the solitude, schedule some private moments during the day instead.

Learn to function on less sleep when you need to.

Use what energy you have to reset both your mood and your schedule. "Give yourself permission to rearrange your day," says Kathryn Lee, a sleep researcher and professor of nursing at the University of California at San Francisco. "Tell yourself, 'I just won't do what I planned.'" If you can, postpone difficult brain work for days when you're most rested.

Don't give up.

The alliance that you build with sleep requires understanding, acceptance, flexibility, and commitment. Sleep perhaps may demand more of you than you like sometimes—but, after all, what worthwhile relationship doesn't? ✳

Dorothy Foltz-Gray is a Health *contributing editor.*

kinder, gentler sleeping pills

Sleeping pills have long suffered a bad reputation: They can be habit-forming and leave you dopey. But the newest pills, Ambien and Sonata, claim to sidestep some of these problems. If sleep is a struggle, should you try one of them?

Perhaps, says Joyce Walsleben, director of the New York University Sleep Disorders Center. "In the right situation and for the right person, they're very helpful."

Chronic insomniacs should probably steer clear. They need to address their sleep problems on a more global level, says Walsleben. For people who may need to be alert during the night—single parents, for example—the new pills are an improvement over the old, but still aren't recommended. They're worth a try as a short-term fix—if you've been losing sleep during a crisis or you need to conquer the effects of jet lag or a new work shift.

Sonata and Ambien both target the same receptors in the brain as older drugs, such as Halcion, but with greater precision. Because they slip in and out of your system faster than the older meds, they're less likely to leave you feeling hungover. Ambien is metabolized in six to eight hours, making it an effective pill to see you through the night. Sonata lasts just four hours, so while it may usher you to dreamland, you may not stay there as long as you would with Ambien. Sonata, however, may be the drug to turn to if you find yourself wide awake at 2 a.m.

If you're inclined to try pills, consult a sleep expert first. If you do take them, here are a few rules to bear in mind:

• SCHEDULE your trial run for a weekend night. If the medication leaves you groggy, you can take it easy the next day.

• GO STRAIGHT TO BED as soon as you've taken your pill; the new drugs take effect very quickly.

• DON'T RAISE THE DOSAGE if a pill doesn't seem to be working. Instead, ask your doctor to suggest a different medication.

• AVOID TAKING THESE MEDICATIONS for any longer than four weeks at a stretch. While the new pills are less habit-forming than the older ones, experts caution that there is still some risk of psychological dependence.

SHORT-CIRCUIT A COLD SORE

Why is it that cold sores crop up the night before your 20th high school reunion or that trip to Paris? Fortunately, with a little know-how and the right medication, unsightly sores no longer need to cause a social crisis.

Afflicting an estimated 40 million Americans, cold sores result from a herpes simplex virus that lies dormant inside a nerve in the upper jaw. Stress, sunlight, extreme temperatures, and other infections (including colds) can kick the virus into action.

The key to stopping the sore is to inhibit the reproduction of the virus. Oral prescription medicines, such as Zovirax and Valtrex, work the fastest to accomplish this goal, says Roy S. Rogers III, professor of dermatology at the Mayo Medical Center. A topical solution, Denavir, works the same way and is an option for those who can't take an oral antibiotic or want to improve the sore's appearance immediately.

Chronic sufferers should invest in a prescription, but if your flare-ups are rare, try a less potent over-the-counter fix. Pure Lip Remedy uses zinc to slow down viral reproduction and ease the pain. The remedy comes in a daily maintenance formula to ward off outbreaks and a healing version for flare-ups.

A little prevention—wearing an SPF lip balm when you're outside, treating other infections immediately, and lowering your stress level—goes a long way.

A simple injection can stop your husband's snoring

The number of solutions speaks volumes about the problem. If you're trying to quiet a snorer, you have 300 patented devices—mouthpieces, neck collars, straps, and pillows—to choose from. A new injection may put them all to rest.

Snoring's distinctive nocturnal rumble is the fluttering of soft tissues at the back of the mouth—the palate and uvula. Effective current treatments employ electric needles or lasers to stiffen the area, but these methods tend to be painful and costly. None met the needs of U.S. Army Captain Scott Brietzke, an otolaryngologist at the Walter Reed Army Medical Center, who wanted an inexpensive remedy to keep recruits quiet in their bunks after taps. Brietzke tried injecting a substance called sodium tetradecyl sulfate into the palate. The chemical, already approved for the treatment of varicose veins, hardened the floppy tissue and muffled the snoring. The procedure retains its effectiveness for at least a year, says Brietzke, at which time it can be redone. Patients' only complaint was a mild sore throat for two to three days following the injection. "It's safe and costs about a hundredth as much as laser treatment," says Brietzke. "And I can get you out of there in 15 minutes."

Dubbed injection snoreplasty, the treatment may not be available at your local ear, nose, and throat specialist's office for a year or two. By the way, it can't solve more serious snoring disorders like sleep apnea. But if you or your spouse suffers from the maddening sound of sawing logs, this injection might just bring sweet dreams.

Headaches in the bedroom

If your bedroom techniques make your partner scream, it could be more than just an indicator of your sexual prowess. For a half-million Americans (more men than women), sex-related headaches can turn nighttime pleasure into bedtime agony. The cause of these headaches, which usually strike at the moment of orgasm, is still unknown.

Taking over-the-counter remedies or anti-inflammatory drugs before sex may help prevent the pain. "But some people become afraid to have sex," says Seymour Diamond, M.D., of the Diamond Headache Clinic. "These headaches can impact a marriage."

While most sex-related headaches are not cause for alarm, if the I've-got-a-headache excuse comes up often, seek medical care to rule out the possibility of a more serious illness.

TEST YOURSELF
How to avoid a cold

THE POLITICIANS SAY the Cold War is long over, so why does it start again every winter? Take this test to find out if you know how to win the battle of the sneezes this flu season.

1. Bundle up: Cold conditions bring on the sniffles.
   True or False?

2. If you're stressed out, you're more likely to get a cold.
   True or False?

3. Which of the following has been proven to prevent a cold?
   - a) Antibiotics
   - b) Vitamin C
   - c) Echinacea
   - d) None of the above

4. Washing your hands is the best way to avoid a cold.
   True or False?

ANSWERS

1. False. Colds are caused by viruses, not weather.

2. True. Relax. If you don't take a deep breath now, you may not be able to breathe later. Running ragged and losing sleep weaken the immune system.

3. D. None of the above. Antibiotics will treat a bacterial infection, not a virus. Although many people swear by popping vitamin C and taking echinacea to ward off a cold, the evidence that these remedies work is spotty.

4. True. Cold bugs can live for up to three hours—we're talking dirty doorknobs and filthy phones. After you touch something—or someone—take time to disinfect your hands.

Snooze—or You'll Lose

Lack of sleep may mean more than a rough morning.
A study presented at the American Diabetes Association's annual meeting showed that people who regularly sleep less than six and a half hours a night may become less sensitive to insulin, the hormone that regulates blood sugar. Insulin resistance can lead to obesity, high blood pressure, and diabetes.

don't let cold air spark an asthma attack

Cold air can worsen asthma. When you step out for a jog, wrap a scarf around your neck so that it also covers your mouth and nose. This warms the air you breathe in, lessening the chance of an attack. If it's just too chilly to hit the streets, take your workout indoors. Shopping malls are an ideal place for a power walk and are easy on an asthmatic's lungs.

got a sore throat?

If your tonsils start giving you trouble, just nuke 'em. Mansoor Mandani, M.D., director of Pennsylvania's Center for Corrective Surgery, has developed tonsillar coblation, a procedure that uses microwave-like radio frequency probes to reduce the size of the tonsils. The upside? Unlike a traditional tonsillectomy, which usually involves general anesthesia and some post-surgery bleeding, patients getting a "microwave tonsillectomy" need only a local anesthetic and experience little to no bleeding. The downside? The $2,100 procedure isn't covered by most insurance companies yet. Call 800-206-2000 or visit www.snorenet.com for more info.

Integrative
Medicine
blending the best of traditional therapies and alternative cures

Take cutting-edge medicine and fill in the gaps
with age-old alternative therapies. The result may just
be the future of American health care.

BY PETER JARET

Plagued by symptoms for much of her life, Carrie Carlson-Scoglio was diagnosed 12 years ago with fibromyalgia, a condition that causes joints and tendons to ache almost constantly—and for which there is no quick cure. She's willing to try almost anything for relief. "Frankly, I don't care if it's conventional, alternative, or something in between, as long as it works," she says.

But many of the people she has turned to for help do seem to care. After trying alternative treatments, such as herbal remedies and homeopathy, and such traditional prescription drugs as anti-inflammatories and steroids, the 37-year-old registrar at the Corcoran College of Art and Design in Washington, D.C., found an array of conflicting advice. "You get doctors who say that alternative approaches are nonsense and alternative practitioners who tell you that you're being poisoned by the drugs doctors prescribe. After a while, you wonder if any of them really know what they're talking about," she says.

Steven Rosenzweig, M.D., understands Carlson-Scoglio's frustration. "There are still plenty of physicians out there who are uninformed, uninterested, or even hostile when it comes to alternative and complementary approaches," says Rosenzweig, director of the Center for Integrative Medicine at Thomas Jefferson University Hospital in Philadelphia. "At the same time, alternative practitioners are often overly suspicious and uninformed about conventional medicine. Patients are the ones who get caught in the cross fire."

Fortunately, that seems to be changing. Rosenzweig is part of a growing band of maverick health-care providers trying to draw the two sides together and fashion a lasting peace. The new approach, called integrative medicine, seeks to combine the best of what medicine has to offer—conventional, alternative, and in between. Over the past three years, it has gained

If you have a health problem that seems to defy a speedy and simple solution—arthritis, fibromyalgic tendinitis, back pain, or chronic fatigue syndrome, for instance—the integrative approach may offer real benefits.

A 1998 study found that only one-third of patients who use alternative therapies talk to their doctors about them, which can spell trouble when alternative remedies interact with conventional treatments.

widespread acceptance, even in the bastions of mainstream medical care. Integrative medicine centers now exist at more than a dozen of the country's leading medical institutions, including George Washington University in Washington, D.C.; the University of Arizona in Tucson; and the Memorial Sloan-Kettering Cancer Center in New York City. Many more are being planned around the country. Supporters of integrative medicine think it will fundamentally change the way patients are treated.

"What we're doing is part of a grand experiment—combining scientifically based Western medicine with the more holistic approach represented by Eastern and alternative medicine," says Martin Sullivan, M.D., director of the Duke University Center for Integrative Medicine in Durham, North Carolina. "The idea may seem simple. But if we can manage to combine the best of what these two systems have to offer, we'll be creating a radically new kind of health care. Many of us, in fact, think that this is what the medicine of the future will look like."

Jennifer Wilson has glimpsed that future, and she likes what she sees. A year ago, the 27-year-old pianist-in-training was diagnosed with Graves' disease, a serious condition that shifts the thyroid gland into overdrive. An endocrinologist at George Washington University treated the illness, but Wilson was still plagued by pain, hand weakness, and other symptoms, which no one seemed able to cure. Then she heard about George Washington University's Center for Integrative Medicine.

"During my first appointment, I sat down with a physician who asked me about everything that was going on, my health, and other things in my life: work, the fact that I was getting married, the stress of being diagnosed with Graves' disease," Wilson says. "For the first time, I really felt as if they were interested in treating me, rather than just the disease I happen to have."

After Wilson's initial interview, a team (that included a medical doctor and experts in a range of alternative therapies) met to decide exactly what blend of treatments—conventional and alternative—might work best for Wilson. In addition to the drugs her endocrinologist had prescribed, the team recommended acupuncture to help relieve the pain in her hands and arms. Within six weeks, she was able to play the piano again. This spring, Wilson was feeling well enough to resume her intensive music studies.

The most obvious benefit of integrative medicine, of course, is that patients can take advantage of both conventional and alternative options, supervised by a single group of medical experts. That means greater access to a wider array of therapies—and less risk. A team that includes both physicians and alternative practitioners is more likely to be alert to potentially dangerous interactions among treatments—a growing problem, experts say, as patients seek out alternative approaches on their own.

Just as important, integrative medicine centers promise to shed light on what works and what doesn't.

Many experts are convinced that the blended approach offers hope to many patients who haven't been helped by either conventional or alternative medicine alone.

"We know that some alternative therapies help patients and some don't. We also know that some are downright dangerous," Rosenzweig says. "We have to be open-minded. But we also have to demand real evidence that a treatment is safe and effective. That's why it's so important that many of these centers are being created at academic medical centers and teaching hospitals, which have a commitment to research."

Even integrative medicine has its limits, though. Carrie Carlson-Scoglio says that after a few months of success with an integrative approach, the pain from her fibromyalgia is back. "When you've got a condition like mine, which is pretty much a mystery anyway, it's always a crapshoot," she says.

So integrative medicine is no magic bullet. But many experts are convinced that the blended approach will offer hope to many patients who haven't been helped by either conventional or alternative medicine alone.

If that sounds like you, here's what to consider.

Chinese herbs:
taking their measure

Chinese herbal remedies are tailored to fit a particular person's needs at a single point in time, so they're difficult to evaluate by Western standards. Still, some intriguing studies suggest that they offer real benefits. It's also clear that some of them carry real risks, so if you're turning to Chinese herbs for more than an occasional upset stomach, it's best to see a trained herbalist or a licensed Chinese medicine practitioner, who can guide you to the proper dose of a safe preparation. Here's what Chinese medicine practitioners and Western scientists say about some of the tradition's most widely prescribed herbs.

GINSENG is given to help the body cope with stress and achieve balance and strength. It's often prescribed to older people suffering from fatigue after a serious illness. Controlled studies have been equivocal: In Mexican research, older adults who took ginseng with a multivitamin reported an improvement in the quality of their lives not seen by those on the multivitamin alone. But other studies have shown no greater physical stamina in healthy people on ginseng.

GINGER is thought to liven up sluggish parts of the body. Known for its warming powers, it is used to soothe an upset stomach and to improve circulation. It's also given to women to regulate the menstrual cycle. Most well-designed studies have looked at its effect on nausea, and it does indeed work: A Swiss study found it prevented motion sickness better than an antinausea drug.

LICORICE is used to mask the taste of bitter herbs and to "harmonize" the effects of other herbs. It's believed to strengthen the endocrine, immune, and nervous systems and is often recommended for ulcers. Practitioners are onto something here: In one double-blind study, licorice extract greatly reduced ulcer size in 16 patients.

DONG QUAI is often called a woman's tonic. It's believed to increase circulation to the uterus and is blended with other herbs to combat painful or irregular menstruation, hot flashes, and night sweats. Analysis has shown dong quai is rich in vitamin E, so it's likely to be a mild blood thinner. It also contains compounds known as coumarins that ease cramping and regulate blood flow. However, no Western studies show the herb works.

ASTRAGALUS ROOT is said to strengthen qi, the body's vital energy; it is given to boost the immune system and fortify lung qi in people with frequent colds or bronchitis. Practitioners believe that it increases blood flow to the heart and can help control sweating. Test-tube research shows that compounds in it may have antiviral properties, but there have been no trustworthy studies on people.

SCHISANDRA, known as the five-flavor berry, tastes like turpentine laced with lemon. Its main use is to strengthen the endocrine system. It is also called on to reverse liver damage caused by pollutants, viruses, or alcohol and to relieve allergy symptoms. As with astragalus, no reliable studies have been done using people.

For reliable info about integrative care, see www.nci.nih.gov or www.nih.gov.

Who can benefit: If you have a medical problem that a quick course of antibiotics or another prescription drug will solve, you don't need integrative medicine. But if you have a health problem that defies a speedy and simple solution—arthritis, fibromyalgia, tendinitis, back pain, or chronic fatigue syndrome, for instance—the integrative approach may offer real benefits. Integrative medicine can also ease some of the side effects associated with conventional treatments. (Acupuncture, for example, has been shown to help cancer patients deal with some of the effects of chemotherapy.) If you're already combining conventional and alternative therapies on your own, it's worth seeking out a center that offers integrative medicine—especially if you have a chronic medical condition. That way, you'll have a team of experts supervising the treatments you take, so you'll run less risk of adverse reactions.

What to look out for:
Unfortunately, as "integrative" becomes the latest buzzword in medicine, many clinics are adopting the name. Don't be fooled: Make sure you find a center that offers actual integrated care, incorporating both conventional and alternative approaches. A genuine integrative medicine center should employ trained medical doctors as well as experts in a variety of alternative disciplines.

At the best centers—such as those associated with teaching hospitals and academic medical centers—physicians oversee all patient care. That's important. Alternatives used to be touted as perfectly safe because they're "natural," but it's now clear that's not always true. Having a physician monitor your case can reduce the risk of dangerous interactions between conventional and alternative approaches.

Of course, the quality of alternative practitioners is just as important; both training and professional experience can vary widely. If you're considering integrative care, ask how the center screens and evaluates the practitioners it recommends. "At the moment, you've got practitioners who've gone through several years of education and training and others who have taken a mail-order course and nothing else. Unfortunately, it's very difficult for patients to know which is which," says John C. Reed, M.D., medical director of American WholeHealth, a firm that advises insurance companies on alternative approaches.

What you'll find: Every center offers its own selection of alternative therapies. Most include acupuncture, chiropractic, herbal medicine, massage, nutrition counseling, meditation, and other stress-reduction techniques. The doctors on staff tend to be primary-care physicians, although some centers specialize in treating patients with cancer, back pain, or other specific conditions.

Patients are typically asked to fill out a detailed questionnaire about themselves and their medical history. Then they meet with a physician for an initial office

Having a physician monitor your case can reduce the risk of dangerous interactions between conventional and alternative approaches.

visit. Afterward, the center's team of physicians and alternative practitioners discusses the case and recommends treatment. In many of the best integrative centers, the team meets regularly to talk about how patients are doing and to fine-tune their therapy.

What you won't get: Experts in integrative medicine don't have all the answers, especially when it comes to therapies that haven't been tested in clinical studies. "A lot of patients come to us saying, 'What do you think of this? What do you think of that?' Often we have to tell them that we simply don't know because there's insufficient evidence," Rosenzweig says.

Even where there is evidence of real benefits, don't expect miracles. Many complementary and alternative therapies can help ease symptoms. Others may even speed recovery. But none, so far, is a cure-all.

If you can't find an integrative medicine center: A growing number of medical centers around the country offer integrative medicine clinics. But if there

how to get started

Interested in the integrative approach? We've rounded up some of the best books, Web sites, and contact numbers to help you learn more.

On the Web

• **www.wholehealthmd.com**

This comprehensive site, operated by American WholeHealth, has a useful list of alternative approaches organized by condition. It also has an A-to-Z reference library on alternative medicine, including potentially dangerous interactions.

• **www.nccam.nih.gov/nccam**

The National Center for Complementary and Alternative Medicine offers helpful tips on how to evaluate alternative therapies and therapists, as well as information about clinical trials of leading alternative approaches.

• **www.cancer.org**

The American Cancer Society provides critical evaluations of dozens of alternative therapies for cancer patients, including mind/body approaches.

Off the Shelf

• *Integrative Medicine: The Patient's Essential Guide to Conventional and Complementary Treatments for More Than 300 Common Disorders,* by Alan H. Pressman, Ph.D., and Donna Shelly, M.D. (St. Martin's Press, 2000).

• *Comprehensive Cancer Care: Integrating Alternative, Complementary, and Conventional Therapies,* by James S. Gordon, M.D. (Perseus Publishing, 2000).

• *The Alternative Medicine Handbook: The Complete Reference Guide to Alternative and Complementary Therapies,* by Barrie R. Cassileth, Ph.D. (W.W. Norton & Co., 1999)

To contact centers in this story

• Thomas Jefferson University Hospital's Center for Integrative Medicine; Philadelphia, PA; 215-879-5121

• George Washington University's Center for Integrative Medicine; Washington, D.C; 202-994-8870

• Duke University Medical Center's Center for Integrative Medicine; Durham, NC; 919-660-6801

• Memorial Sloan-Kettering Integrative Medicine Service; New York, NY; 212-639-8629

isn't one in your area, don't despair. You can still piece together an integrative program of your own, if you're willing to do a little extra work (see "How to Get Started," at left).

First, if you're interested in complementary or alternative approaches, find a primary-care physician or other doctor who shares your interest. Then collect all the information you can. There's plenty on the Internet, of course, though it ranges from scientifically reliable to downright silly. Always check the source; if a Web site that touts alternative therapies also stands to make a profit from them, beware. You can find good, reliable information about many popular alternatives at Web sites run by the National Cancer Institute (www.nci.nih.gov), the National Institutes of Health (www.nih.gov), and by patient advocacy groups like the American Cancer Society (www.cancer.org). A growing number of books offer advice about combining conventional and alternative treatments.

No matter what you choose, talk to your primary-care doctor before you begin an alternative therapy, especially if it involves pills, herbal supplements, or vitamins. A 1998 study found that only one-third of patients who use alternative therapies talk to their doctors about them, which can spell trouble when alternative remedies interact with conventional treatments. Finally, keep your doctor posted on how you're feeling. To assess how well an alternative approach is working, some experts recommend keeping a symptom diary. That way, you and your doctor will know whether acupuncture is really easing your pain or whether those herbs are truly revving your energy. ✳

Ask the Doctor—*Online*

There's a wealth of useful info on alternative treatments for dozens of ailments at www.onebody.com. Staffed by experts from such institutions as the Stanford University School of Medicine, this site has everything from a comprehensive herb guide to a library on various treatments. The section on stress-relieving yoga poses, with easy-to-follow animated instructions, is a *Health* staff favorite.

are you
poisoning
your home?

Most American homes are polluted with toxins and contaminants. But the war against dirt doesn't have to threaten your health. With a few changes, you'll leave those domestic demons in the dust.

BY RICK CHILLOT

Don't be offended, but your body is polluted. And so is your neighbor's, and your rabbi's, and your paperboy's. In fact, everybody is contaminated with such metals as lead and mercury, with chemicals that have tongue-busting names like diethyl phthalate, and with the nasty by-products of pesticides, nicotine, and car exhaust.

How did people become such walking chemistry sets? For many, the answer lies in the way you clean and beautify your home. Ask a toxicologist about the average person's exposure to chemicals, and one category of offenders rises to the top of the list: cleansers and solvents. The products you use to make the toilet sparkle, dissolve hairballs in the drain, and tint the walls a nice robin's-egg blue can, if used carelessly, expose you to toxic substances that would make mutant sewer rats flee in terror.

Yet in all of this, there is good news. Your exposure to household chemicals is within your control. Unlike some other contaminants, such as leaded gasoline, what you put in your drains and on the walls is completely your decision. Good choices about your home can translate into good choices about your health.

What's so bad about cleansers and solvents? Problems range from eye and skin irritation to allergic reactions to long-term health problems, such as liver damage and cancer. In addition to substances known to be hazardous, many of these products also contain phthalates, a ubiquitous class of chemicals also found in some cosmetics and plastics. Studies have detected cancer in animals exposed to high concentrations of phthalates, and some are suspected to affect the sexual development of children.

According to a study released earlier this year, the Centers for Disease Control (CDC) discovered phthalates in thousands of urine samples. The study, which was designed to represent the demographics of the American population, measured the presence of about two dozen environmental chemicals. The samples they studied create a snapshot of some of the

> **There's no need to clean** with something that smells like a chemistry experiment when hot water, soap, and a little elbow grease will work just as well.

Always label homemade formulas and keep them away from children.

chemical schmutz found in the veins and tissues of the average American—including some heavy metals, nicotine, pesticides, and phthalates (see "The Inside Story: A Chemical Report Card" at right for more findings).

As with most of the substances in the CDC's report, "it's the first time phthalates have been measured in a population that's representative of the whole United States," explains Julie Fishman, associate director for policy at the CDC's Environmental Health Lab in Atlanta. The first studies that will measure the effects in humans are just getting started, so it is too soon to know if the levels of phthalates detected in the study are high enough to be a health threat.

But why wait for the results of new studies or for a government-recommended cleanup plan? You can begin limiting your exposure to these chemicals now by doing something most people don't: reading labels and following directions. "See what the health warnings are. If it says to use gloves, use gloves," says Alan Hedge, Ph.D., director of the Human Factors and Ergonomics Laboratory at Cornell University's Department of Design and Environmental Analysis. Same with protective clothing and eyewear. Adequate ventilation is also crucial, since many substances release toxic chemicals slowly over time. Use the recommended ventilation time on the label as a starting point; let the room air out longer if possible, especially during cold weather. "Evaporation is slower when it's cold," Hedge says—a good reason to plan major cleaning projects for the warmer months.

An even wiser solution might be to break off relations with these personal pollutants altogether, and admit they're not as indispensable as you think. Face it: The real reason you stock your closets with chemical weapons is that their hyperpotency allows you to put off cleaning until you're shin-deep in grime. "Very few people dust and vacuum every day," Hedge notes. "Most people don't do anything for weeks. Then they clean like blazes." Give your house the once-over more frequently, and you may eliminate (or at least reduce) your dependency on chemical solvents. Regardless of

the inside story: a chemical report card

Sure, there are some chemicals in your blood that don't belong there, but the news about these contaminants that have become part of your body—or not—isn't all bad. When the Centers for Disease Control (CDC) released its National Report on Human Exposure to Environmental Chemicals in March 2001, it provided information on the U.S. population's exposure to 27 chemicals. The lowdown:

• **Nonsmokers' exposure to tobacco smoke is falling dramatically.** The levels of cotinine, a marker of nicotine exposure, have dropped by 75% since similar measurements were made in the late 1980s.

• **Exposure to lead has been dropping for some time.** "This data confirms the decline is continuing," says Julie Fishman of the CDC's Environmental Health Lab. For information on checking your home for lead, take a look at the CDC's Childhood Lead Poisoning Prevention Program at www.cdc.gov/nceh/lead/lead.htm.

• **Mercury bears watching.** "We looked at children ages 1 to 5 and women ages 16 to 49," Fishman says. "We didn't find any cases where mercury exposure reached dangerous levels, but in a small number of cases exposure did come within a factor of 10 of the dangerous levels. "That suggests a need to keep an eye on mercury exposure to make sure that there's no increase, she says. (See "Which Fish Are Safe—and Which Aren't" on page 245 for how to avoid mercury in your diet.)

• **Pesticides are present.** The CDC measured six pesticide by-products, representing exposure to 28 pesticides. "We know a lot about what these chemicals do to the pests they kill, but not what they do to humans," says Alan Hedge, Ph.D., of Cornell University. However, you may not want to wait for more information to take action. Start with your lawn: The pesticides typically used on lawns often get tracked into the house, where they can persist for much longer than they would outdoors. Choose chemical-free pest control, and you'll lower exposure inside.

how fastidious you are, though, you probably reach for a bottle of something that smells like a chemistry experiment when some hot water, soap, and elbow grease would work just as well. But what if you need more firepower to get rid of a stubborn stain? There are plenty of alternatives to harsh chemical cleansers, says Annie Berthold-Bond, author of *Better Basics for the Home* (Three Rivers Press, 1999) and other books containing her nontoxic formulas for everything from pesticides to wallpaper paste. She developed many of them out of necessity. "In 1980, I was poisoned by a gas leak at a restaurant; it wasn't until I learned to live without chemicals that I got better," she says. Here are some of her key strategies for fighting the nontoxic fight. (Remember to always label homemade formulas and keep them away from children.)

• **Use baking soda** as a nonabrasive cleaner for countertops, sinks, and tubs. Just sprinkle some on a damp sponge or cloth and wipe.

• **Try lemon juice** to dissolve gummed-up gunk, battle tarnish, and remove dirt from wood surfaces.

• **For a home-brewed window cleaner,** fill a squirt bottle with a combination of vinegar and water (2 cups water plus $1/4$ cup white distilled vinegar). Add $1/2$ teaspoon of liquid soap the first time you use it; this removes the fine wax residue left on the glass by commercial window cleaners. Vinegar also makes a good antibiotic to spray on cutting boards, bathroom surfaces, and other germ havens. (The smell will fade in a few hours.)

• **Fight mold and mildew with tea tree oil.** Mix 2 teaspoons oil with 2 cups of water in a spray bottle and spray it on the offending fungus. (Tea tree and other essential oils are available at health-food stores.)

Staying on top of cleaning, dusting, and vacuuming might take time away from really important activities, but these household tasks effectively remove contaminants that can blow into your home from the outside, like lead (left in the soil from the days of leaded gas) and pesticides (used on your lawn or your neighbor's). And if you employ cleaning tactics that are less toxic, it just might save you from becoming a casualty of domestic chemical warfare. ✳

Pennsylvania-based freelance writer Rick Chillot writes regularly about health and other topics.

COFFEE AND INCONTINENCE

If you're a person who knows the location of every rest room in town, a recent study has a bit of advice: Put down that cup of coffee.

Conventional wisdom has it that caffeine may exacerbate a condition called "unstable bladder," which creates major problems for many older women in the form of a split-second need to pee. Younger women too, sometimes find themselves with a kind of precursor condition that demands frequent pit stops (we'll call it "impatient bladder"). But it hasn't been clear whether a coffee sacrifice was really worth making. So urologist Lily Arya looked closely at a group of women with unstable bladders and found a strong piece of evidence: They were dedicated coffee drinkers who downed more than four cups a day on average. It's well known that caffeine is a diuretic, Arya says. But few people realize the chemical also increases bladder irritability, sometimes triggering spontaneous contractions of the muscle. And that's what causes the urgency and the incontinence.

Arya says the study doesn't connect all the dots between sip and slip. But the findings suggest, she says, that women with urinary incontinence should cut back on caffeine or steer clear entirely. That means avoiding not just coffee but other caffeinated drinks, such as colas and black teas. And to avoid a problem later, younger women who find themselves taking frequent bathroom breaks should probably keep coffee consumption below two cups daily. As for the woman with a bladder like a camel's, she can stick to her regular caffeine routine without much concern.

Q+A
Remedies for poison ivy and oak

Are there any good treatments for poison oak, ivy, or sumac? My eyes were swollen nearly shut during my last outbreak.

The next time you have such a severe reaction, get to the doctor right away. It's likely that she'll want to prescribe a steroid cream, pills, or even an injection to get your symptoms under control.

The smartest strategy is to keep the rash from raging in the first place. Your itching, oozing, and swelling are part of an allergic reaction to urushiol, an oil common to the "poison" plants. If you know you've brushed against a plant and can get the oil off your skin quickly, your chances of an outbreak drop drastically.

One recent study showed that washing skin with an oil-removing product called Goop within two hours of exposure could cut the severity of a reaction by more than half. (Goop is marketed as a hand cleanser for mechanics; look for it in automotive stores.) A lotion called Tecnu, sold for combatting urushiol, also works well, as does Ultra Dial dishwashing liquid. Some experts also recommend lifting the oil off with rubbing alcohol, then rinsing with water.

To soothe a mild rash, soak in Aveeno bath powder or smooth on calamine lotion. Taking aspirin every few hours can reduce inflammation, especially in the early phases. And try not to scratch!

THE EASY WAY TO PREVENT INFECTIONS
(that some of us neglect)

Take just 15 seconds to soap up, and you can rid your hands of 99 percent of all germs.

A new survey reveals the real dirt on Americans: When it comes to hand washing, it seems that few of us have the right to a clean conscience.

Researchers at the American Society for Microbiology asked 1,000 adults over the phone whether they were scrupulous about washing their hands after using the bathroom: 95 percent said they always scrubbed down at the sink. Yet when the scientists decided to check first-hand on people's diligence (the researchers loitered surreptitiously in the public rest rooms of five U.S. cities), they found that only 67 percent of adults actually took the time to stop at a sink on the way out.

Judy Daly, a microbiologist with the society, says she can't stress enough the importance of washing away germs. "In just 15 seconds, you can eliminate 99 percent of whatever is on your hands," says Daly. "Even if you can't see these little guys, they can certainly make you sick."

Here's a guide to which urban dwellers you can shake hands with and which you'd be better off waving to.

handwashers

Group	Percent who washed hands
Chicagoans	83
San Franciscans	80
Atlantans	64
New Orleanians	64
New Yorkers	49
Women overall	75
Men overall	58

For women with allergies, black cats are bad luck.

Don't let one cross your path if you have allergies. Dark-hued kitties seem to trigger more sneezing and wheezing than fair-haired felines.

Self-Care: Solving Swimmer's Ear

If your vacation plans include rafting down a lazy river or sinking into a hot spring, don't be surprised if you emerge with an unseemly souvenir: swimmer's ear. This outer-ear infection stems from bacteria in dirty water or your own natural bacteria that have gone out of whack. You know it's the culprit if your ear is itchy, red, and tender, or if you wince from tugging gently on your lobe. Need help? Lend an ear:

• Pop ibuprofen or acetaminophen every four to six hours to minimize discomfort.

• Rest the achy ear against a warm heating pad or lukewarm hot-water bottle until pain subsides.

• Vanquish mild infections with over-the-counter antiseptic eardrops or use a homemade brew of equal parts rubbing alcohol and white vinegar (alcohol to dry the ear canal, vinegar to restore pH levels). Rest your head to the side, dribble several drops into the infected ear, and stay put for five minutes. Then, holding a towel against the ear, tilt your head up and to the opposite side to help the liquid roll out. Repeat twice a day for up to three days.

• Keep it dry. In the shower, put a cotton ball coated with petroleum jelly just inside your ear (off-the-shelf earplugs may trap water). If water happens to creep in, a well-aimed hair dryer (set on low heat only) will take care of it.

When to see a doctor

Swimmer's ear is nothing to pooh-pooh. Left untreated, it can lead to a perforated eardrum, hearing loss, even life-threatening infection. See your doctor right away if:

• your symptoms intensify, last more than three days, or

• if you have diabetes or a compromised immune system.

She'll want to examine the ear and remove any wax buildup. Most likely, she'll prescribe antibiotic eardrops to stomp out the infection.

Four Tips to Ease Earache Pain

Listen up. Earaches can be a real pain. Fortunately, you can take steps to ease the agony and prevent a recurrence.

• Pop ibuprofen or aspirin for the pain—for up to three days.

• Place a warm towel or hot water bottle on the ear for about 15 to 30 minutes several times a day.

• Be alert to temporomandibular joint disorder (TMJ). If you don't notice any stuffiness or hearing loss in the ear but it hurts to open your mouth, you most likely have TMJ, a pain in the jaw that can radiate to your middle ear. Rest your chops by avoiding hard, chewy foods for a week or two.

• Prevent earaches when flying by taking an over-the-counter decongestant pill and using a nasal spray about an hour before the plane lands.

When to see a doctor

Contact your physician immediately if you also have a fever, a severe headache, or tingling or numbness in your face. Although the chances are slim, you may have meningitis or a neurological problem. If you experience hearing loss or ringing in the ears, call a doctor. If you have any drainage or bleeding from the ear, you may have an infection, warranting antibiotics. Finally, if the earache fails to improve after two to three days, you may want to see an ear, nose, and throat specialist.

homeopathy eases earache in children

It's one of the first rigorous studies to find results with homeopathy: Pediatricians at the University of Washington gave kids with middle-ear infections either homeopathic remedies such as German chamomile and windflower or a placebo. Those who got homeopathy reported less ear pain and had lower fevers than the placebo group.

end jaw and face pain
once and for all

TMJ can make you miserable, causing jaw pain and headaches. But some surprisingly simple measures can offer real relief.

BY CATHERINE GUTHRIE

n 1984, a jaw-straightening procedure left Patty Kaczmarek's mouth so swollen and stiff that talking and chewing reduced her to tears. After Kaczmarek endured many pain-filled months, her dentist told her she had temporomandibular joint disorder (TMJ, aka TMD). Kaczmarek was hopeful: Now that her agony had a name, surely she would find a cure.

Her optimism was short-lived. Kaczmarek spent the next year hopscotching from dentist to physical therapist to chiropractor—but no one could ease her misery. Finally, her original dentist recommended the treatment du jour: jaw-joint implants, synthetic devices that would replace the cartilage-like disc that serves as a cushion between the skull and the jawbone. The implants were suppos-edly capable of withstand-ing the jaw's intense pressure and would cure Kaczmarek's TMJ. She readily agreed to the surgery, only to fall into the black hole that can separate theory and practice.

Her first implant caused trouble from the start; after two months of struggling to open and close her mouth normally, Kaczmarek had it removed. She tried a different implant. This one disintegrated slowly, causing pain, inflammation, and—combined with the aftereffects of the surgeries—nerve damage

Jaw-joint implants of past decades have caused many people no end of pain and suffering. Today, such radical procedures are considered only as a last resort.

that has left part of her face and tongue paralyzed. She continues to endure debilitating migraines, a burning sensation in one ear, and numbness in her left arm and leg. Looking back, the 35-year-old Kaczmarek longs for the days when she had only TMJ.

Official neglect

How did this nightmare happen? Well, simply put, Kaczmarek—and about 150,000 other people who received similar jaw-joint implants—was the victim of shoddy government regulation.

Until the mid-1970s, there was no oversight what-soever of medical devices. When Congress gave the job to the Food and Drug Administration (FDA) in 1976, the agency was suddenly responsible for ensuring the safety of thousands of implants, ranging from heart valves to hip replacements. "It was an enormous undertaking," admits former FDA com-missioner Jere Goyan. "The agency had staff who were good at the tradi-tional mission—food, drugs, cosmetics—but even today there aren't many materials people."

Overwhelmed, the FDA allowed those devices already on the market to stay. And it created a loophole for future ones: If manufacturers could prove their invention was related to one that was on the books before 1976, they could leapfrog certain testing barri-ers. The makers of jaw-joint implants simply laid claim to a distant relative, and the devices squeaked through virtually untested.

Tragically, manufacturers failed to take into account the complexities of the jaw, and the FDA failed to make them do so. As it turns out, the implants were made of materials that could not hold up under the significant pressure the jaw brings to bear. It was enough force to overwhelm the flimsy devices: Some split in half, while others crumbled.

Eventually the FDA caught wind of the situation, and in 1990 the agency issued a safety alert about the worst offender. By 1999 every manufacturer had taken its faulty implants off the market.

Some aspects of the TMJ landscape have scarcely shifted in the years since the implant debacle. Many women, like Kaczmarek, still cope with the devastating effects of the flawed devices. TMJ is no longer dismissed as "a condition afflicting suburban housewives in bad marriages," as a doctor once opined, but it can be baffling to patients and health-care providers, with no clear-cut cause or cure.

Still, the plight of TMJ patients has improved. Patients are no longer isolated: Kaczmarek and others have formed networks offering support and advice to people who have been diagnosed with or think they might have TMJ. Several clinics now specialize in the disorder, and in 2000 the National Institutes of Health organized a panel of experts to discuss holistic treatments for TMJ. Most important, patients and dentists now pin their hopes on noninvasive, reversible therapies, several of which appear to bring relief.

Why does it hurt?

Jaw pain is TMJ's calling card, but it can bring a host of other symptoms, ranging from the conspicuous (popping, clicking, and locking of the jaw) to the more covert (headaches, earaches, facial pain, and shoulder tension). Most of us experience—and more or less ignore—the occasional stiff or noisy jaw, but about 10

don't suffer in silence

If you have a temporomandibular joint disorder or if you are coping with the aftereffects of joint implants, you can get emotional support and advice from the TMJ Association at 414-259-3223 or www.tmj.org.

million Americans, 90 percent of them women, seek treatment for TMJ's more debilitating symptoms.

There's rarely a single explanation for jaw pain. In some cases, it results from damage to the disc in the jaw joint. If that wears down, the joint's alignment can be thrown off. This eventually strains the connecting muscles, causing tension and pain throughout the head and neck.

For some people, the delicate balance is upset by osteoarthritis or a blow to the jaw; for others the cause is as mundane as poor posture or too much gum chewing. Rarely, as in Kaczmarek's case, a failed orthodontic procedure is the culprit. Many experts believe that stress, especially when it takes the form of teeth grinding (bruxism) and clenching, is a significant factor.

Because it's often difficult to know just what's causing the pain, it can be tough to figure out how to relieve it. "In one part of the country, dentists favor one method of treatment, and in another area they're doing something completely different," says H. Clifton Simmons, president of the American Academy of Head, Neck, and Facial Pain. "The situation is changing, but for a long time dentists knew very little about TMJ."

Detecting the cause and finding a cure are especially frustrating when stress is part of the picture. "Most dentists aren't trained to ask a patient what's going on in his or her life," says Jeffrey Okeson, a TMJ expert and director of the Orofacial Pain Center at the University of Kentucky. "They'd rather just do the dentistry."

This has led to some misguided treatments. For example, Okeson notes, experts used to think that the disorder stemmed from upper and lower teeth that refused to fit together properly. "We'd throw an appliance at everybody, adjust everybody's bite," he says. But several studies indicate that a bad bite isn't the offender after all. "Today, if I had jaw pain and a dentist told me I needed extensive orthodontics," says Okeson, "the first thing I'd say is, 'I need a second opinion.' "

Fortunately, for most people with TMJ, radical procedures like surgery are now considered only as a last resort. A newly designed jaw-joint implant approved by the FDA last year is recommended for patients whose joints have been damaged by previous implants or cancer, but the average patient is advised to think positively and proceed with caution.

Your best bet

No single remedy has been proven 100 percent effective, but a combination of approaches will likely help.

Pain management. According to Okeson, it's important to reduce pain for a couple of reasons. First, you'll feel better. Second, when you're not hurting, your muscles start to relax and the cycle of pain is interrupted. Aspirin and ibuprofen are usually effective, as is moist heat, although some people find that ice works better.

You can also minimize discomfort by minimizing jaw use. That might mean changing some eating habits by taking small bites, chewing slowly, and choosing softer foods. And toss that pack of gum.

Relaxation. Experts agree that relaxation is a crucial part of the nonaggressive approach. "With a $6 tape you can learn how to quiet your system, how to understand your body better," says Okeson.

If calming your entire being sounds overwhelming, start with relaxing your teeth and tongue. Your upper and lower teeth should meet only for the time it takes to chew and swallow food—a maximum of just eight minutes a day. "The main thing we tell our patients is 'Lips together, teeth apart,' " says Okeson. "Puff some air between your lips and then seal them. The tongue should be kept on the floor of the mouth. Keep that position and you won't load your joints. The important thing is to be aware.

"These methods are cheap and easy," says Okeson. "And you can't get into trouble with any of them."

Physical therapy. This treatment works best when the problem is in the facial muscles rather than in the joint. It usually includes a combination of relaxation exercises, biofeedback, ergonomic adjustments (e.g., don't cradle a telephone receiver between your shoulder and jaw), and posture training. The latter may be particularly helpful; TMJ researchers in Texas reported significant improvement in study subjects who corrected their faulty head-forward posture.

Splints. Many chronic teeth grinders find that splints—which are sometimes referred to as mouth guards—protect the teeth and ease jaw tension. Custom-made splints can run more than $1,000. Athletic versions and drugstore knock-offs are cheaper, but a one-size-fits-all philosophy may not cut it; wrap your lips around a horseshoe and chances are you'll not only lose sleep but also aggravate sore muscles. Clenchers may want to steer clear: Some people clench more with a splint than without.

"No matter what you do, be very cautious," says Okeson, "and do the most conservative thing first." ✳

Is what you're eating good for your teeth?

Remember your mother condemning sweets for the sake of your incisors? Well, she was right (did you have any doubt?), and recent dental research shows that some foods may affect your teeth's health more than even Mom imagined. You should still go easy on the sugar bowl, but look at what you should—and shouldn't—bite into:

• Eating fresh cranberries interrupts the bonding of oral bacteria before they can form damaging plaque.

• Calcium and vitamin D supplements have been shown to decrease the risk of tooth loss in the elderly.

• Cheese packs a burst of calcium that mixes with plaque and sticks to the teeth. The sticky mixture protects teeth from the acid that causes decay and helps rebuild tooth enamel on the spot.

• A balanced meal can help. If you are eating sugary or carbohydrate-rich foods as part of a larger meal, the body produces more saliva than digestion demands, which washes away more food and helps neutralize harmful acids before they mount an attack.

• Just because it's good for you doesn't mean it's necessarily good for your teeth. Sticky foods, including nutritious choices like raisins, dates, and dried fruit, hold acid against the teeth longer than other foods.

yoga

nonsurgical treatment to ease pain of carpal tunnel syndrome

If CTS is crippling your life, take off those splints and try a treatment with a twist.

BY CHRISTIE ASCHWANDEN

Imagine wrist pain so intense that typing is torture. Imagine your garden strangled by weeds because pulling them is an exercise in agony. Imagine your morning coffee sloshing to the floor as your wrist gives way under the weight of the mug. Kathie Greenacre doesn't have to imagine such scenarios. Until recently, carpal tunnel syndrome (CTS) had turned the 58-year-old Philadelphia physician's life into a cruel obstacle course.

Greenacre doesn't know what brought it on, but her CTS first hit in 1984. "The tingling was just intolerable," she says. "My hands were so weak that it was difficult to do ordinary things like writing or lifting a cooking pot." She gave up her practice in pulmonary medicine, which put inordinate strain on her wrists, and became a part-time internist. But her pain persisted, despite treatments ranging from wrist splints to surgery.

In 1998, her doctor told her about intriguing research that he and several other rheumatologists had recently conducted—research that suggested Greenacre might benefit from an unconventional therapy. The study, he told her, had yielded tantalizing evidence that a combination of yoga poses could provide CTS sufferers a level of relief unmatched by more traditional treatments.

Almost 4.5 million Americans live with carpal tunnel syndrome, at least 60 percent of them women. It can strike anyone, but many cases are thought to be job-related, provoked by repetitive hand movements, such as lifting, typing, and operating a cash register. Because it is a tough beast to tame, CTS can spell the end of a normal work life for people whose careers depend on these activities. Indeed, the pain and disability it entails can spell the end of normalcy for anyone.

Nine tendons and the median nerve travel from arm to hand through the carpal tunnel, a narrow passage created by the bones of the wrist and the carpal ligament. If one of the tendons gets inflamed, it puts pressure on the nerve, causing numbness and

After eight weeks, the pain and tingling had improved so much that I abandoned my wrist splints. Now I'm back to gardening and sewing, and I'm fitter than ever before. —carpal tunnel sufferer Kathie Greenacre

Go to the first yoga class early, and tell the instructor you have CTS. A good teacher will help you adapt each routine to fit your needs and abilities.

tingling, especially at night. Left untreated, CTS can result in permanent weakness and atrophy of the hands.

Typically, doctors dole out wrist splints to their CTS patients, advising them to limit the offending wrist motions and take aspirin or ibuprofen for pain. If those don't do the job, corticosteroid injections can help, at least temporarily. In extreme cases, doctors often recommend surgery to reduce pressure on the median nerve; the outpatient procedure is successful 75 to 99 percent of the time.

But Greenacre had been through two surgeries when her doctor sent her to his colleague Marian Garfinkel, who led the research showing yoga's beneficial effects on CTS. A researcher in the department of rheumatology at the University of Pennsylvania School of Medicine, she is also a yoga instructor in downtown Philadelphia. For almost three decades Garfinkel has spent several weeks a year in India studying with guru B.K.S. Iyengar, whose eponymous method of yoga she teaches in her studio.

In the early 1990s, Garfinkel, who wrote her doctoral dissertation on osteoarthritis of the hands and finger joints, conjectured that Iyengar yoga, by stretching and strengthening the muscles and tendons in the wrist and upper torso, might help reduce the inflammation and pain of CTS.

Eager to test her theory, she applied for a grant from the state of Pennsylvania. "I believed in yoga, but I needed data," she says. She received only a fraction of the money she requested; to make up the rest she borrowed equipment and donated her time.

Photograph by Misha Gravenor

The most effective poses are those that stretch and strengthen the upper body.

Garfinkel's experiment was simple. She and her colleagues, among them four rheumatologists from the University of Pennsylvania School of Medicine, rounded up 42 volunteers with CTS. The subjects were split into two groups. People in one group stayed on their prescribed course of treatment, including painkillers and wrist splints. Members of the other group put away their splints and pills and attended an Iyengar yoga class twice a week. At each session Garfinkel led the yoga group through 12 modified Iyengar asanas, or poses, that help stabilize the joints in the upper body.

After two months, the volunteers in the yoga group reported a 42 percent drop in wrist pain, and their grip strength had increased by about 16 percent. The group that had stuck to traditional treatment reported no significant improvement in either category. One of only a handful of yoga studies ever to appear in an established medical journal, Garfinkel's research was published in the *Journal of the American Medical Association* in 1998.

Garfinkel believes the most effective poses are those that stretch and strengthen the upper body, but she says there's no one magic pose. "You need to progress through the whole program," she says. "By learning to lengthen your spine, open your shoulders, and spread your knuckles, you'll increase your strength, range of motion, circulation, and flexibility—all keys to reducing the pain of CTS."

Yoga may not be in the medical mainstream, but Garfinkel's work is inspiring at least some physicians to advise their CTS patients to strike a pose. "I've found that yoga can be a very important part of a successful treatment program," says Christopher D'Arcy, a rheumatologist at the University of Washington in Seattle. "Surgery will still be necessary in some cases, but yoga may be the best option, especially for people in the early stages of CTS. I regularly suggest it to my patients—and I get positive reports back."

Garfinkel says yoga's benefits start with pain relief, but go much further. For one thing, yoga can ease the anxiety that often accompanies CTS. "It brings order to chaos," she says. "When everything around you is crumbling, yoga helps you find peace within yourself."

What's more, she says, the practice is empowering. "Yoga teaches you to have a positive attitude and to do what you can for yourself first. You don't have to run to the doctor and get an operation right away." D'Arcy concurs. "Through yoga, patients gain a beneficial sense of control over their bodies," he says. "They learn to breathe and relax—and that's crucial to the reduction of pain."

If you want to give your wrists a yoga twist, look for an experienced instructor. Some poses may do more harm than good, so you need someone who knows the ropes. Go to the first class early, Garfinkel advises, and tell the instructor you have CTS. A good teacher will help you adapt each routine to fit your needs and abilities.

The B.K.S. Iyengar Yoga Association can help you find a certified Iyengar instructor in your area; call 800-889-9642 or log on to www.iynaus.org. A more interactive site is www.iyengar-yoga.com. There you can find CTS-related articles and testimonials—or even take a virtual trip to India and chant with B.K.S. himself.

Garfinkel hopes to demonstrate yoga's healing powers in other arenas. She's now in the initial stages of a study that will explore the effects of yoga on people suffering from osteoarthritis of the knee.

Greenacre, for one, needs no further evidence of the benefits yoga can provide. "It didn't work overnight," she says, "but after eight weeks, the pain and tingling had improved so much that I abandoned my wrist splints. Now I'm back to gardening and sewing, and I'm fitter than I've ever been before." ✳

Christie Achwanden is a Health *contributing editor.*

Q+A
end indoor pollution—with houseplants

Can houseplants really purify air? Do some do a better job than others?

It sounds New Agey, but it's true: Decorating a room with lots of plants can get rid of nasty toxins floating about your house.

Here's why. You may think the air in your house is clean, but it probably contains traces of chemicals like formaldehyde, benzene, and trichloroethylene, which can seep into the air from cleaning products, dry-cleaned clothes, and your ventilation system. Some scientists think that when low levels of these chemicals combine, they can contribute to an allergy-like syndrome called multiple chemical sensitivity.

Certain houseplants, researchers have learned, actually like to suck these chemicals out of the air and eat them like candy. The leaves of these plants release moisture into the air, and as they do, they pull in chemicals—along with airborne bacteria and viruses—and shoot them down to their roots. The results of a NASA experiment, for instance, showed that areca palms cleared a room of 99 percent of its formaldehyde in just four hours.

But one lone plant isn't enough to do the trick. Studies show that it takes at least two to three plants per 100 square feet to start bringing down chemical levels in the average home. Some of the best air cleaners are:

- areca palm
- lady palm
- Boston fern
- English ivy
- rubber plant

Here's one more tip for you: To keep the plants from growing mold, which only seems to muck up your air all the more, cover the top of your potting soil with a couple of inches of pebbles or aquarium gravel.

FAST HELP FOR SPRAINED ANKLES

Ankle sprains are the most common injury in the United States. One sideways slip off those groovy platforms is all it takes to leave you with an angry ankle. When gravity gets the best of you, here's what to do.

ELEVATE the injured ankle so that it rests above your heart. This minimizes swelling and bruising by diverting blood flow away from broken blood vessels.

APPLY AN ICEPACK to the injured joint—20 minutes on, 30 minutes off. Icy temperatures shrink blood vessels and curb bleeding, but don't get the area too frosty (blood flow increases to ward off frostbite). Repeat four to eight times a day for up to three days.

WRAP AN ELASTIC BANDAGE around the injury, starting at the ball of the foot. Make two or three turns, then begin a figure-eight pattern, alternately encircling the ankle and the instep. Leave the heel exposed. Be careful not to cut off circulation: If you can't slip a finger under the bandage, it's too tight.

WHEN TO SEE A DOCTOR: If you can't move your ankle or walk more than four steps without intense pain, see a doctor right away. If the sprain is severe, the ligaments may be badly stretched or torn, and you could need a special boot or cast to immobilize the joint. An X-ray is sometimes required to rule out broken bones.

Play bridge to boost your immune system

Next time you feel yourself coming down with a bug, forget echinacea—play bridge. A recent study suggests that the brain-stimulating card game may give your immune system a lift. Researchers at the University of California at Berkeley found that after playing for an hour and a half, elderly women showed significant increases in the number of immune-boosting cells in their blood.

Q+A
What it really means when your back cracks

My back and neck crack easily if I move and stretch a certain way. It feels good, but does it mean I might have a back problem?

No. A spontaneous pop now and then is simply your body's way of readjusting itself. It feels good because it relieves tight muscles. The pop you hear is actually nitrogen gas being released from the blood into a vacuum (caused by the stretch) in the joint. You might even crack your back on purpose by stretching or twisting to relieve tension. But use your common sense. If a gentle stretch doesn't result in a pop, don't go overboard by having someone press (or even walk!) on your back. You might overstretch your joints and end up with chronic discomfort.

Be careful if touching your toes or doing a split has always come easily. This kind of super-flexibility may allow you to overstretch your ligaments if you repeatedly pop your joints. Your muscles will tighten to compensate for the loose joint or ligament, exacerbating muscular tension.

The best antihistamine? *a good laugh*

Could a good laugh be just what the doctor ordered for allergy-sensitive skin? Japanese researchers exposed 26 allergic people to cat hair and dust, first while they watched a Charlie Chaplin film and again while they gazed at a weather video. The results: A good chortle cut the patients' reaction to irritants by as much as 75 percent.

TEST YOURSELF
Are you good to your feet?

WHEN TEMPERATURES RISE, it's time to set those toes free. Take this test to learn how to get off on the right foot in sandal season.

1. It is unsafe to file off corns.
   True or False?

2. Which of these will help stinky feet?
   a) Drying them with a hair dryer
   b) Applying antiperspirant to them
   c) Soaking them in tea
   d) All of the above

3. Athlete's foot can spread to your hands.
   True or False?

4. Your feet get bigger as you get older.
   True or False?

ANSWERS
1. False. Corns are bumps of thickened skin. As long as you're not diabetic and, thus, vulnerable to foot ulcers, take a nail file or pumice stone and carefully sand away.

2. D. All of the above. Most foot funk is caused by bacteria, which thrive in damp places. So keep your tootsies dry. A hair dryer (on a low setting) does a more thorough job than a towel, and antiperspirant works as well on soles as underarms. Black tea contains tannic acid, which may keep overactive sweat glands in check. But beware: tea does stain, so soak just your soles.

3. True. The fungus easily insinuates itself into any moist environment. So it can start on the locker-room floor and end up in the hiding places between your toes. Scratch too much, and it can wind up under your fingernails—and from there go anywhere you scratch, including your hands.

4. True. But the actual length may not change. Typically, the food widens and the arch settles. As if that's not bad enough, the pads under the heel thin.

Got a migraine?
maybe it's cold outside

Autumn's crisp weather can spell trouble for some migraine sufferers. Research presented at the 10th International Headache Congress (a biannual meeting for specialists in the field) suggests—contrary to popular belief—that cold, dry conditions are the most common weather-related migraine triggers. Don't buy a one-way ticket to the Bahamas just yet, though, as other culprits can include high temperatures and humidity, as well as air pressure changes. If you think your migraines may be weather-sensitive, keep an eye on the forecast and your meds at hand.

Heal Your Aching Heels

The chronic heel pain known as plantar fasciitis accounts for 15 percent of all foot complaints; it can make a walk in the park excruciating. Healing takes time, and involves over-the-counter painkillers, stretching, shoe inserts, and lots of rest. Now a shock-wave treatment called Ossatron may speed recovery. When podiatrists zapped ailing feet, patients reported feeling better right away. The therapy seems to ease inflammation.

a site for sore eyes
Whether you're seeking chic specs or info about your eyesight, take a look at www.allaboutvision.com. You'll find the lowdown on computer vision syndrome and LASIK surgery, as well as tips on choosing frames that flatter your face. Plus, a resident ophthalmologist can answer your questions.

Comparison shopping can help you find relief when pain gets the best of you. But read this before you let anyone rub, manipulate, needle, or operate on your back.

cure your aching back

BY CHRISTIE ASCHWANDEN

Penny Rickhoff remembers exactly when her pain started. "I was on the tennis court finishing up a set," she recalls. "The next thing I knew, I was in the doctor's office." The 55-year-old interior designer has had two surgeries in the 15 years since that first episode, but she still faces daily discomfort.

She's not alone. Fully 80 percent of all Americans will experience back pain at some point. "The people who never have pain are the weird ones," says psychologist Dennis Turk, who's on a renowned team of pain researchers at the University of Washington.

Luckily, things are looking up for the aching millions. The last decade has brought a silent revolution in back care, says physician Richard Deyo, also at the University of Washington, who's led some major studies of back pain. This shift has fundamentally changed how experts try to explain, diagnose, and treat this vexing condition.

These days, the experts offer tough love. Back when Rickhoff had her front-court collapse, the standard advice was to stay in bed. "We now know that's the worst thing you can do," says Deyo. In fact, he argues, lying around actually boosts your risk of developing back pain. "We gave people this idea that they're walking on eggshells and their back is going to snap at any moment," he says. "But that's just not true. Your spine is strong and resilient."

Though it might seem odd, physicians are also less likely to offer a diagnosis than they used to be. When Jean Lacocque's back gave out, the 46-year-old Chicagoan went from doctor to doctor in search of help. "I felt like I'd been hit with a sledgehammer," she says. Alas, none of them could tell her what was wrong. Lacocque's doctors may have been as frustrated as she was. For years, specialists have tried to pinpoint the cause of their patients' pain, convinced that a diagnosis was required for proper treatment.

Today, the experts say a diagnosis frequently isn't necessary. "There are a million diagnostic labels for back pain, but often they just cover up the fact that we don't know what's causing it," says Michael Von Korff, a back researcher at Group Health Cooperative in Seattle. "In the end, it doesn't matter. As long as you've excluded serious disease, the treatment is the same." Turk estimates that only 15 percent of the walking wounded have pain with an obvious cause.

Of course, there's no shortage of theories to explain the remaining 85 percent. The back is a complex system that includes bones, ligaments, muscles, and nerves—and it's not hard to find a specialist who can make a persuasive case to pin your pain on problems with one or more of these structures.

Many chiropractors point the finger at vertebrae that have become immobile due to injury or swelling. Physical therapists often say it's poor flexibility, posture, and body mechanics. Just about everyone believes that pain and mobility problems can arise from weak muscles in the back and torso or from muscles or tendons that are inflamed, tight, or pulled.

Medical doctors are in the mix too. They typically attribute back pain to intervertebral discs, shock absorbers that sit between the vertebrae, preventing them from grinding together and allowing the spine to bend. Debilitating aches and spasms emerge, the logic goes, when ruptured, herniated, or slipped discs (take your pick, they mean the same thing) start pushing into nearby tissues or nerves. In the past, many people had surgery to correct that kind of problem.

But experts now say that going under the knife is often a mistake. Eugene Carragee, an orthopedic surgeon at Stanford University, analyzed the MRIs of 96 people who had risk factors for disc degeneration. Many did have damaged discs, but those with obvious problems were only slightly more likely to report pain during activity than those without them. Even more startling, tests revealed disc irregularities in 25 percent of the subjects who experienced no pain at all.

"These imaging techniques can be misleading," says Deyo. "They see all sorts of nasty-looking things, even in people with no pain."

Yet the sufferers in Carragee's study had one surprising thing in common. "When we looked at who hurt the most, the best predictor was a psychological problem like depression," he says.

Carragee and other experts are not saying the problem is in your head. No one denies that the pain is

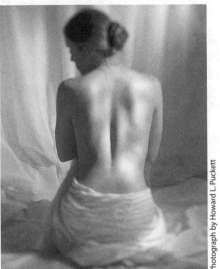

Photograph by Howard L. Puckett

What's the recommended treatment for common back ailments? Nothing. Most back pain goes away on its own.

real. But they say people's attitudes about the discomfort play a major role in how they cope—and how fast they heal. "People get back pain and become anxious or fearful. Then they limit their activities and that makes it worse," says Deyo. "It can be a downward spiral."

So if back specialists aren't going to tell you to take it easy or try to reassure you with a diagnosis, much less offer you some old-fashioned aggressive treatment, what are they suggesting you do? Not much, say the experts. And that's a good thing. "Virtually all back pain goes away on its own," says John Loeser, a neurosurgeon at the University of Washington.

The key, researchers say, is not to expect a simple diagnosis and an easy cure. Instead, find ways to manage your pain and prevent flare-ups.

You've got plenty of choices. The vast majority of people can get relief with one or two of the most common treatments. Studies show that folks recover most quickly when they take the approach that best fits their lifestyle and that they believe in the most. Pick one you think will work for you and it probably will. Here are eight back-pain busters worth trying.

Self-Care

You spent Sunday morning hefting boxes, and your back is begging for mercy. Doctors call these intense attacks acute pain. When misery strikes, you can take immediate action.

For starters, try an over-the-counter pain medication like ibuprofen, aspirin, or acetaminophen. (If you have recurrent back pain, you may want to get a prescription medication to have on hand for your next bout with acute pain. Since such agony usually subsides quickly, the risk of addiction is low.) Then, ice the area that hurts for 15 minutes at a time, three to five times per day. A bag of frozen peas makes a great ice pack.

If the pain persists more than a few days, many experts say you should substitute a heating pad for those 15-minute periods. In the meantime, remain as active as you can. The pros say staying in bed for more than a day or two will only make things worse.

It doesn't sound like much, but the experts say such simple steps work just as well as more complicated—and certainly more costly—treatment options. "Taking action to control your pain will likely do more for you than seeing a doctor," says Turk.

To prevent further flare-ups, try to make your environment more back friendly. Sleep on a firm mattress and curl up on your side with a pillow between your knees. Choose chairs that support your lower back.

Rethink those activities and behaviors that exacerbate your woes. Kim Hedberg, a 41-year-old business consultant from Boulder, Colorado, controls her pain in part by avoiding things like sitting still for extended periods, lifting heavy objects, and stressing out—all of which can bring on an attack. "Every little thing helps," she says.
COST: One bag of peas, under $2; bottle of 50 aspirin, $5; finding ways to eliminate stress, priceless.
RESOURCES: James E. Moore's *The Back Pain Helpbook* (Perseus Book, 1999) is an informative guide.

Exercise

Though you might feel inclined to moan in bed, experts say regular exercise may be the best thing you can do for back pain. The only time you should avoid

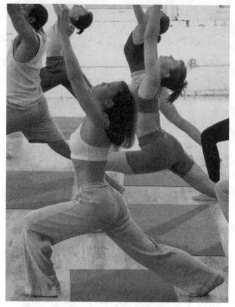

Aerobic activities—like walking and such exercises as crunches and back extensions that strengthen back and stomach muscles—are important to having a strong and healthy back. A trainer at any gym can show you moves that will be right for you.

working out is during the first day or two of an acute attack. "Studies show that people who do as many active things as they can are the ones who recover best," says Carragee.

Hedberg is a believer. "If I don't exercise for two or three days, I'm going to get a flare-up," she says. She relies on weight lifting, aerobic exercise, and stretching to stave off attacks.

Experts agree that no single workout will erase your pain, but they say two categories are important: aerobic activities like brisk walking and such exercises as crunches and back extensions that strengthen your back and stomach muscles. A trainer at any gym can show you moves that will be right for you.
COST: Walking, free; gym memberships, typically about $50 per month and up.
RESOURCES: For a primer on relevant exercises and other back pain topics, check out www.spine-health.com.

Relaxation Techniques

"Fighting daily pain takes a lot of energy. You have to do something to unwind," says Penny Rickhoff. For her, that something is tai chi, which she practices every day. "The relaxation I get can diminish the pain," she says.

Many scientists also are fans. Stress and anxiety can cause your body to tense up, worsening your back pain, says Deyo. Relaxation techniques aim to break this cycle by helping you to relax and to focus your attention inward, letting go of tensions that might be

Exercise may be the best thing you can do for an aching back. Studies show that people who are the most active are the ones who recover best.

Attitude is key to coping with back problems. Researchers warn not to expect an easy cure. Instead, find ways to manage the pain and prevent flare-ups.

triggering your pain. In a landmark 1995 report, a panel of multidisciplinary experts assembled by the National Institutes of Health (NIH) concluded that techniques like meditation and hypnosis can ease chronic pain. Scientists say that these activities seem to mellow out your nervous system, which appears to blunt your body's sensitivity to pain.

Some relaxation techniques like yoga and tai chi have the added benefit of including exercise, but the key is to focus your attention on the area that's causing your pain. For this reason, yoga varieties that emphasize meditative breathing and relaxation may work best.

COST: Meditating at home, free; classes, $5 to $25 per session.

RESOURCES: The American Yoga Association; call them at 941-927-4977 or visit their Web site at www.americanyogaassociation.org.

Massage

Few would argue with the idea that massage feels really good. But that's not the only reason to give it a try. A massage therapist can target both the back and surrounding areas. For some people, results are immediate. The rubbing, pushing, and kneading seem to work by increasing circulation to the back and by relaxing tense muscles.

Massage comes in many flavors. A recent study suggests that neuromuscular massage therapy—a vigorous technique that targets specific pressure points—is especially effective for back pain, but any technique that makes you feel good may offer relief. At the very least, you'll feel splendid while it lasts.

COST: $50 an hour and up.

Hypnosis and relaxation techniques like yoga can ease chronic pain. Scientists say these activities ease stress and anxiety and may blunt your body's sensitivity to pain.

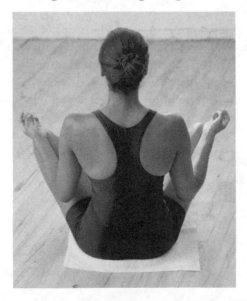

RESOURCES: The American Massage Therapy Association (call 847-864-0123 or www.amtamassage.org).

Acupuncture

Jean Lacocque swears by the benefits of this ancient Chinese technique. It's helped control pain she's had for years. "It works best for me," she says.

Here's what to expect: An acupuncturist will have you lie down or sit up on a table. Once you're comfortable, she'll gently insert a series of extremely thin needles into your skin. The needles are placed at specific points on lines, or meridians, along your body that, according to Chinese medicine, conduct energy between the body's surface and internal organs. Though the acupuncturist will likely put needles in your back, she may also place them in other areas. Most people feel little or no pain when the needles are inserted. Some even report feeling relaxed or energized by the experience.

And it really seems to work. A few years ago, an NIH panel concluded that acupuncture is indeed helpful for treating low back pain. The World Health Organization has endorsed it as well. Research suggests that acupuncture spurs the release of your body's natural painkillers and may speed the flow of these substances to the spots that hurt.

In one study, medical acupuncturists reported that about two-thirds of their patients said they were pleased with the results. Most people feel at least some benefit after the first visit. If the technique is going to help you, you should notice a clear response by the fifth or sixth treatment.

Acupuncture seems to be an effective and pain-free treatment for back pain.

Research suggests that acupuncture spurs the release of your body's natural painkillers and may speed the flow of these substances to the spots that hurt.

COST: At least $45 to $100 per session. Many insurance companies will cover the treatment.
RESOURCES: The American Association of Oriental Medicine can help you find a local acupuncturist (888-500-7999 or www.aaom.org.). Or the American Academy of Medical Acupuncture can supply a list of physicians who practice acupuncture (800-521-2262 or www.medicalacupuncture.org.).

Physical Therapy

Blair Hurst went to a New York pain clinic in desperate shape. "My back was so bad I could barely stand," the 53-year-old Californian recalls. Luckily, a physical therapist (PT) at the clinic helped her get back on her feet again. The therapist showed her stretching and strength exercises that have diminished her pain—and taught her new ways to move around without injuring herself.

That's the point. Physical therapy's goal is to decrease discomfort, to restore and maintain normal movement, and to prevent pain through exercise and treatment, says Annie Sirotniak, a physical therapist at the University of Colorado's Wardenburg Health Center in Boulder. A physical therapist can teach you how to do exercises to eliminate alignment problems or muscle weaknesses and imbalances that might be aggravating your pain; she can also show you kinder, gentler ways to do movements such as lifting and bending. A PT may even visit your office or home to help you make back-friendly adjustments to your environment.

Recent research suggests that all this stretching and strengthening works. In particular, studies have demonstrated that the technique speeds up people's return to work after a back injury.
COST: Typically $85 to $150 for the first session, $40 to $100 thereafter. Most insurance plans will cover the therapy.
RESOURCES: The American Physical Therapy Association (800-999-2782 or www.apta.org/Consumer).

Chiropractic

Chiropractors were long perceived as back-cracking hacks. Those days are over, say experts. Studies and a report from a prestigious government panel suggest that manipulations—whether done by a chiropractor or a doctor of osteopathy—can bring relief to an aching back.

The theory behind the manipulations is simple. Chiropractors and osteopaths say that swelling, joint irregularities, or muscle spasms can immobilize your back joints, limiting your range of motion and causing chronic pain. By moving these joints with their hands, they say, they can relieve tension and allow them to move again. "It's like a concentrated exercise in the joint," says chiropractor Daniel Hansen at the Texas Back Institute. Hansen says that manipulations can also stimulate your body to release endorphins and other natural painkillers.

Here's how it works. First, a chiropractor or osteopath will take your medical history and perform a brief physical exam. Then if it's appropriate—and it's not if you're experiencing severe acute pain—the practitioner

Physical therapy aims to restore normal movement and prevent pain through exercise and treatment.

Research shows that all the stretching and strengthening works.

will proceed to the manipulations. While you lie on a table, the practitioner will gently maneuver your spine with his hands, then make some harder thrusts. Note that these movements should not be painful. It's normal to feel a pop during the process. "It's like cracking a big knuckle," says Hansen. If you're nervous, ask the provider to explain what's happening.

COST: $50 to $150 and up per visit, depending on the treatments. Many insurers offer coverage.

RESOURCES: The American Chiropractic Association (800-986-4636 or www.amerchiro.org) and the American Osteopathic Association (800-621-1773 or www.aoa-net.org).

Surgery

The rate of back surgery in the United States is two to eight times that in other developed countries. Experts believe a fair number of these surgeries are unnecessary. Deyo says there are only four reasons to consider surgery: a herniated disc that's been causing pain below your knee for a month; a spinal stenosis (narrowing of the spinal canal); a vertebra that's displaced, a condition called spondylolisthesis; or a tumor or other life-threatening problem. Only

about 2 percent of all back-pain patients are appropriate candidates for surgery.

Despite the cautionary approach taken by most researchers, surgeons are still out there performing a slew of procedures or patients. And new methods are being touted many in journals. Deyo and other experts urge people to be wary about going in for the newest surgery. "Many patients rush into the latest thing, and five years later we discover that it's worthless—or worse," says Deyo. If, after getting a second opinion, you've decided that the scalpel offers your best chance at relief, look for an experienced surgeon, and be sure you're clear on what kind of recovery and long-term outcome you can expect.

> Despite new surgical techniques, many experts now believe that going under the knife for back surgery is often a mistake.

COST: Likely tens of thousands.

RESOURCES: The American College of Surgeons has a series of general-interest pamphlets called *When You Need an Operation*. They're available online at www.facs.org/public_info/operation/wnao.html. For specific spinal procedures, the American Academy of Orthopaedic Surgeons offers a number of helpful fact sheets at orthoinfo.aaos.org. ✳

Christie Achwanden is a Health *contributing editor.*

IS HIGH BLOOD PRESSURE GIVING YOU A BAD BACK?

An aching back can bring you to your knees again and again, without offering so much as a clue as to what could be causing such agony. Now researchers may have discovered an unexpected explanation: problems in your blood vessels.

In the largest and longest study of its kind, Nicholas Ahn, the chief resident in orthopedic surgery at Johns Hopkins University, sifted through medical records of 1,300 people

spanning more than 50 years. His goal was to see which health risk factors were associated with chronic low back pain. Ahn found that smoking, high cholesterol, and high blood pressure all increased a person's chances of developing an achy back. In fact, patients with high blood pressure were nearly twice as likely to have a problem as those who didn't.

What's the connection? Ahn suspects clogged or constricted blood

vessels are the culprits, since hypertension, high cholesterol, and smoking are known to cause such problems in the arteries. "This may slow the blood flow to the lumbar spine, which can cause back pain," says Ahn.

It all adds up to yet another reason to quit smoking, eat a low-fat diet, and get more active. "People should realize that the same things they can do to prevent heart disease may help them avoid low back pain too," says Ahn.

from massage to movement therapy

a guide to
BODYWORK

More and more people are trying therapies such as
Alexander Technique and Feldenkrais Method for creaky joints
and aching backs. Here's the straight story.

BY PAULA DRANOV

Complain often enough about a stiff shoulder or a bad knee, and chances are that a friend, a co-worker, or the guy making your latte will recommend bodywork. Not just massage: That feels great, but eventually you have to get off the table. The really enthusiastic suggestions will come from converts to educational methods such as Feldenkrais, Hellerwork, and Alexander Technique. With these approaches, you learn to shrug off the bad posture and awkward movements that supposedly cause your ailments. Get your body in balance and, voilà, no more pain.

It's a seductive idea. The popularity of body education has been soaring, buoyed by legions of satisfied customers. In the past five years, the number of trained Feldenkrais

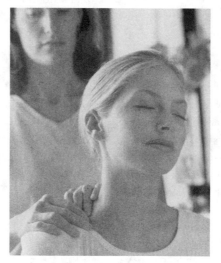

Get your head
into the right position
over your spine,
Alexander said, and
you'll relieve a constant
source of muscle
tension and gain
energy.

practitioners has doubled, says Andrea Wiener, assistant director of the Feldenkrais Guild of North America, in Portland, Oregon; in 2000, it topped 2,000. The demand has even convinced some tightfisted insurers to cover visits to practitioners or to offer classes.

Unfortunately, there hasn't been much research on these methods. The concept underlying such therapies—that there are both right and wrong ways to stand and walk—has yet to be proven. Orthopedists (doctors who specialize in muscle and joint problems) point out that many people with abnormal strides and stances can move with ease, while others with picture-perfect posture suffer from crippling joint or back pain.

How are bodywork practitioners able to satisfy clients? Perhaps in the same way a masseuse can find your cricks and knots, they can intuitively identify overworked muscles and stressed joints in your body and suggest ways of moving that ease the strain on these areas.

Whatever may be behind the treatments, some sufferers of low-back pain, knee pain, muscle aches, headaches, stress—even some people with cerebral palsy, multiple sclerosis, or lupus—claim to have found relief with one or another of these methods. Is there a bodywork treatment that will turn you into a true believer? Here's a guide to help you decide.

Feldenkrais Method: Mend Your Moves

During World War II, Moshe Feldenkrais spent most of his time aboard a ship in the British Navy. All that rocking to and fro turned a nagging knee injury into a near-crippling infirmity. After the war, the Polish-born physicist came up with his form of body education while teaching himself to walk without pain. The goal is to rewire the body, in effect. Feldenkrais believed the brain and nervous system will choose the simplest, most energy-efficient way of moving if presented with that option. Examine the way you look over your shoulder, he said. Break down the motion, repeating small parts of it to increase your flexibility and find the path of least resistance, and eventually the easiest means of glancing over your shoulder becomes ingrained.

TYPICAL VISIT: The Feldenkrais Method is taught in both classes and in one-on-one sessions. In individual sessions, you either lie or sit on a massage table while the instructor gently guides your limbs through small parts of motions; ideally, you'll learn to feel the difference between your usual patterns and the effortless ones.

SESSION LENGTH: 45 to 60 minutes.

COST PER VISIT: $60 to $90.

For more information, call the Feldenkrais Guild at 800-775-2118 or find them on the Web at www.feldenkrais.com.

Alexander Technique: The Posture Prescription

In 1900, an Australian actor named F. Matthias Alexander began struggling with his voice during performances. He studied his posture in a mirror and determined that he habitually tilted his head back as he spoke, straining his neck. "Unlearning" the tic, he restored his voice and developed a theory: One could treat a number of problems, such as shoulder pain and even fatigue, by getting the head, the neck, and the spine into proper alignment. The head must be in a position that requires almost no effort on the part of the neck or back muscles to support it. Find that magic spot, Alexander said, and you'll relieve a constant source of muscle tension. You'll gain energy and be able to address other habits that have led to, say, your tennis elbow.

TYPICAL VISIT: The plan is to relearn every position you find yourself in: sitting, walking, lying down, jumping. In one-on-one visits or as part of a class, you'll go through the motions of daily life while the instructor watches the way you carry yourself, noting how your head position relates to, say, a hitch in your step, a chronically tensed shoulder, abbreviated arm swings, an unconscious slouch, or any other physical habit that restricts motion. As you move, the instructor will offer suggestions and guide your limbs.

SESSION LENGTH: 30 to 60 minutes.

COST PER VISIT: $35 to $75.

For more information, call The American Society for the Alexander Technique at 800-473-0620 or find them on the Web at www.alexandertech.org.

Trager Approach: Rock Away Rigidity

Milton Trager, a boxer who later became a physician, stumbled on his technique when he offered to give his trainer a massage. The man was impressed, so the 18-year-old Trager went home and set to work on his father, whose low-back problems had made his legs numb. After two sessions, Dad was better. By 1959 Trager had started a regular practice doing his special brand of bodywork. This may be the most relaxing form of body re-education: Practitioners jiggle, cradle, rock, and vibrate the muscles and limbs of reclining patients. Trager believed the feeling of freedom and lightness you experience while this is done could break patterns of tension and rigidity that stem from old injuries, daily stresses, or emotional trauma. Your nerves, muscles, and brain retain that feeling, he said, so you can move without tension and pain.

TYPICAL VISIT: After the therapist enters a meditative state referred to as "hooking up," he or she tugs gently on your limbs and musculature. This therapy has homework, as well—a set of light exercises that you perform on your own to reinforce the subconscious lessons learned during visits.

SESSION LENGTH: 60 to 90 minutes.

COST PER VISIT: $40 to $100.

For more information call Trager International at 216-896-9383 or find them on the Web at www.trager.com.

Aston-Patterning: Reshape Your Environment

Aston-Patterning is an offshoot of the deep-tissue massage called Rolfing. Biochemist Ida Rolf believed physical and emotional stress cause the fascia, the tough tendons and ligaments that tie the skeleton and muscles together, to become inflexible. This rigidity causes pain and limited mobility; the treatment is vigorous massage. In 1977, dancer Judith Aston combined her own teachings, which are much like an ergonomics lesson, with a gentler version of Rolfing. She believes the progress achieved during the massage must be reinforced by repetitive exercises and an ergonomically sound workplace and home.

TYPICAL VISIT: An Aston-Patterning session begins with an evaluation of your fitness, home and work environments, and movement habits—the way you stand, walk, sit, bend, and reach. With this information, along with your detailed physical measurements, the practitioner suggests ways to improve your environment, such as adjusting your chair or sleeping position. After the massage, you'll be coached through drills to help you learn effortless ways of

moving based on the configuration of your body.

SESSION LENGTH: 90 to 120 minutes.

COST PER VISIT: $75 to $130.

For more information, call The Aston-Patterning Training Center at 775-831-8228 or find them on the Web at www.astonenterprises.com.

Hellerwork: Tame Your Emotions to Heal Tension

Like Aston-Patterning, Hellerwork combines Rolfing-style massage with ergonomics. But the key contribution of Joseph Heller, former aerospace engineer and one-time president of the Rolf Institute, is to delve into emotional issues that he believes express themselves in muscle and joint pain. Just as stress can lead to an aching back, Heller thinks attitudes and emotional trauma can lead to unconscious muscle tension, which in turn causes injury or chronic pain.

TYPICAL VISIT: As with Aston-Patterning, Hellerwork requires a thorough assessment of your movements and environment, and you'll receive advice on ways to improve both. Then the instructor will probe for emotional stress and conflict that may be exacerbating your problems and will encourage you to address those issues. Finally, there's deep-tissue massage.

SESSION LENGTH: 60 to 90 minutes.

COST PER VISIT: $75 to $150.

For more information, call The Hellerwork Institute at 800-392-3900 or find them on the Web at www.hellerwork.com. ✳

---

if a massage is enough

A quick way to find a certified practitioner is via the American Massage Therapy Association. Visit its Web site at www.amtamassage.org or call 888-843-2682.

---

f i t   t o   c o p e
Ninety-six percent of women agree that if they feel fit and healthy,
they're better able to handle other areas of their lives.
—*Health* Women in Motion study, 2001

FOR DEPRESSION, EXERCISE WORKS BETTER THAN DRUGS

People go on and on about the mood lift they get from working out. That ain't the half of it: In treating depression, exercise works as well as drugs.

Psychologists and exercise physiologists alike have toyed with the idea that regular workouts can beat the blues. After all, studies show that depression seems less likely to strike people who exercise. But that could just mean happy people like activity, while depressed people prefer to sit.

So recently, Duke University psychologists decided to tackle the matter head on. They recruited 156 men and women age 50 and older who suffered from major depression. One group walked or jogged for 30 minutes, three days a week. Another group took the antidepressant Zoloft, and a third bunch both exercised and took the medication.

Though the patients who were getting medication began to respond sooner than the exercise-only folks, at the end of four months all three of the groups were markedly better.

Without question, regular workouts were an effective treatment. But exercise takes commitment, and depression is a tenacious malady. Would the patients relapse?

The researchers checked back six months after the study concluded to see how people were faring on their own.

The news was mixed: In the combination group, 31 percent of the subjects had fallen back into depression; in the Zoloft-only group, 38 percent. But among the exercisers, just 8 percent saw their symptoms return.

"Exercise is a viable alternative to drugs," says lead researcher James Blumenthal. "It may not be for everybody, but if a patient's motivated, the chances of beating depression may actually be better."

Protect yourself from the FDA

Lotronex was touted as a breakthrough drug for irritable bowel syndrome. But as reports of side effects spread, including links to at least five deaths, the Food and Drug Administration (FDA) was forced to ponder regulatory action. In the end, the manufacturer pulled Lotronex from the U.S. market, only 10 months after its release.

Sadly, it's a too familiar story. Between 1997 and 2000, the FDA either banned or pressured manufacturers to withdraw 10 prescription drugs. Together, the drugs were implicated in hundreds of deaths.

Why the crisis? Some experts say that as the FDA approves more drugs, more withdrawals will come. But critics say that the agency, by expediting the review process, has let standards slide. Either way, you're left in the lurch.

Here's how to help yourself.

LOOK FOR ALTERNATIVES. New drugs are rarely your only option. Duract, for example, which the FDA banned in 1998, was just one of many available painkillers.

ASK QUESTIONS. Why has your doctor recommended a particular drug? What's the approved dosage? Are there serious side effects to watch for? Do your doctor and pharmacist know about any other drugs you're taking?

BE WARY. To win FDA approval, a manufacturer must submit evidence of a drug's safety and effectiveness. But often, fewer than 2,000 people have taken the medication—not enough to uncover many problems. "We approve drugs based on clinical trials," says Alastair J. J. Wood, a professor of medicine at Vanderbilt University. "Then we run an experiment to see if they're safe and effective in the real world."

"The most dangerous drugs are the new ones," says Larry D. Sasich, a pharmacist with the consumer watchdog group Public Citizen. He advocates waiting until a drug has been available for at least five years unless it's a "breakthrough" medicine. If you have cancer, the risk of a promising new drug may be worth it. If you have chronic diarrhea, though, it's a completely different story.

slowing down the progress of
Alzheimer's Disease

It's terrifying and, for now at least, incurable. But we just might be able to slow this brain-ravaging disease.

BY JAMIE TALAN

It wasn't until she reached her early 70s that Anne Rosen began having trouble remembering the plots of movies she'd just seen and the characters from novels she'd just read. "I thought I was simply getting old," the retired bank secretary recalls thinking. "It never occurred to me that it might be serious."

Rosen's husband and children, however, grew concerned about her increasing forgetfulness and suggested she see a doctor. To her shock, tests revealed that areas of the brain associated with learning and memory had begun to shrink. Rosen's doctor told her what she was totally unprepared to hear: Rosen had Alzheimer's disease.

But the day-to-day reality of the diagnosis has not been as earth-shattering as Rosen had expected. Because the disease was identified so early, she's been able to take steps to slow its progress. By availing herself of the treatments that provide modest benefits in later stages of Alzheimer's, she's fended off the worst symptoms for the past four years.

"My short-term memory hasn't improved much," says Rosen, "but I can still play with my grandchildren and have discussions with my husband about archaeology and history."

Without treatment, Rosen's story might well have unfolded quite differently; typically, people who have had Alzheimer's for as long as she has have already begun to show dramatic changes in personality and behavior and are unable to meet the basic demands of daily life. Rosen's experience lends support to a theory that is gaining ground among those who study aging and dementia: The sooner people with Alzheimer's get medical care, the better are their chances for living longer and fuller lives.

Forgetting names and numbers is normal at any age—but sometimes it can be an early warning of dementia.

There's still no cure for the frightening and mystifying disease that afflicts 4 million Americans and will claim 360,000 more each year. But new focus on earlier diagnosis and treatment may significantly delay its course. What's more, researchers are testing various medications in people as young as 55 who show signs of Alzheimer's. Results aren't in yet, but if these remedies work, the world of aging could be dramatically different from what it is today.

The key to early treatment, of course, is early detection. While the only indisputable diagnosis can be made after death, when an autopsy reveals the havoc wreaked on the brain, researchers have recently made tremendous strides in recognizing Alzheimer's in living patients. Some diagnostic methods are high-tech; magnetic resonance imaging (MRI), for example, can show whether the brain structures associated with memory are shrinking—a sign that Alzheimer's has taken hold. Positron-emission tomography (PET) scans can reveal changes in the way glucose is metabolized in parts of the brain that tend to be most affected by Alzheimer's. Using these and other tools, neurologists can diagnose Alzheimer's accurately up to 90 percent of the time.

One study suggests that Alzheimer's can be reliably predicted well before an MRI or PET scan delivers its verdict. In 1986, Ronald Petersen, director of the Mayo Clinic Alzheimer's Disease Center in Rochester, Minnesota, began tracking the brain function of 1,200 people over age 65, using tests that measure memory, comprehension, and verbal skills. Over time, Petersen's team noted that about 150 people were having significant memory problems but showed none of the other classic signs of dementia. Aside from their abnormal forgetfulness, they were functioning and competent—they drove, wrote checks, cooked, lived alone. Petersen labeled their condition mild cognitive impairment (MCI), which he says is a distinct transitional state that occurs between regular aging and Alzheimer's.

"It's normal to have occasional memory lapses—to forget where you parked the car or where you put the keys," says Petersen. "But people with MCI forget important things, like doctors' appointments or dates with friends. The family begins to suspect something's wrong."

That suspicion usually is correct. Petersen found that 12 percent of the MCI group progressed to a diagnosis of Alzheimer's every year—compared with 1 to 2 percent of the control group. Within six years, 80 percent of the MCI patients were suffering the effects of Alzheimer's.

"Given that high percentage, we believe that when we see MCI we're seeing the earliest observable signs of dementia," says Petersen, who published his results in 1999. "Now that neurologists know how to identify MCI, we can test the belief that medical intervention can delay the progress of Alzheimer's."

As researchers learn how Alzheimer's works, they've also learned more about how it might be held in check. It's known, for example, that the neurons that produce acetylcholine, a chemical that helps us learn and remember, are among the first to die when Alzheimer's sets in. Three related drugs—Cognex, Aricept, and, most recently, Exelon—work by increasing the brain's store of acetylcholine. These are the only medications currently approved for the treatment of Alzheimer's; they are now being tested in people diagnosed with MCI.

Scientists suspect that inflammation may also contribute to the demise of some brain cells. A study conducted at Johns Hopkins School of Public Health found that the incidence of Alzheimer's was lower among people who frequently used nonsteroidal anti-inflammatory drugs (NSAIDs), such as Advil, Aleve, and Motrin, than it was among those who took Tylenol or no painkillers. The National Institute on Aging is currently studying 320 people ages 55 and over who are diagnosed with Alzheimer's to see if NSAIDs slow the disease.

Researchers also think that neurons can fall victim to free radicals—unstable molecules that damage cells—and they are looking at vitamin E as a potential antidote to these toxic substances. Scientists at Columbia University College of Physicians and Surgeons reported that antioxidants such as vitamin E helped Alzheimer's patients stay out of nursing homes seven months longer than those who took a placebo. Scientists are also studying the brain-protecting capacity of estrogen, which can work as an antioxidant and an anti-inflammatory, as well as a promoter of acetylcholine. Initial results show it's probably not effective once Alzheimer's has taken hold, but the hormone may be useful as a preventive.

> Early detection and treatment may put the brakes on Alzheimer's, but some experts question the value of telling a patient there's a train wreck ahead.

Petersen's research on MCI prompted a study that researchers hope will shed even more light on the value of early treatment. In 1999, the federal government (and two pharmaceutical companies) embarked on the Memory Impairment Study at more than 70 medical centers in the United States and Canada. The three-year study will test dementia-delaying powers of Aricept and vitamin E on 780 volunteers, ages 55 to 90, who meet Petersen's criteria for MCI.

Petersen stresses that these possible remedies are still in the testing stage—and that they are not cures. "We know some drugs can alleviate the symptoms of Alzheimer's, but none of them stop or reverse the disease," he says. "And we still don't know how long it would be safe to take them or for how long they would even work."

Then too, there are the psychological considerations. Early detection and treatment may put the brakes on Alzheimer's, but some experts question the value of telling a patient there's a train wreck ahead. Is it useful to tell someone she's going to have full-blown Alzheimer's in 10 years when there's no cure and the long-term effects of most treatments are unknown? Other experts answer that it's crucial for patients to have as much time as possible to prepare themselves and their families and to participate clear-headedly in the decisions that affect their futures so profoundly.

For Rosen, the diagnostic label is irrelevant. Every day she takes her many pills: an anti-inflammatory, estrogen, Aricept, vitamin E, and an experimental drug she gets from a pharmacy in Germany. Once or twice a week she and her husband attend meetings of the Early Alzheimer's Club at the Long Island Alzheimer's Foundation. There, Rosen and 12 others share stories of coping, hear experts speak on the latest research developments, and joke about their own faltering memories. "It's reassuring to know that other people with brains still have Alzheimer's," she quips.

"It doesn't matter to me if what I have is mild cognitive impairment or early Alzheimer's," she says. "The important thing is that I keep busy and my mind is always active. I travel. I spend time with my family. I laugh." ✳

other memory stealers

You're at the market and forget what you came to buy. Worse, you run into your neighbor at the checkout line and can't recall her name. Are you losing it? Don't panic. It's normal to blank on names no matter how old you are, and spacing out on what you're doing is really no big deal either—as long as you don't get lost on the way home or consistently overlook vital matters like turning off the stove. If you're under 65, you probably don't have Alzheimer's—plenty of other culprits can rob your memory bank, and most of them are treatable. Here are a few.

STRESS can mess with short-term memory in at least two ways, according to Paul J. Rosch, president of the American Institute of Stress. First, it increases the production of free radicals, which accelerate shrinkage of the hippocampus, a crucial part of the brain's memory loop. Second, people under prolonged stress have high levels of the hormone cortisol, which also causes the hippocampus to shrink. Just one more good reason to find ways to let off steam and lighten your load.

DEPRESSION, like stress, is associated with high cortisol levels, but some experts think depressed people experience memory problems because they are unable to concentrate; it's not a matter of forgetting but of not paying attention. Some antianxiety drugs and certain drug combinations can have similar effects.

MENOPAUSE and forgetfulness often seem to go hand in hand, but it's not clear that they have a cause-and-effect relationship. Some experts speculate that because menopausal women are frequently overtired—a result of shifting hormones—they're not as sharp as they once were.

HYPOTHYROIDISM causes every cell in the body to slow down and can, thus, hinder mental focus. A blood test will determine if your thyroid's on the blink.

EXCESSIVE DRINKING can impair memory even when the drinker is sober. Alcoholics are short of vitamin B-1, a deficiency that over time hinders memory.

SUDDEN DAMAGE TO THE BRAIN, such as a head injury or stroke, can cause irreversible short-term memory loss. See your doctor if you experience an abrupt, dramatic loss of memory.

hypnosis:
drug-free pain relief

Long regarded as mental voodoo, hypnosis is going
mainstream and winning respect, treating everything
from asthma to labor pain. Should you try it?

BY KELLY JAMES-ENGER

Lisa Parker, 38, had a somewhat unusual
pregnancy with her second child. In
addition to the typical high-potency
vitamins, OB-GYN exams, and childbirth
classes, she practiced hypnotism. "I'd had a long,
hard labor with my first daughter, and didn't
want to go through that again," says the Virginia
Beach, Virginia, mother.

Seven months into her pregnancy, Parker visited
Donald Lynch, M.D., a urologist who uses hypnotic
suggestion in his practice at the Sentara Cancer Institute at Eastern Virginia School of Medicine. He
taught her two techniques to help her during delivery:
He had her imagine she was alone in a swimming pool,
beginning in the shallow end. The deeper she went
into the pool, the more relaxed she would become.
Then he said to visualize a series of numbered dials,
each controlling a part of her body—head, back,
stomach, and so on. By selecting a dial and turning

it backward, the doctor suggested, she could reduce
the intensity of her contractions.

Parker practiced the techniques at home during the
last trimester of her pregnancy, so she was ready when
her water broke. In the delivery room, she used both
the pool imagery and the pain dials throughout her
eight-hour labor. It worked: She delivered baby
Taylor without so much as an Advil—and she could
talk during the most intense contraction. The only
discomfort she experienced was a "feeling of pressure" as the baby crowned. "My husband said if he
hadn't sat there and watched it, he would never have
believed it," Parker says.

Parker is one of a growing number of people using
hypnotic techniques as part of treatment for an array
of medical conditions from asthma to cancer. "When
I entered practice 25 years ago, I'd get two or three
calls a year about hypnosis," Lynch says. "Now I get
two or three a week."

Hundreds of published studies have helped educate
doctors about the health benefits of hypnosis, and

Some believe hypnosis is just a form of relaxation, but advocates
say it's a powerful adjunct to traditional medical care.
Research shows the body undergoes a series
of physiological changes under hypnosis.

medical schools including Stanford, Tulane, UCLA, and Temple University offer hypnosis courses to their medical students and residents. Lynch and other medical experts attribute the newfound appreciation to the groundswell of support for alternative medicine among both patients and physicians. "There is a growing sense on the part of patients to take more control of their own care, and complementary and alternative medicine is one way that they can do that," he says. "Hypnosis is one of the more refined and acceptable forms of alternative medicine."

Conventional medicine is exploring the technique: Medical schools at Tulane, Stanford, and UCLA teach hypnosis.

If you have ever watched the Sci-Fi Channel, you probably have a good mental image of the stereotypical scene of hypnosis: the hypnotist—usually a rather villainous character—intoning, "You are getting sleepy, sleeeepy," as he dangles a pocket watch back and forth before the "victim's" eyes. That portrayal, Lynch says, has perpetuated the idea that hypnosis is a form of mind control, when in reality the person being hypnotized is the one in charge. The hypnotist simply guides the person to what Lynch calls "a state of enhanced imagination," in which she has better control of her perceptions and responses in certain situations than she does otherwise. That means a stage hypnotist can't

Move Over, Prozac!

In a survey by Harvard investigators, more than 50 percent of people who said they suffer from severe depression or anxiety attacks reported having tried some form of alternative treatment—whether it was acupuncture, laughter therapy, herbs like Saint-John's-wort, or hypnosis. Half of those who had sought alternative treatment said it was very helpful, a satisfaction rate about the same as reported for conventional medicine. Among the 2,000 participants, relaxation techniques and spiritual healing were the most common choices.

actually compel you to bark like a dog at the sound of a doorbell under hypnosis, unless you somehow allow it to happen. Granted, a talented stage hypnotist can make it seem as if he is controlling the guinea pigs who dare to volunteer from the audience. But in most cases volunteers do not want to disappoint the audience or their peers and, while in a trance, respond to the hypnotist's suggestions to play along.

The same "suggestibility" can make hypnosis an effective medical tool. Patients can experience a number of physiological changes while in trance, the deep state of relaxation triggered by hypnosis. Heart rate and breathing slow, blood pressure drops, and levels of the stress hormones cortisol and adrenaline may also decrease. These physical effects may explain why hypnosis can be helpful in the treatment of disorders aggravated by stress and anxiety, such as asthma. In fact, asthma, particularly in children, is one of the most promising areas for hypnotic

One OB-GYN says his patients who practice hypnosis need less medicine in labor and have lower C-section rates.

treatment. A recent review of 20 published articles on the effects of hypnosis on asthma found that in 16 studies, the practice reduced or eliminated asthma symptoms. For many asthma sufferers who try hypnotic methods, the treatment involves learning self-hypnosis, where a doctor might have the asthmatic induce and overcome an attack while in a trance state to teach how to alleviate asthma without medication.

Researchers have also found that under hypnosis, pain-related neurological signals to the brain are blocked, and blood flow to specific body parts decreases. That may be why women like Lisa Parker could make it through labor and delivery without medication, and why hypnosis sometimes proves effective in pain management after surgery and during cancer treatment. In one recent study on pregnant teenagers, those who used hypnotic techniques had fewer complications during delivery and were released from the hospital earlier than those who didn't. With hypnosis, "instead of the contractions controlling the patient, the patient controls the labor process," says Larry Goldman, M.D., an OB-GYN in Fort Myers, Florida, who uses the technique with about a third of his patients. He asserts that women who use hypnosis during labor and delivery need less pain medication than those who don't, and have a much lower rate of cesarean sections—5 percent compared with 15 percent.

Whether hypnosis would work for you as well as it did for Lisa Parker, though, depends on whether you're able to be hypnotized at all. Ten percent of people are not susceptible to hypnosis, according to a review of surveys published by the American Society of Clinical Hypnosis. About a quarter of the population is considered "highly responsive," and everyone else falls somewhere in between.

If you decide to try it, you can expect to begin with a simple interview. Most hypnotherapists spend the first session asking you questions to determine whether you're a good candidate. During subsequent meetings, the hypnotherapist uses a variety of techniques to help you relax. One common method is "fixation induction," in which you focus on a particular point in the room or close your eyes and imagine yourself in a peaceful, pleasant place. As you do, the hypnotherapist encourages you to relax until your heart rate and breathing slow. On average, it takes about 20 minutes to slip into a trance.

The hypnotherapist then leads you through visualizations, perhaps asking you to picture a favorite vacation spot or relive happy memories. If you're preparing for surgery, you might imagine yourself awakening afterward feeling comfortable and secure in the knowledge that the procedure went well. Most sessions last about an hour, and often the therapist will record them so you can practice at home.

You should know, however, that some physicians don't consider hypnosis a valid form of medical treatment. Self-described "hypnosis skeptic" Robert A. Baker, Ph.D., professor emeritus of psychology at the University of Kentucky and author of *They Call it Hypnosis* (Prometheus Books, 1990), claims there is no such thing as a hypnotic trance. He says that any benefits associated with it are due to the subject's state of deep relaxation or an attempt to please the hypnotherapist. " 'Hypnosis' is just using relaxation and suggestion to help people," Baker says. "We really ought to change its name and call it 'relaxation therapy.' "

Brian Berman, M.D., director of the complementary medicine program at the University of Maryland School of Medicine, notes that hypnosis has not yet reached its full medical potential. "In a 1997 national survey, approximately 50 percent of primary-care physicians considered hypnosis to be a part of mainstream medical treatment," Berman says. "In the future, it will probably become more and more mainstream, particularly with pain-related conditions." ✳

Freelance writer Kelly James-Enger lives in Downers Grove, Illinois, and writes about health, fitness, and nutrition.

HOW TO FIND A
hypnotherapist

Because there aren't any national certification or licensing standards for hypnotherapists, don't just go with the first one you find in the phone book. The best bet is to ask your physician for a referral or contact the American Society of Clinical Hypnosis (630-980-4740 or www.asch.net) for a list of medical professionals in your area who use hypnosis in their practices. As with all alternative treatments, make sure you tell your primary-care physician if you decide to use hypnosis.

how to choose the best
pill for your pain

Choosing wisely can mean less risk—and more relief. Here's what to reach for when you hurt.

BY JAN GREENE

If your head didn't already throb like the dickens, the effort of choosing a pain reliever would bring on one doozy of a headache. Advil, Bayer, Tylenol, Aleve: Who has the brain space to keep them straight? You've heard that one is best for cramps, another might give you an ulcer, and a third doesn't do a thing for muscle aches. And here you are with Costco's grande bottle of your favorite pain reliever, the one you use for whatever ails you. Isn't that good enough?

It's true that despite the array of choices, it often doesn't matter which pain reliever you take. But more frequently than you might think, choosing wisely can mean the difference between blessed relief and discomfort that grinds on unabated—or even a new pain caused by medicine that was supposed to help. It's time to open your mind and your medicine cabinet. Here's how to make sure you find relief on its shelves.

Do I need a different pain reliever for different aches and pains?

There are three main types of pain relievers, and each has its time and place. There's good old aspirin (Bayer and Ecotrin, for example, and their generic pals); acetaminophen (Tylenol, for instance); and finally, the NSAIDs—aka, nonsteroidal anti-inflammatory drugs—which include ibuprofen (Advil and Motrin, among others), naproxen sodium (Aleve), and ketoprofen (Actron and Orudis).

For fever and run-of-the-mill headaches, it usually doesn't matter which one you take. But remember

Aspirin helps protect against blood clots, heart attacks, and strokes. If you're at risk of heart disease, your doctor may suggest a daily "low-strength" aspirin.

this key difference between the groups: Aspirin and especially the NSAIDs can reduce inflammation, while acetaminophen can't. That means any NSAID is better able to ease joints inflamed by arthritis or swollen after running on a hard surface. They're also your best bet for menstrual cramps. In fact, downing a 400-milligram dose before cramps occur can stave them off completely.

On the other hand, if you think NSAIDs will reduce your pain after one too many steps on the Stair-Master, think again. Studies have shown that anti-inflammatories aren't effective at relieving muscle soreness. That's because inflammation isn't the only problem behind this kind of discomfort. Exercise tears muscle fibers, and the body, worried that invaders may be causing damage, responds by unleash-ing immune chemi-cals known as histamines (the substances that make people with allergies feel congested when pollen proliferates). In fact, one researcher is studying antihistamines to see if they might make overworked muscles feel better.

When should you favor acetaminophen over other options? If you get headaches often, it's probably the best remedy, as it can be taken regularly without risk-ing the side effects that can crop up with frequent use of aspirin or NSAIDs.

Finally, sometimes nothing but aspirin will do. By preventing platelets from sticking together, it helps protect against blood clots, heart attacks, and strokes. If you're at risk of heart disease, your doctor may suggest a daily "low-strength" aspirin.

Which pain reliever is the safest?

All are quite safe when taken as directed, but no drug is risk free. Acetaminophen is the least likely to cause side effects when used properly, but in some cases, people who consume more than three drinks a day have wound up with liver failure or gone into a coma after taking a higher-than-recommended dose of the drug. If you're a heavy drinker, check with your doctor before taking acetaminophen.

The anti-inflammatories, including aspirin and NSAIDs, can cause upset stomachs or ulcers in people who take them all the time or who have underlying gastrointestinal problems. The side effects are directly related to how these drugs work. They inhibit fatty acids known as prostaglandins, some of which play a role in pain and inflammation. The problem is, other prostaglandins safeguard the gastrointestinal system by increasing protective mucus in the stomach lining and reducing acid production. Restraining the "bad" prostaglandins also reduces the "good" ones. (Prostaglandins are responsible for the ache of menstrual cramps too, which is a good reason why women who are plagued with them should keep NSAIDs within easy reach.)

If you're popping a pill more than three times a week, you should work with your doctor to find and treat the cause of the pain.

Keep in mind that regularly taking a pill for recurrent headaches can actually make them worse.

Most people with a chronic stomach disorder, such as gastroesophageal reflux disease, should steer clear of aspirin and NSAIDs. If you're generally healthy, take these pain relievers with milk or a meal to avoid minor stomach upset. If you have a reaction, don't simply add an antacid to the mix; you may just mask the pain until your stomach's really in trouble. Instead, switch to acetaminophen and check with your doctor.

It's also important to realize that aspirin increases the risk of Reye's syndrome—which can be fatal—when taken by a child or teen suffering from the flu or chicken pox.

No matter what pain reliever you take, remember: Just because it's over-the-counter (OTC) medication doesn't mean you can up the dose willy-nilly. Maybe you've doubled up when you've had an especially painful menstrual period and nothing bad hap-pened. But serious side effects can pop up without warning. If the standard dose isn't cutting it, ask your doctor how much you can safely take.

What's best when I really hurt?

Aleve's active ingredient is especially long lasting; that can be helpful for the all-day ache of arthritis, though it may be overkill for a minor tension headache. And extra-strength versions of OTC remedies have more of the active ingredient than their regular-strength cousins, so they cut down on the number of pills you must pop to soothe a big ouch.

Your doctor may prescribe a higher-octane model of one of the OTCs if you've had minor surgery, say, and need some stronger pain relief; this too contains the same active ingredient as the drugstore remedy, only more of it. The advantage to using prescription pills is that both your pharmacist and your physician can keep tabs on your intake and any side effects.

A new class of prescription pain relievers known as Cox-2 inhibitors (Vioxx, Celebrex) is also on the market. They work like the NSAIDs but more judiciously: They single out the prostaglandin that causes pain and don't mess with the ones that protect the lining of the stomach and intestines. Because Cox-2 inhibitors are new and much more expensive than over-the-counter drugs, doctors are reserving them for people with chronic illnesses such as osteoarthritis whose daily pills have caused stomach problems.

Do I need to worry about interactions with other drugs?

It's worth keeping an eye out. One of the most common problems is that people can double up on pain relief. Many cold remedies, for instance, include acetaminophen or aspirin, either of which could be enough to give you an overdose if you're also taking a

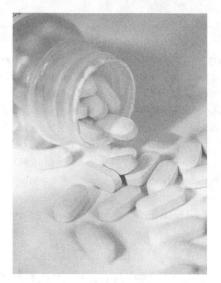

The advantage to using prescription pills is that both your pharmacist and your physician can keep tabs on your intake and any side effects.

pill specifically for your headache. Other problem pairings: Aspirin interferes with the ability of blood to clot, so anyone taking a blood-thinning medicine (such as Coumadin) should avoid it. So should people taking steroids or other drugs for arthritis, diabetes, gout, or cancer, because the combination can trigger bleeding in the stomach.

Can I take these drugs long-term?

Yes, but if you're popping an over-the-counter pill more than three times a week, you should work with your doctor to find and treat the underlying cause of the pain and to avoid side effects.

Keep in mind that regularly taking a pill for recurrent headaches can actually make them worse. Daily or near-daily use of analgesics shuts down the body's production of its own pain-fighting chemicals, making headache sufferers more vulnerable to pain once the medication wears off. Some folks even have to be hospitalized to get weaned from the drugs.

Bottom line: You don't want to pop pain relievers like candy. But you know they're more precious than that. Treated wisely, they're the treasure in your medicine chest that can vanquish a headache or cramps and make life worth living again. ✳

---

go ahead and save

Some drugs just don't seem the same in generic form. If you're on thyroid hormone, for instance, and switch to generic, you need to be retested. But with pain relievers, the only difference you'll feel is in the weight of your wallet.

the 7 medical tests
EVERY WOMAN
should have

A new study highlights the most important preventive measures for women. Are you missing out?

BY PETER JARET

ourtney Michaels wouldn't describe her-self as wild, exactly. But at 22, she has had a few sexual relationships. Something she's not sure she's ever had, however, is a test for chlamydia, a common sexually transmitted disease that can cause sterility in women if left untreated.

"I'm embarrassed to say this, but I'm not even sure how the test is done," says Michaels (her name has been changed), a manager with a telecommunications company in Denver. "Maybe my doctor has done it as part of a regular exam. But I wouldn't have known to ask for it."

The fact is that Michaels can't neces-sarily count on her doctor. A recent study of more than 1,200 health-care providers in Colorado found that only 54 percent regularly tested their patients for chlamydia—despite the fact that the U.S. Preventive Services Task Force recommends testing all sexually active women under age 25 for the disease, which typically causes no noticeable symptoms and often goes undetected.

Unfortunately, this is not the only medical test that women aren't getting as often as they should. In June 2001, the Partnership for Prevention, a nonprofit

coalition of the top preventive-care experts in the country, released a report showing that many of the tried-and-true procedures that can reduce illness and often save lives are not being used frequently enough. "In some cases, effective preventive tests or treatments weren't reaching even half the people who should be getting them," says Ashley Coffield, a senior research fellow with the Partnership for Prevention and author of the report.

To help doctors and patients zero in on the ones that matter most, Coffield and her colleagues ranked preventive services on a scale of I to IO, according to how well they work in averting unnecessary illness or

A surprising new study shows that in some cases, effective screening tests aren't reaching even half the women who could benefit from them.

death. Some of the high scorers come as no surprise. Childhood vaccinations topped the list; programs that help smokers kick the habit weren't far behind. But the list also included several surprises—particularly for women. Here are seven of the top-scoring tests, plus everything you need to know before you schedule one of them.

Pap Smear

Cervical cancer, once the leading cancer killer among women—now ranks seventh, thanks in large part to early detection. Still, one in five women don't receive Pap tests as often as recommended—and among the poor, that number is even higher. Every year, almost 13,000 women are diagnosed with cervical cancer; more than 4,400 will die from it. Most of those deaths could be prevented.

Who should get it: Women 18 and older should get a Pap smear at least once every three years. Some experts believe that annual testing could prevent even more deaths.

How it's done: A sample of cells scraped from the cervix during a vaginal exam is placed on a glass slide and examined in a laboratory for signs of abnormalities that could indicate cancer.

About one-fourth of American women
with high blood pressure don't know they have it. Nationwide, average readings are on the rise.

Blood Pressure Test

Twenty-five percent of American women with high blood pressure are not aware that they have the condition, which significantly increases their risks of heart disease and stroke. What's more, after years of falling, the nation's average blood pressure readings are now on the rise—just one more reason that the test is so important. If you find out that you have high blood pressure, do something about it: Less than one in three women with the condition are successfully controlling it, according to the National Heart, Lung, and Blood Institute.

Who should get it: Everyone, at least once a year, according to the National Institute on Aging.

How it's done: Blood pressure is measured using an adjustable cuff that wraps around your arm. A consistent blood pressure reading of 140/90 mm Hg or higher is considered high blood pressure.

Flu Vaccination

For most people, a case of the flu means a week at home feeling rotten; but during an outbreak of this

Twenty percent of all women
aren't tested regularly for cervical cancer. **Are you one of them?**

disease, as many as 175,000 Americans may land in the hospital—and up to 40,000 die from complications related to influenza. The vaccine can reduce the risk of contracting the flu by up to 90 percent. Yet a recent study found that less than half of high-risk women ages 50 to 64 were routinely vaccinated; only 32 percent of men in the same age range were.

Who should get it: The fatality rate from influenza begins to rise at around age 45—especially among people who have lung disease, heart disease, or diabetes. For that reason, the American Academy of Family Physicians recommends that both men and women 50 years and older receive an annual influenza vaccination.

How it's done: A simple shot in the arm is all there is to it. You may experience some soreness at the injection site for a day or two afterward. The vaccine is incubated in eggs, so if you are allergic to them, talk to your doctor before getting the shot. The best time to get vaccinated against influenza is in October and November, just before the virus begins to circulate. But even during the peak of flu season, a shot can protect you—as long as you haven't already developed symptoms.

Colorectal Cancer Screening

The tests doctors use to screen for cancer of the colon and rectum may not be pleasant, but they can save lives. Almost 136,000 Americans are diagnosed with colorectal cancer every year, and 57,000 die of the disease, making it the second deadliest cancer in the United States. By indicating trouble in time to begin treatment, two screening tests—fecal occult blood testing and sigmoidoscopy—can significantly lower the risk of death from colorectal cancer. Harvard Medical School experts recently showed that screening is particularly effective in increasing the life expectancy among women. Unfortunately, a survey conducted last March by the National Colorectal Cancer Alliance found that only 28 percent of women over the age

Getting regular mammograms can't
prevent breast cancer, but it can catch the disease before
it becomes a serious threat to your health.

of 50 planned to get a colorectal cancer screening in the next year.

Who should get it: Women and men over age 50. Experts recommend getting a fecal occult blood test every year and a sigmoidoscopy every five years.

How it's done: For the fecal occult blood test, a stool specimen is tested at doctor's office or lab for traces of blood.

Sigmoidoscopy requires the insertion of a flexible, narrow tube that allows the doctor to see inside the rectum and colon in order to check for abnormalities.

Cholesterol Test

Cholesterol clogs arteries and can lead to heart attacks and stroke. Lifestyle changes, such as a lower fat diet, and cholesterol-lowering drugs can bring sky-high numbers back into the safety zone. And studies show that every 1 percent drop in cholesterol can lower heart-disease risk by 2 to 3 percent. But first, of course, you have to know where your blood cholesterol levels stand.

Who should get it: According to the National Cholesterol Education Program, all adults ages 20 and over should have their blood cholesterol checked at least once every five years. The recommended test measures total cholesterol as well as the levels of both "good" and "bad" cholesterol.

How it's done: A blood sample is drawn from your finger or from the inside of your elbow and sent to a lab for analysis. A desirable total cholesterol reading is anything under 200 milligrams per deciliter. Ideal LDL levels are under 100 mg/dL; over 130 is high.

Chlamydia Screening

An estimated 3 million cases of chlamydia occur in the United States every year, making it the country's most commonly reported infectious disease. But 75 percent of infected women and 50 percent of infected men don't even know they have the disease, which can easily be treated with antibiotics. If it is left untreated, the infection can cause pelvic inflammatory disease in women and may lead to reproductive problems. And recent research finds that infected women are three to five times more likely to acquire HIV if exposed to the virus that causes AIDS.

Who should get it: All sexually active women and men age 25 or younger should be tested annually.

How it's done: Doctors typically use a urethral swab to test for chlamydia in women. Men can be tested using a urine sample.

Breast Cancer Screening

In the United States, women get breast cancer more often than any other form of cancer. Screening cannot prevent the disease, but it can reduce the risk of dying from it. For women in their 40s, regular mammograms reduce the risk of dying from breast cancer by 16 percent. For women ages 50 to 69, screening with mammograms can cut breast cancer deaths by 25 to 30 percent.

Who should get it: The National Cancer Institute recommends mammograms for all women ages 40 to 69, every one to two years.

How it's done: A screening mammogram is an X-ray of the breasts that detects changes in the tissue that may signal cancer. The test usually involves two X-rays of each of your breasts. If the test is positive, your doctor may recommend a follow-up mammogram or even a biopsy. ✳

Peter Jaret is a contributing editor.

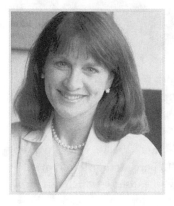

Good Question
about Wellness
by Nancy Snyderman

How Long Flights Make Feet Swell

I've noticed that every time I take a long airplane flight, my feet swell. What causes this? Is it dangerous?

You might have heard about the tragic case of the woman who, during a flight from San Francisco to London, collapsed on the plane and died from a blood clot that had traveled from her legs to her heart and lungs. That's the extremely rare result of the process that causes in-flight foot swelling.

Everyone's feet swell a little on long flights. It's sheer physics: If you're sitting for an extended period of time and you can't put your legs up, the fluids in your legs pool in your feet. The change in air pressure only makes it worse. The fact that your shoes feel tighter and your ankles aren't as shapely may not seem like a big deal, but you should keep close watch, especially if you have circulation or blood-clotting problems. If blood isn't circulating properly, you could develop a clot.

Here's the good news, though: It's easy to keep the swelling to a minimum. When the captain turns off the fasten-seatbelt sign, don't just feel free to move around the cabin—do it, especially if your flight is longer than three hours. Walk a little bit, stretch, and get your heart pumping.

What to Do if Your Doctor "Tunes Out"

I have an injury that won't heal, and my doctor seems to be getting tired of me. What should I do?

Unfortunately, it's very easy to end up in the category of "difficult patient" when you have an intractable problem. The fact is, many doctors don't like to admit they're stumped, so they'll either dodge the issue or make you feel like you're asking for too much. A good physician will exhaust all the possibilities and have helpful conversations with you each step of the way. At the very least, he should let you know when he feels there's nothing more he can do for you—and suggest some other specialist. If you're not even getting that, it's time to look for a new doctor.

That said, you are in a tricky position because even though your frustration is justified, you can scare off a new doctor if you come on too strong. It's not a good idea, for instance, to say, "I've seen 12 doctors already, and no one's been able to help me!" The new doctor may roll his eyes internally and think, "Well, I'm just number 13. What can I do?" And try to avoid bad-mouthing your other doctors.

Stick to the facts: Tell the doctor how long you've been hurting and describe any treatments you've tried that have or haven't helped. The key is to trust your instincts. You're entitled to a doctor who cares about you and will do his or her best, and if you feel like yours has tuned out, that's good enough reason to move on.

Forgetful? This Common Condition Could Be Why

A friend says my high blood pressure can make me forgetful. Is that true?

Heart attacks and stroke are the real killers associated with hypertension, but it looks like high blood pressure can also affect memory. And losing our minds is certainly worrisome.

A recent study followed nearly 1,000 Swedish men for 20 years and found that high blood pressure at age 50 was an excellent predictor of mental decline at age 70. A French study that examined about 1,400 people ages 59 to 71 uncovered a similar connection.

It all comes down to blood flow. High blood pressure basically means your blood vessels are constricted, so you've got less blood flowing through them. And whatever organ is on the receiving end can suffer. In the brain, cells get knocked off and you end up forgetting the name of that book you just read or where you left your keys.

It's not that simple, of course, but the point is that you don't want to let high blood pressure go untreated, even if it's just considered borderline. The first step is to adopt a heart-healthy lifestyle that includes four things: a healthy diet, exercise, weight loss if you're heavy, and stress reduction. If those don't work, excellent drugs that control or reduce blood pressure are available. See your doctor for advice about which one's best for you.

Answers for Restless Leg Syndrome

As soon as I get in bed at night, I feel a strange itching or pulling sensation in my legs. It's keeping me up—I haven't had a good night's sleep in months. It is driving my husband crazy too. What's going on?

That sounds like restless leg syndrome (RLS)—a central nervous system disorder that makes people feel as if they literally can't keep still. If you watch these sufferers in bed at night, they look like cats chasing rabbits! RLS is unpleasant, but it usually doesn't indicate any underlying problem (unless you're also feeling numbness, pins and needles, or radiating pain down your legs, in which case you might have a pinched nerve). Generally, the biggest annoyance is the sleep deprivation RLS causes and, as you've discovered, the strain it can put on your relationship with the person who shares your bed.

Unfortunately, drug remedies are less than satisfactory. There are several medications you can try, especially if you have a severe case, but finding the right one requires trial and error. Luckily, many get relief from simple lifestyle changes.

Since anything that improves circulation can help, you should get regular exercise—including lots of stretching—and try having a hot bath before bed. Cut back on caffeine and alcohol and consider taking one ibuprofen tablet before turning in; that may alleviate any crampiness or pain that's keeping you awake. You should also ask the doctor for a serum ferritin test, since there seems to be some association between RLS and low iron levels in the blood.

Why Anger Makes Your Nose Run

My nose is often stuffy, and, strangely enough, it gets worse when I'm angry. What's going on?

The fact that anger exacerbates your congestion makes me think of nonallergic rhinitis. The symptoms are pretty much the same as those of allergies (or allergic rhinitis)—congestion, sneezing, runny nose—but the causes and treatments can be different, so it's important to know which you've got.

With allergies, it is contact with a particular item—pollen, say—that triggers a systemwide immune response, including a massive outpouring of histamines, the chemicals that cause all the nasty symptoms. That's why antihistamines are helpful. But some people with classic allergy symptoms come up negative on allergy tests, and doctors often don't know what to do with them.

That's where nonallergic rhinitis comes in. With this condition, certain triggers cause a reaction just in the nose; blood vessels swell, which leads to excess mucus production. Temperature changes, perfumes, smoke, and spicy foods can all spark this physiological reaction, but surprisingly, so can anger and other strong emotions.

If this is what you have, try a nasal antihistamine spray, like Astelin, or a nasal steroid, such as Vancenase or Rhinocort. These sprays target inflammation in the affected area rather than flooding your body with unnecessary medication.

Nancy Snyderman, M.D., is a medical correspondent for ABC News and author of *Guide to Good Health for Women Over Forty* (Harvest Book, 1996).

VITAL STATS

64

Percentage of men who say they don't make plans in advance for Valentine's Day

4.5 million

Number of cesarean deliveries per 100 births in 1965

22

Number of C-sections per 100 births in 1999

700

Percentage increases in scooter-related injuries since summer 2000

50

Number of teens who get a weekly allowance

50

Average number of dollars in that allowance

19

Pounds of apples consumed per capita in 1998

25

Pounds of candy consumed per capita in 1998

Unless otherwise noted, statistics apply to the United States.

Leave Me **Alone**

Sixty-one percent of women say they prefer to be alone when in pain.

—*The Gallup Organization*

TEST YOURSELF
What's your eye-Q?

Take this quiz to find out if your optical knowledge is 20/20.

1. Was your mother right? Sitting too close to the television will damage your eyes.
   True or False?

2. Reading fine print for a long period of time will damage your eyes.
   True or False?

3. Cataracts are age-related.
   True or False?

4. Eating carrots will improve your vision.
   True or False?

ANSWERS

1. False. Many people sit too close to the TV because they can't see well to begin with, but doing so won't make their eyesight any worse.

2. False. Fine print may give you eye fatigue but won't cause permanent damage. To rest your eye muscles, look at something as far away as possible—ideally out a window.

3. False. Young adults and even children can develop cataracts, and people who've suffered an eye injury or have diabetes are particularly prone.

4. False. While carrots are an excellent source of vitamin A, an overall healthy diet is more essential to good vision.

Diabetes: Get tested in the morning

Rapidly rising diabetes rates have been grabbing headlines lately, a sure sign that more people need to be tested for the disease. If you're one of them, make sure you nab a morning appointment. That's the word from a new study that found an afternoon test could miss one of every two cases of diabetes.

Researchers at the National Institutes of Health compared the blood sugar levels of approximately 13,000 men and women, half of whom were tested in the morning after an overnight fast and half in the afternoon after a daytime fast.

When the test results were reviewed, the afternoon group averaged significantly lower blood sugar than the morning patients, perhaps due to hormonal shifts that occur naturally during the day. Problem is, the test wasn't designed to account for that difference.

chapter 6

food and nutrition

savor the health

experts agree:
the best diet has a
Mediterranean
flair

Confused by all the conflicting news about how you're supposed to eat? The nation's top nutrition expert has it all figured out—and *you'll love it.*

BY PETER JARET

RECIPES BY VICTORIA ABBOTT RICARDI

Throwing a dinner party these days is a little like brokering a truce in the Middle East. Moira's avoiding potatoes because they do a number on her blood-sugar levels. Russell's fine with potatoes, but no red meat, please—he's worried about his cholesterol count. Allison's sworn off dairy products, while Will has given up white flour. The Stantons are slowly turning into vegetarians—or is it vegans?

And so it goes. We all want to eat right, of course, but what we need is someone to tell us what's officially on—and off—the menu. You'd think the nation's top nutritionists, the very people who've done the research and drawn the conclusions, would be the ones to try to set us straight. In fact, a handful have done just that, publishing impressive books that in the past few years have reshaped the way we think about food. Each promises to reveal, once and for all, the secret to good health.

Take *The Omega Diet* (HarperCollins, 1999), by Artemis Simopoulos, a physician who for nine years headed a key nutrition committee for the National Institutes of Health. If anyone knows her stuff, Simopoulos should. And she doesn't pull any punches. Her book offers a diet plan that she says fights heart disease and cancer, boosts immunity, and even chases away depression.

The omega in the title refers to certain types of essential fats. According to Simopoulos, we're not as healthy as we could be because we don't get enough omega-3 fats, the kind found mostly in fish. We eat far too many omega-6s, the kind in corn, safflower, and sunflower oils. Ideally, the ratio of omega-3s to 6s should be about even, says Simopoulos.

Happily, her advice seems simple: Ease up on the omega-6s and fill your plate with foods rich in omega-3s, including fish, walnuts, canola oil, flaxseed, and leafy greens. One of Simopoulos's favorites happens to be purslane, a vegetable rich in omega-3s.

Canola and olive oils are rich in monounsaturated fats, which actually help fight off heart attacks. Canola is also a great source of omega-3s, unlike other cooking oils.

I figure I can learn to love purslane, as soon as I find a market that carries it. But when I dip into a second book, *The Glucose Revolution* (Marlowe & Co., 1998), I notice that it never mentions purslane. Or omega-3s. The authors are Jennie Brand-Miller, Thomas M. S. Wolever, Stephen Colagiuri, and Kaye Foster-Powell—leading nutritionists from Canada and Australia who together have enough Ph.D.s and M.D.s to start a small university. The real problem, they say, is that we help ourselves to too many foods that send our blood sugar through the roof. The result is an epidemic of obesity, diabetes, and heart disease.

Their solution is simple too: Choose low-fat foods that keep your blood sugar steady. To make that easy, their book includes a handy list, or "glycemic index," that ranks various foods by their effect on blood-sugar levels after a meal. White rice, white bread, and baked potatoes come in for hard knocks. Lentils, barley, and vegetables win praise. Most esteemed is chana dal, an obscure little legume that happens to have the lowest blood-sugar impact of all.

Okay. I can live with chana dal. Maybe I can find a recipe for chana dal on a bed of purslane. But when I turn to Kilmer McCully's *The Heart Revolution* (Harper Perennial Library, 2000), guess what: no mention of chana dal or purslane. Or the glycemic index. McCully is a pathologist at the Veterans Affairs Medical Center in Providence,

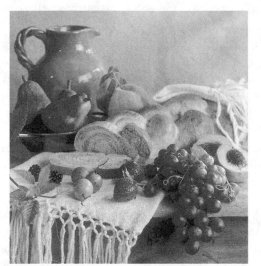

Rhode Island, but his claim to fame is having been the first scientist to notice a link between heart disease and levels of homocysteine, an amino acid in the blood.

To McCully, the key to good health, or at least robust arteries, isn't stable blood sugar or omega-3s; it's folic acid and other B vitamins. When we fall short on these key nutrients, he explains, homocysteine levels climb. That in turn injures the arteries and leads to heart attacks and strokes.

McCully's idea of a great diet is one loaded with foods rich in those vitamins, including fish, green leafy vegetables, nuts, and beans. Liver even makes his list, since it's packed with folic acid, B-6, and B-12.

Before I start spreading spinach leaves with liverwurst, though, I dig into Gerald Reaven's *Syndrome X: Overcoming the Silent Killer That Can Give You a Heart Attack* (Simon & Schuster, 2000). Barely a mention of homocysteine or the glycemic index. Nary a word about omega-3s. The renowned Stanford researcher, in fact, comes up with an altogether different reason why we're not as healthy as we should be: a potentially deadly mix of factors that includes insulin resistance, low HDL, high triglycerides, obesity, and elevated blood pressure.

For people with this scary condition, Reaven says, the American Heart Association's low-fat, high-carb diet may actually increase heart attack danger. He admonishes adherents to eat more fat—around 40 percent of the calories they consume instead of the widely accepted 30 percent—while suggesting a cutback in carbohydrates.

Healthy eating is a joy when you cook dishes inspired by traditional diets of the Mediterranean region, made with ingredients you'll have no trouble finding at your local supermarket.

Wait a minute. Doesn't *The Glucose Revolution* say we should be cutting back on fat and loading up on carbs? And if Syndrome X is so important, why doesn't McCully mention it? What about omega-3s? Aren't they supposed to be the secret to healthy eating? Four books, a batch of leading experts, and one very confused and hungry food-lover.

"Help!" is my plea to Kathy McManus, head of the nutrition department at Boston's Brigham and Women's Hospital. McManus doesn't have a book with her name on it, but she's widely regarded as one of the nation's top nutrition scientists. More to the point, for 20 years she's been in the business of telling people what they should eat to be hale and hearty.

So, Kathy McManus, I say, laying my stack of tomes on the table, what *should* we be eating? She laughs, then she sighs. "It's easy to see why anyone reading these would come away thinking, geez, do even the experts know what they're talking about?" she says. "It's true, each of these books has its own theory. Each has its own little hobbyhorse to ride."

But when you get beyond the fancy explanations, highfalutin hypotheses, and purported breakthroughs, she says, the picture changes. "What all four of these books say we should be eating, in fact, looks remarkably the same."

McCully waits till near his book's end, then offers that his eating plan is very much like the traditional diets of the Mediterranean region. Simopoulos declares right up front that her program is "based on the diet of the island of Crete." *The Glucose Revolution*'s authors never say it straight out, but almost every recipe they include—minestrone, tomato-basil soup, tortellini salad, pasta primavera—would be right at home in an Italian trattoria. Even Reaven recommends fettuccine and seared scallops one night and linguine and clams the next.

What gives? The meal plan suits McCully because it's rich in B vitamins. Simopoulos believes classic

Lemony Lentil-Rice Salad with Toasted Walnuts

SERVES 12
PREPARATION: 10 MINUTES
COOKING: 40 MINUTES

1 cup brown lentils
$1/2$ cup medium-grain white rice
$1 1/2$ tablespoons olive oil, divided
1 medium onion, chopped
3 cloves garlic, minced
1 (10-ounce) package frozen artichoke hearts
$1/2$ cup chopped fresh parsley
$1/2$ cup nonfat plain yogurt
1 lemon
3 tablespoons chopped walnuts, toasted in a hot skillet

1. Place 3 cups water and lentils in a large saucepan. Bring to a boil, reduce heat, and simmer, partially covered, 30 minutes or until tender. Drain; let cool. Meanwhile, in a medium saucepan, boil $1 1/2$ cups water. Add rice, and reduce heat. Simmer, covered, 15 minutes or until tender. Fluff with a fork; let cool.
2. Heat $1 1/2$ teaspoons oil in a nonstick skillet over medium heat. Add onion and garlic; sauté 6 minutes or until golden.
3. Cook artichoke hearts according to package directions. Drain; let cool. Cut into quarters.
4. Place lentils in a salad bowl. Add rice, onion mixture, artichoke hearts, parsley, and yogurt. Grate rind of lemon over bowl; stir in 3 tablespoons lemon juice along with walnuts and remaining oil. Season with salt and pepper to taste.

Per serving: Calories 134 (20% from fat), Fat 3 g (0 g saturated), Protein 7 g, Carbohydrate 21 g, Fiber 7 g, Cholesterol 0 mg, Iron 2 mg, Sodium 33 mg, Calcium 48 mg

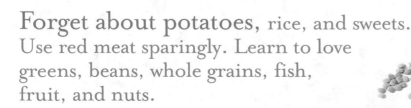

Forget about potatoes, rice, and sweets. Use red meat sparingly. Learn to love greens, beans, whole grains, fish, fruit, and nuts.

Swiss Chard with Golden Raisins and Black Olives

SERVES 4
PREPARATION: 10 MINUTES
COOKING: 10 MINUTES

1¹/₂ pounds Swiss chard, rinsed but not dried

2¹/₂ teaspoons olive oil

¹/₃ cup golden raisins

3 tablespoons pitted oil-cured black olives, quartered

4 cloves garlic, minced

¹/₄ teaspoon red pepper flakes

Salt to taste

1. Strip leaves from Swiss chard stalks, and set leaves aside. Trim stalk bottoms; slice stalks lengthwise into ¹/₄-inch-wide strips, then chop crosswise into ¹/₄-inch dice.

2. Heat oil in a large nonstick skillet over medium heat. Add chard stems; sauté 3 to 5 minutes. Coarsely chop chard leaves. Stir in raisins, olives, garlic, red pepper flakes, and chopped leaves. Cover pan, and cook over low heat 6 minutes, stirring occasionally, or until chard is tender. Season with salt to taste.

Per serving: Calories 124 (35% from fat), Fat 6 g (1 g saturated), Protein 4 g, Carbohydrate 19 g, Fiber 3 g, Cholesterol 0 mg, Iron 3 mg, Sodium 573 mg, Calcium 105 mg

Pan-Seared Tuna with Tomato-Mushroom Ragout

SERVES 4
PREPARATION: 15 MINUTES
COOKING: 20 MINUTES

4¹/₂ teaspoons canola oil, divided

2 ounces prosciutto, diced

3 cloves garlic, minced

1 medium leek, white and light green parts only, chopped

10 ounces cremini or button mushroom caps, thinly sliced

4 plum tomatoes, cored and diced

4 cups torn fresh spinach

1 cup torn fresh basil

4 (6-ounce) tuna steaks

Salt and freshly ground black pepper to taste

1. Heat ¹/₂ teaspoon of oil in a small nonstick skillet over low heat. Add prosciutto; sauté 5 minutes or until crispy. Stir in garlic; turn off heat. Heat 2 teaspoons oil in a large nonstick skillet over medium-high heat. Add leek and mushrooms; sauté 8 to 10 minutes or until golden. Stir in tomatoes; season with salt and pepper to taste. Stir in spinach, basil, and prosciutto-garlic mixture. Cover; keep warm.

2. Season both sides of tuna steaks with salt and pepper to taste. Heat remaining 2 teaspoons oil in a medium nonstick skillet over medium-high heat. Add tuna; cook 3 minutes on each side for medium rare or 4 minutes on each side for medium. Spoon ragout onto 4 plates; top with tuna.

Per serving: Calories 342 (25% from fat), Fat 10 g (1 g saturated), Protein 49 g, Carbohydrate 17 g, Fiber 5 g, Cholesterol 86 mg, Iron 5 mg, Sodium 415 mg, Calcium 127 mg

Greek Penne with White Beans, Tomatoes, and Lamb

SERVES 6
PREPARATION: 10 MINUTES
COOKING: 20 MINUTES

1 teaspoon olive oil

1 medium onion, chopped

2 tablespoons fresh chopped oregano

¹/₂ pound lean ground lamb

2 (14.5-ounce) cans diced tomatoes with basil, garlic, and oregano

1 (19-ounce) can cannellini beans, drained

2 cloves garlic, minced

¹/₂ cup chopped fresh mint leaves

1 pound uncooked penne pasta

¹/₂ cup (2 ounces) crumbled feta cheese

1. Heat oil in a large nonstick skillet over medium heat. Add onion, oregano, and lamb; sauté, breaking lamb into small pieces with a spoon, until meat is lightly browned, about 6 minutes. Stir in tomatoes, beans, and garlic; simmer.

2. Turn heat to low, and cook 10 minutes. Stir in mint. Cover and keep warm. Cook pasta according to package directions. Drain.

3. Divide pasta among 6 shallow bowls. Top with equal portions of sauce and feta cheese.

Per serving: Calories 482 (14% from fat), Fat 7 g (2 g saturated), Protein 24 g, Carbohydrate 78 g, Fiber 7 g, Cholesterol 34 mg, Iron 3 mg, Sodium 995 mg, Calcium 130 mg

Forget flip-flopping diet news and expert advice. Stick with these eight basic principles for a healthy diet.

Italian and Greek foods prevent heart disease because they deliver the ideal mix of omega-3s and 6s. The ancient diet of Crete and southern Italy also happens to offer the precise ratio of fat, carbohydrate, and protein that Reaven touts—and it's plentiful in foods low on Brand-Miller's glycemic index, so it tends to tame blood sugar.

"No matter what your theory about the healthiest way to eat," says McManus, "the Mediterranean diet seems to fit the bill"—which is splendid, except that each of the other experts insists we shop for dinner wearing his or her own special goggles, making for some weirdly distorted views.

Fortunately, clarity is coming in a new book: the *Harvard Medical School Guide to Healthy Eating* (Simon & Schuster, 2001), by Walter Willett, a Harvard University epidemiologist who is perhaps the country's leading expert on nutrition and health. (He's helped run the famed Nurses' Health Study for 20 years, for starters.) His book wraps up several decades of research and works it into a levelheaded plan based in part on the Mediterranean model. "It's a wonderful blueprint for healthy eating," says Willett. "And it's a blueprint that can be adapted to suit almost any taste."

With Willett as our guide, we can forget all the flip-flopping diet news. We can even ignore the government's Food Guide Pyramid, he says, since it rests on the idea that all carbs are healthy and all fats dangerous, and other outmoded notions. Instead, stick with these eight principles.

1. Replace bad fats with good fats. Don't

sweat the amount of fat you eat as much as the type, Willett says. Saturated fat—the kind abundant in fatty cuts of meat and full-fat dairy products such as butter, cheese, and whole milk—is the undisputed bad guy. But just as damaging to your arteries, it turns out, are trans fats, the hydrogenated kinds that show up in margarine and loads of baked goods, including most crackers and cookies. Instead of spurning fat, sauté your veggies and brush your bread with olive or canola oil, or use trans-free canola margarine. Canola and olive oils are rich in monounsaturated fats, which actually help fight off heart attacks. Canola is also a great source of omega-3s, unlike other cooking oils. And because it's essentially flavorless, it's a good choice when olive oil would come on too strong—in muffins, say.

2. Use meat sparingly. The healthiest traditional cuisines, in both the Mediterranean region and Asia, have long used red meat as a savory accent—slim slices of beef in a stir-fry, for instance, or bits of flavorful cured pork in a tomato sauce. You don't have to cut out meat entirely; just take in less saturated fat by choosing lean cuts and by eating meat less often. Not only will you protect your heart, there's good evidence you'll cut your cancer risk too.

3. Learn to love beans and nuts. Both are terrific sources of vegetable protein, which experts now agree can benefit a body as much as protein from meat or milk. Nuts are rich in heart-healthy oils. Beans have lots of fiber. And both can turn a meatless dish—such as a stir-fry with cashews or a casserole with chickpeas—into a satisfying meal.

4. Eat fish twice a week. True omega-3 believers go as far as grinding their own flaxseed for a nutty topping in which the healthy fats are abundant. But for most of us, seafood remains the most appetizing source. Salmon and other fatty fish are richest, but tuna—canned or fresh—is also good, whether stacked in a sandwich or tossed in a salad or with pasta.

5. Load up on greens and veggies. The people of Crete have been found to eat as many as 70 kinds of wild greens. Simopoulos thinks that's behind their good health: Leafy greens are abundant in omega-3s. McCully backs them because they're loaded with B vitamins, including folic acid. Brand-Miller smiles on their large supply of fiber, which keeps blood sugar steady.

6. Kick the potato habit. It may be America's favorite vegetable, but that starchy baked potato (white rice too) really makes blood sugar surge, many experts agree, upping the risk of diabetes and heart disease. You don't have to spurn all spuds—the less-starchy small red ones are better since they're digested more slowly—but it's wise to think of potatoes as a treat, not a staple. Sweet potatoes, brown rice, bulgur, and couscous all rank lower on the glycemic scale (as do spaghetti and other dry pastas, for obscure reasons).

7. Go for whole grain. It's likewise smart to lighten up on baked goods made with refined white flour. Modern processing robs grains like wheat and rye of much of their goodness. "Removing the wheat germ pulls out vitamins and unsaturated fats," says Willett. "Whacking away the branny outer layer removes fiber, magnesium, and more vitamins." What's left is easily digested, so, like baked potatoes, it sends blood sugar soaring. Trade those bagels and white breads for dark breads made with whole wheat, rye, and oats. If you're a breakfast-cereal lover, choose one made with whole grains. Diets rich in whole grains have been shown to lower the risk of heart disease, diabetes, many forms of cancer, and intestinal troubles like diverticulitis.

8. Satisfy your sweet tooth with fruit. Apart from being high in fiber, which helps keep blood sugar in check, fruit is also a great source of antioxidants such as vitamin C, which may protect against cancer, heart disease, and age-related ills like macular degeneration, a leading cause of blindness. Mediterranean meals traditionally end with grapes, figs, nectarines, or other fruit—orange juice still appears regularly on dessert menus in parts of Spain.

I'm dreaming of a dinner. First, a green salad with walnuts and pears, then salmon on a bed of couscous, spinach sautéed in olive oil, crusty whole grain bread, and for dessert, a small glass of juice squeezed from the most delicious oranges I can find. It's a menu to satisfy a world full of nutritionists—and a roomful of persnickety friends. ✻

Peter Jaret is a Health *contributing editor.*

Looking for healthy snacks? Try these five guilt-free treats.

If you're eager to be an even more virtuous snacker, you've got plenty of options. Here are a few vice-free finger foods.

JUST VEGETABLES The brainchildren of Just Tomatoes, Etc., a small company in central California, these dehydrated niblets of corn, carrots, peas, tomatoes, and bell peppers make eating veggies almost as satisfying as scarfing popcorn. There's nothing added, so all you get is phytochemicals, fiber, and vitamins A and C—plus a mild, slightly sweet flavor. Find them at natural foods stores or log on to www.justtomatoes.com for a store near you.

DRIED FRUIT Here's a snack that's packed with potassium, antioxidants, and fiber. Granted, dried fruit is high in sugar, but that actually makes it a good choice when you need a little pick-me-up. Just Tomatoes, Etc., has applied its crunchy touch to fruit too: You can munch a cup of dried blackberries and take in just 90 calories and a whopping 9 grams of fiber.

EDAMAME A traditional snack in Japan, edamame, or blanched soybeans in pods, are becoming increasingly available in the United States. The sweet, nutty-tasting beans are loaded with soy protein, which has been shown to help lower cholesterol. A half cup of shelled beans has 125 calories and 4 grams of fiber. Look for unsalted edamame in the frozen foods section.

SLICED RAW VEGETABLES Make your own mini-party platter with sweet red peppers, baby carrots, celery, and a bit of hummus. The fiber in the veggies and creamy bean dip will fill you up—without loading you down with calories.

RICE CAKES Whole grains are the prize here. A slew of recent studies have linked diets rich in whole grains to a reduced risk of diabetes and some cancers. Unsalted rice cakes can be cardboardy; if you're eating them unadorned, opt for ones with a little salt. Quaker's Lightly Salted rice cakes are satisfyingly crunchy and are made with only two ingredients: whole grain brown rice and salt. Two cakes deliver 70 calories and a scant 30 milligrams of sodium.

the
all-natural
way to reduce
cholesterol

The new breed of drugs are potent, but why pop pills when diet and exercise may be just as powerful?

BY PETER JARET

For starters, give yourself a little pat on the back. In the years since the nation first declared war on cholesterol, Americans have steadily lowered their levels of the artery-clogging gunk by almost 5 percent—enough to make a significant dent in the average person's risk of heart disease and stroke. That's great, the experts say, but not nearly good enough.

Last May, federal health officials at the National Cholesterol Education Program (NCEP) announced a new set of more aggressive guidelines for lowering cholesterol. They warned that as many as 53 million Americans still have dangerously high levels. In fact, a majority of those—36 million—are at such a high risk for heart disease that they should probably begin taking the newest generation of cholesterol-lowering medications. Pronto. Some researchers think that people with even slightly elevated cholesterol levels could cut their risk of heart disease by taking the new medications. If they're right, half of all U.S. adults might do well to begin popping a pill every day.

There's good reason researchers are so gung ho about the new drugs, which are called statins. Before the latest pills came along, even the best medications lowered cholesterol levels only by about 10 percent. Statin drugs, which work by blocking the liver's ability to produce cholesterol, can bring those levels down by 40 percent or more.

But amid all the hoopla over cholesterol-fighting pills, it's only natural to wonder what happened to all the other ways that experts have touted to lower cholesterol over the years. What about a low-fat diet and regular exercise? Weren't they supposed to help keep our arteries free and clear? What about the cholesterol-lowering power of oat bran or soy powder? Have the experts given up hope that most people can use diet or exercise to bring cholesterol down to a safe level?

Most people can reach their cholesterol goal without taking a pill every day. As remarkable as the new drugs are, exercise and a healthy diet are still the best ways to lower LDL and the risks of heart disease.

It's a question worth asking, especially now that new, tougher cholesterol guidelines have been released—the first change in the official recommendations since 1993. The guideline for total cholesterol hasn't changed; experts still say most people should aim for 200 milligrams per deciliter or less. The big change is a new focus on what researchers say is the culprit behind coronary artery disease: low-density lipoprotein, or LDL.

The new guidelines set three upper limits for LDL, depending on individual risk: 160 milligrams for healthy people free of heart-disease risks such as smoking, excess weight, and high blood pressure; 130 for folks with two or more risk factors; and 100 for people already diagnosed with heart disease or diabetes.

"Unfortunately, many of us have a long way to go to get our LDL down to a healthy level," says James Cleeman, M.D., who coordinates the NCEP. One in three American adults has an LDL level high enough to be at significant risk of developing heart disease.

These folks are likely to end up taking cholesterol-lowering drugs. Luckily for them, new findings show that the medications not only lower heart-attack risk but also save lives.

But everyone else, Cleeman says, can reach the new goal without taking a pill every day for the rest of their lives. As remarkable as the new drugs are, a healthy diet and exercise are still the best ways for most people to lower LDL and heart-disease danger, he insists. One good reason: Most drugs—statins included—are not without side effects. In fact, Bayer Pharmaceutical Division voluntarily withdrew the statin drug Baycol from the market in August 2001, due to reports of potentially fatal muscle reactions. The Food and Drug Administration had received reports of a number of

statin drugs: a comparison

If a healthy diet and regular exercise aren't enough to tame high cholesterol, most doctors recommend cholesterol-lowering drugs called statins. Studies show these powerful pills are already reducing the risk of heart attacks. Here's a comparison of the five leading kinds of statins. Keep in mind that the effect of statins on HDL and LDL levels vary from person to person. Prices also vary widely. Which drug your doctor recommends will depend, in part, on your cholesterol profile. And not all insurance plans cover all versions of statin drugs.

Name (generic)	Starting dose	Lowers LDL by (at max. dosage)	Raises HDL by (at max. dosage)	Average monthly cost of starting dose
Lescol (Fluvastatin)	20mg	34%	0%	$40
Lipitor (Atorvastatin)	10mg	60%	6%	$60
Mevacor (Lovastatin)	20mg	40%	0%	$70
Pravachol (Pravastatin)	20mg	34%	0%	$70
Zocor (Simvastatin)	20mg	47%	11%	$115

Statins are good news for people with high cholesterol; the medication can lower LDL levels by 40 percent or more.

deaths associated with Baycol in the United States at the time it was recalled.

Unless your cholesterol levels are sky-high and you are already a candidate for heart disease, most doctors advise that you begin with an exercise and diet plan—lifestyle changes—to see if they can bring your numbers into line.

Low-Fat Diet ↓15%–37%

When the anti-cholesterol campaign began, the target was dietary cholesterol—the kind in foods like eggs and shellfish. While it's still wise to keep dietary cholesterol levels down to less than 300 milligrams a day, a far more serious risk comes from saturated fat and trans fat. Saturated fat shows up in meat and poultry, whole-milk dairy products, and some tropical oils. Trans fats—vegetable oils modified to create

Drastic cuts in fat yield the best results. But even moderately low-fat diets can bring LDL back into the comfort range.

solids—show up in all kinds of processed foods, from crackers and chips to ice cream. The trouble is, both saturated fats and trans fats cause the liver to churn out cholesterol, especially the artery-clogging LDL variety.

How far are you likely to bring your level down by cutting back on bad fats? The most encouraging answer comes from research done by University of California at San Francisco heart-disease expert Dean Ornish, M.D., who tested an extremely low-fat, vegetarian diet on men who had already suffered a heart attack. After a year on Ornish's program, which included an improved diet, increased physical activity, and stress reduction, volunteers lowered their LDL cholesterol by a whopping 37 percent—results right in line with what statin drugs can offer.

"But there's a catch," says Robert Rosenthal, M.D., professor of medicine at Baylor University Medical Center in Dallas. "The Ornish diet does away with meat, cheese, eggs, vegetable oil, and butter. And frankly, not that many people are willing to make such a drastic change in their diet, even to save their lives."

The American Heart Association (AHA) offers a less-restrictive, more-palatable diet, which recommends getting no more than 30 percent of calories from fat and only 10 percent from saturated or trans fats, has been shown to bring LDL cholesterol down by an average of 15 percent. That's short of Ornish's results, but it's

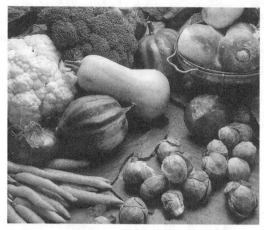

Power food: Fruits, veggies, and even nuts are good first-line defenses against high cholesterol.

good enough to bring borderline high cholesterol back down into the comfort zone.

If you're already at risk for heart disease, the NCEP recommends keeping saturated and trans fats down to no more than 7 percent of your total calories. Reach that level, studies indicate, and you might bring LDL levels down by as much as 20 percent.

High-Fiber Diet ↓33%

By filling their plates with high-fiber foods such as fruits, vegetables, and nuts, most people can coax LDL levels down even more than on a low-fat diet alone. In findings published earlier this year, University of Toronto researcher David Jenkins, Ph.D., showed that a diet that gets more than a third of its calories from fruit, vegetables, and nuts can lower LDL cholesterol by an impressive 33 percent. What's more, the numbers fell within the first week of starting the diet.

If you don't prowl the produce aisle as much as you should, another option is to add a fiber supplement. Last year, researchers at the Veterans Affairs Medical Center and the University of Kentucky reviewed eight studies that looked at the LDL-lowering power of psyllium, a seed husk rich in soluble fiber that's used in dietary fiber supplements. Volunteers who added 10 grams of psyllium a day cut their LDL levels by an average of 7 percent. What makes that finding all the more encouraging is that many of these volunteers were already following the AHA diet—suggesting that a fiber

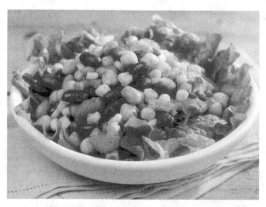

Here's the scoop: Eating high-fiber foods such as legumes can help lower cholesterol by as much as 33 percent.

supplement added to an already-healthy diet can yield additional benefits.

Cholesterol-Lowering Margarine or Salad Dressing ↓11%

These spreads and dressings are laced with substances derived from plants, called sterols and stanols, which have been shown to prevent cholesterol from being absorbed into the blood. The latest studies suggest that most people can expect to lower their LDL as much as 11 percent by adding just 2 to 4 grams a day. The two leading brands of cholesterol-lowering margarine are Benecol and Take Control.

Exercise is better at raising HDL than it is at lowering LDL, which is particularly important for women.

Regular Exercise ↓7%–10%

When volunteers in a Stanford University study switched to a low-fat diet, their LDL levels fell by 7 to 11 percent. Those in the study who followed the same diet plus exercise—walking or jogging 10 miles a week—had numbers that fell almost twice as far. That's impressive. But the real benefit of exercise is its ability to keep heart-protective high-density lipoprotein, or HDL, cholesterol levels high. That's particularly welcome news since some of the same low-fat, high-carbohydrate diets that are recommended for dropping total and LDL cholesterol levels also tend to drag HDL levels down.

"Regular exercise keeps HDL levels up even when total and LDL cholesterol are falling," says Stanford University researcher Marcia Stefanick, Ph.D. In one recent study conducted at Stanford, volunteers who began walking or jogging nine miles a week saw their HDL levels climb 13 percent.

The HDL effect of exercise may be especially important for women, researchers say. The new NCEP guidelines recommend HDL levels of 40 milligrams or higher (compared with 35 milligrams or higher) but women may do well to aim for even more. According to Rose Marie Robertson, president of the AHA, women's risk of heart disease begins to climb when HDL falls below 45 milligrams.

margarine vs. butter: spread softly

Hard bodies, yes. But when it comes to fat, softer is better. That's the final word—or so we think—in the butter vs. margarine debate.

A 1999 study by Tufts University researchers compared the effect of numerous fats on cholesterol levels and found that butter produced the highest levels of the artery-damaging low-density lipoprotein (LDL) cholesterol. The softer products, such as tub margarine and oil, were found to be healthier than stick margarine because they contain fewer trans-fatty acids, which raise cholesterol levels and the risk of heart disease. The study also found that those who ate the softer fats had smaller reductions in beneficial high-density lipoprotein (HDL) cholesterol. How soft should you go? "If you're thinking about butter or margarine, think about using liquid oil instead," says Walter Willett, M.D., chairman of the nutrition department at Harvard University's School of Public Health.

But sometimes the softer fats just don't cut it. Tub margarine, for instance, isn't made for baking—often, only stick margarine or butter will do. And butter fans insist that there's no substitute when it comes to flavor. What to do? In order to stay within the American Heart Association's recommendations of getting 30% of calories from fat and only 10% from saturated or trans fats, try to go easier on the solid fats.

"I'm a chef; I could not live without butter," says Joan Carter, a spokesperson for the American Dietetic Association. "If you like butter or stick margarine, cut back on other animal fats. It's easy to rack up that 10%." The chart below shows how the fats stack up.

per 1 tablespoon serving	total (g)	sat (g)	trans (g)
corn oil	13.6	1.8	0.00
olive oil	13.5	1.9	0.14
liquid margarine	11.5	1.9	0.00
stick margarine	11.4	2.3	2.4
tub margarine	11.2	1.9	1.1
stick butter	10.8	7.2	0.3

Whether you need statins or not, maintaining a healthy lifestyle with diet and exercise is still part of the prescription.

Soy Protein ↓15%

More than a dozen studies have shown that people with elevated cholesterol who consume 25 grams of soy protein a day can lower their LDLs by 15 percent.

The Ideal Combination

Add it all up—low fat, high fiber, cholesterol-lowering margarine, and plenty of physical activity—and what do you have?

Surprisingly, even the experts don't really know how much the ideal combination can achieve in lowering cholesterol. "We've looked at the individual pieces, but so far no one has put it all together," says Jenkins, widely regarded as one of the leading experts on diet and cholesterol. Studies to test the best combination are under way.

But there's good reason to think that combining several cholesterol-lowering strategies can come close to matching what statin drugs offer. "Take the 10 to 15 percent reduction you get from reducing saturated and trans fats; add the 10 to 15 percent that you can get from including high-fiber fruits, vegetables, and nuts, along with a couple of servings of either soy or a margarine made with plant sterols. You're looking at a drop of perhaps 20 to 30 percent," Jenkins says. That's more than enough to bring moderately elevated LDL levels back to a safer range. Add the effect of exercise, and you up the ante as well.

Lifestyle changes won't work for everyone, though; about 20 percent of adults are what researchers call "nonresponders"—their cholesterol levels won't budge even on the best diet and exercise regimen. Another 20 percent will never have to worry about their cholesterol levels no matter what they eat. That

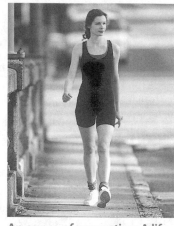

An ounce of prevention: A life-long commitment to regular exercise is particularly important to women who need to reap the benefits of heart-protecting HDL cholesterol.

still leaves 60 percent of the population who can benefit by making a few simple changes in diet and lifestyle.

The fact is, even people whose doctors end up prescribing statin drugs are told to follow the same advice—for plenty of good reasons. The farther you can lower your LDL levels with diet and exercise, the lower the dose of the drug you'll need. And a healthy diet and plenty of exercise offer benefits that go beyond lowering cholesterol.

Even the most optimistic researchers are aware that getting people to make lasting changes is a difficult undertaking. When study participants were spoon-fed every meal, for instance, the AHA's low-fat diet succeeded in lowering their cholesterol levels by as much as 15 percent. But in the real world, where dinners out and lunches on the fly are an inherent part of an average week, people who tried to follow these same guidelines averaged only about a 5 percent reduction in LDL cholesterol.

That's no reason to be discouraged, says NCEP's

A healthy diet and plenty of exercise offer benefits that go beyond lowering cholesterol.

Cleeman. "What numbers like those say is that most of us really can make a difference in our cholesterol levels, but we have to be willing to work at it." For his part, Cleeman thinks it's not unreasonable to expect that most people with elevated cholesterol levels are capable of lowering their LDL levels by 20 percent or more without having to resort to pills. "And when you consider that every 1 percent drop in total cholesterol translates into a 2 to 3 percent reduction in heart-disease risk," he points out, "we're talking about a pretty substantial payoff." ✳

Peter Jaret is a Health *contributing editor.*

WHY SUPPLEMENTS CAN'T REPLACE HEALTHY FOOD

For years, beta-carotene was the hot antioxidant. When people got plenty from their meals, their risk of cancer and heart disease plummeted. But then researchers gave it to people in pills and the protection vanished; in smokers, the tablets actually raised the risk of cancer. Now scientists worry that flavonoid supplements may prove to be similarly risky.

Martyn Smith, a toxicologist at the University of California at Berkeley, reviewed the body of research on flavonoids, a group of potent antioxidants. He found plenty of evidence that in food sources such as fruits, vegetables, grains, and wine, the nutrients help to protect against cancer and heart disease. But there were no studies demonstrating the value or safety of supplements. What's more, in test tube research, scientists discovered that high concentrations of flavonoids—similar to those found in pills—can damage your DNA, which could cause cancer and birth defects.

Consider the flavonoid quercetin, says Smith. Pill manufacturers advise swallowing 500 to 1,000 milligrams daily, roughly 20 times more than a person could get in a well-rounded vegetarian diet. "Take that much daily," he says, "and you might wind up doing yourself more harm than good. Until we know more, stick with flavonoid-rich foods like apples and onions."

The Newest Cavity Fighter:
SUSHI

Few sushi lovers need an excuse to indulge. But here's one anyway: New research shows that wasabi, the spicy green horseradish paste served with sushi and sashimi, may fight cavities.

In test-tube studies, Japanese chemist Hideki Masuda found that the same substances responsible for wasabi's pungent flavor can inhibit the growth of a bacterium that causes tooth decay. Masuda believes these chemicals, which are also found in broccoli and cabbage, can interfere with bacteria's ability to adhere to teeth.

"This certainly sounds promising," says Dan Meyer, associate executive director for science at the American Dental Association. "Still, I'd like to see clinical studies with patients. What works in the test tube doesn't always work in the mouth."

Masuda hopes to study wasabi's real-world effects on human subjects. If the results are good, wasabi toothpaste might soon be in your medicine cabinet (with the requisite adjustments made to mask its sinus-clearing flavor). In the meantime, Meyer says, the best way to keep your mouth healthy is still to eat a balanced diet, avoid sugary foods, and keep brushing and flossing regularly. Of course, enjoying a little extra sushi couldn't hurt.

ECO-FRIENDLY FISH

First came dolphin-safe tuna; now, it's time to start thinking out of the can when you're planning a meal from the sea. The Marine Stewardship Council has begun putting "eco-labels" on packages of fresh salmon from "sustainable" fisheries. Sustainable fisheries offer an environmentally friendly option in seafood, limiting the catch to preserve the population and prevent overfishing. Several outfits have already received certification, and dozens more are working toward obtaining it.

Interested in helping the environment by seeking out eco-labeled fish? Visit www.msc.org to dive into the details.

super foods
from the sea

New guidelines say you should eat more fat, if it's the right kind. Where can you find it? In many of the world's tastiest fish.

BY TIMOTHY GOWER

When it comes to food, we're a nation of landlubbers. The average American scarfs down more than 2 pounds of red meat a week. But order a tuna sandwich for lunch? Or broil a piece of salmon for supper? Not likely. Per person, we eat a mere 4 ounces of fish each week—less than what's in some cans of StarKist.

Ahoy, mates: It's time to take the plunge. Health experts now say that no diet is complete without regular servings of seafood. The American Heart Association (AHA), for one, has issued new guidelines that urge people to eat fatty fish, such as tuna or salmon, twice a week. The AHA's recommendation was based on impressive clinical evidence that consuming fish can help prevent heart trouble.

Impressive indeed. In one recent study, scientists concluded that older adults who ate fatty fish at least once a week were 44 percent less likely to die of a heart attack than those who didn't. Other research has found similar benefits in middle-aged folks. Studies also show that fish can offer hope to people with existing heart disease. In one, heart attack survivors advised to eat fatty fish cut their risk of dying by 29 percent.

For a nation trained to fear fat, these results may seem hard to swallow. But a generation ago, scientists noticed that Eskimos rarely had heart disease, despite their high-fat diets. The source of all that fat likely holds the key: blubbery meat from the seals and whales the Eskimos hunted. Go one link down the food chain, and you see why blubber is so salubrious: Seals and whales subsist mostly on seafood.

Fish, it turns out, is packed with compounds called omega-3 fatty acids, which appear to benefit the heart in several ways. For one, they help maintain a normal heart rhythm, says Penn State nutritionist and AHA spokesperson Penny Kris-Etherton. If this rhythm gets too speedy or erratic, the result can be sudden cardiac death, a condition that kills roughly 225,000 Americans each year. And seafood can make a difference: One major study found that eating fish at least once a week slices the risk of being struck by this killer in half.

Fish is packed with compounds called omega-3 fatty acids, which benefit the heart in several ways.

In one study, older adults who ate fatty fish at least once a week were 44 percent less likely to die of a heart attack than those who didn't.

Omega-3s appear to have other heart-healthy benefits. They seem to lower levels of triglycerides, a blood fat linked with heart disease, says endocrinologist William Connor, of Oregon Health Sciences University in Portland. (Eating fish won't lower your cholesterol, though, and may lead to a slight rise.)

Research also suggests that omega-3s act as a kind of lubricant for the arteries. If your cardiovascular system is well greased with fish oil, the thinking goes, substances in the blood called platelets are less likely to form heart-stopping clots. Omega-3s could also prevent clots from forming in arteries that feed blood to the brain; those clots are the cause of most strokes. A recent study found that women who dined on fish five times a week or more were half as likely to have a stroke as those who ate it less than once a month.

The dietary path to happiness begins at the local fish house, experts say. Depression rates are lowest in nations where seafood is a staple.

Fish may also have broader disease-fighting powers. For instance, omega-3s seem to interfere with the production of substances in the body that cause inflammation. More than 20 studies have shown that fish-oil capsules can provide modest pain relief to people with rheumatoid arthritis. In one trial, patients who added fish oil to their medication regimen had reduced joint soreness and stiffness—a few were even able to quit taking anti-inflammatory drugs.

While you may find joy in a bonbon, some researchers believe the dietary path to happiness begins at your local fish house. Depression rates are lowest in nations where seafood is a staple, those scientists say. They also point to evidence that fish oil can actually give people with mental illness a boost. In a landmark study, patients with manic depression had far fewer episodes of depression and mania if they took fish-oil capsules along with their regular medicines. Researchers speculate that omega-3s may act like the drug lithium in the brain. A theory is also emerging that consuming fish oil may even delay or minimize the debilitating effects of neurological disorders such as Alzheimer's and Parkinson's disease.

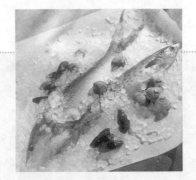

which fish are safe—and which aren't

When the Environmental Working Group, a Washington, D.C.-based advocacy group, reviewed mercury levels, they stacked up fish this way. To cut your exposure to polychlorinated hyphenyls (PCBS), remove skin and extra fat. Women who are not pregnant or planning to become pregnant can safely eat fish several times a week. The same goes for men.

Safe fish for pregnant and nursing women: farmed trout, farmed catfish, fish sticks, summer flounder, shrimp, wild Pacific salmon, croaker, mid-Atlantic blue crab, haddock

Pregnant women should eat no more than one serving of these per month: canned tuna, mahimahi, blue mussels, Eastern oysters, cod, pollock, Great Lakes salmon, wild channel catfish, blue crab from the Gulf of Mexico

Any woman considering pregnancy, already pregnant, or nursing should avoid the following: shark, swordfish, king mackerel, tilefish, tuna steaks, sea bass, marlin, halibut, pike, walleye, white croaker, largemouth bass, oysters from the Gulf of Mexico, sport fish caught from waterways with fish advisories

A note of caution: Catching your own fish isn't necessarily better. Check with your state's fish and wildlife department before you head out to catch your own fish. In many areas, catches from local streams or lakes are highly polluted.

In many studies of omega-3s, subjects have taken fish-oil supplements. Which raises an inevitable question: If I don't like fish, can I get my omega-3s in a pill?

Kris-Etherton takes a guarded stance, urging you to ask your doctor if it's okay to take fish-oil pills. After all, she argues, large doses of omega-3s may cause side effects. Connor feels that's a bit overcautious. "It's safe enough for most people to take one or two grams of fish oil per day," he says, noting that a typical serving of salmon contains about five grams of oil.

What does wahoo taste like? Good question. The answer is just a click away, thanks to a crew of seafood merchants, chefs, and journalists who met to try 57 kinds of fish, from char to dogfish. To view the results—including details about taste, texture, and aroma—visit the flavor guide on www.simplyseafood.com.

Connor declines to use supplements, since he's a big fish-eater. "Pills don't taste good," he says. "But fish tastes great." Unfortunately, the latter message remains a tough sell. Many people don't like fish, and others think that cooking it is a culinary challenge that too often produces a bland, mealy dinner and a smelly kitchen.

But even if you know how to pull off a palate-pleasing seafood dinner, deciding which fish to buy can be tricky. Newspapers are filled with stories about species that are threatened with extinction, because they're either overfished or poisoned from polluted water. Fish farms were supposed to spare salmon and other endangered species, but some experts believe they could make matters worse if the fish escape from their pens and breed in the wild.

What's a green chef to do? It depends on whom you ask. Some experts say the only solution is to stop eating endangered and threatened species. The Monterey Bay Aquarium in California has put a fish-buying cheat sheet for eco-conscious shoppers on its Web site (www.mbayaq.org). But abiding by the chart means avoiding such delights as bluefin tuna, Atlantic cod, farmed salmon, and Chilean sea bass.

That still leaves a lot of fish in the sea. And not all observers take such a hard line. George Liles, spokesman for the National Marine Fisheries Service (NMFS), says you can buy most fish on sale in markets and restaurants with a clear conscience. The NMFS works to ensure that fishermen and fish farmers abide by laws that safeguard endangered species and the environment. "If a fish has been caught legally and you avoid it," says Liles, "you're hurting people who fish responsibly."

So shop for seafood as your conscience permits, but quit angling for excuses to avoid fish. With a little care in the kitchen, anyone can get hooked on these healthful gifts from the sea. ✳

Seafood Savvy
How to Buy and Cook Fabulous Fish

Many Americans—including some skilled home chefs—think buying and cooking great seafood is a kind of black art. But, in fact, fish is tough to screw up, as long as you shop wisely and follow a few simple rules in the kitchen.

• Good, fresh fish is firm, bright, and free of discoloration. If a piece smells like ammonia or, well, fishy, when you get it home, shop somewhere else the next time.

• Prewrapped fish should be tightly wrapped. And don't buy cooked fish if it's displayed next to raw fish; cross-contamination can occur.

• Don't be turned off by the word frozen. Thanks to modern techniques, fish that's frozen at sea can be just as tasty as fresh. The best way to defrost frozen seafood is to place it on the lowest shelf in your refrigerator overnight.

• Cut down on cooking odors by adding a little wine or vinegar to the liquid used to cook or marinate fish. Chef Gary Puetz, who appears on television as the "Seafood Steward," says that white vermouth neutralizes fishy smells better than anything.

• For an easy dinner, Puetz suggests poaching. Bring 2 cans of chicken broth, 1 cup white vermouth, and some peppercorns, crushed herbs, and grated lemon rind to a boil, then reduce to a simmer. Add a salmon fillet and cook for 10 to 12 minutes.

• The old rule stating fish should be cooked for 10 minutes per inch of thickness is a handy start. But be flexible: Fillets of delicate fish such as sole require less cooking time—as do species with firmer flesh like tuna. Rather than watching the clock, cut into the flesh to check if it's opaque. As soon as the fish stops looking raw in the middle, remove it from the heat. You can always use a thermometer; fish is thoroughly cooked at 145° F.

great cancer-fighting
Greens

They're a healthy food-lover's dream: beautiful, delicious, easy to prepare, and more powerful at preventing cancer than almost anything else in the market.

With recipes and cooking tips from the world-famous chefs at Chez Panisse.

BY PETER JARET

On a misty morning in Sonoma, California, Bob Cannard leads me through a field of dinosaur kale—waist-high plants whose crinkly blue-black leaves look as if they really might have been snack food for a stegosaurus. "Feel this," he says, breaking off a frond. "This is what a healthy leaf should feel like—strong and resilient. Have a taste."

I've always loved greens, but this is special—as if the kale has absorbed the loamy smell of the morning itself. I'm here because this field marks the spot where superb food and good health come together. Cannard plunges on, up and down the rows of his 20-acre organic farm, stopping to grab young mustard, watercress, and more. An elfin guy with gray hair flowing from under an old wool cap, he comes off as an eccentric, holding forth on the spiritual life of plants. But he walks

Kale
(aka, cavolo nero or lacinato)
and bok choy are both rich in
natural cancer fighters

among the nation's culinary giants. Almost everything he grows is destined for Chez Panisse, the world-famous Berkeley restaurant that helped establish the joys of green vegetables raised without chemicals and served at the peak of freshness.

While Cannard and the chefs at Chez Panisse have been reshaping our notions of what greens can do for our taste buds, scientists have been redefining what vegetables do for the rest of the body. Leafy greens, it turns out, are laced with substances that may offer more cancer protection than anything else in the produce section. According to findings from the Iowa Women's Health Study, women who eat plenty of veggies of all kinds lower their risk of ovarian cancer. But those who favor leafy greens get an extra dose of protection, cutting their risk by 56 percent compared with the women who rarely toss a salad or wilt a spinach leaf.

In fact, scientists are finding substances in leafy vegetables that can block cancer at almost every step of the way. Some neutralize carcinogens like those in tobacco and grilled meats.

247

Some nutritionists believe leafy greens are part of the secret behind the Mediterranean diet, widely regarded as the world's healthiest.

Others stymie cells that have turned malignant, while still others shut down the growth of such hormone-dependent tumors as breast cancer.

Some nutritionists think leafy greens are a big part of the secret behind the Mediterranean diet, widely regarded as the world's healthiest. Researchers a generation ago noted that the inhabitants of Crete enjoyed unusually long lives, and it may be no coincidence that they devoured more than 80 wild greens, from sorrel and arugula to mustard and borage. In her cookbook *Mediterranean Grains and Greens* (HarperCollins, 1998), Paula Wolfert tells of a physician assigned to a post on Crete by the Turkish sultan. When no one turned up at the doctor's clinic, he sent a message back to Istanbul: "The people here eat only greens, herbs, and olive oil. As a result, they don't need me."

Back then, the islanders foraged for wild greens, of course, while today most of us do our foraging at the market. Here are 10 easy-to-find greens to help keep you healthy, with tips and recipes—from Chez Panisse, no less—for delicious ways to use them.

spinach & chard

For a virtually instant side dish, rinse fresh spinach leaves, drop them still wet into a saucepan with some minced garlic and olive oil, and cook until wilted; serve with a squeeze of lemon. Or, suggests Russell Moore, the café chef at Chez Panisse, strip the leaves from several red, green, and yellow chard fronds, then prepare them as above. Cut the stems into matchsticks and plunge them briefly into boiling water; drain, then toss with a little olive oil and salt, spoon onto a platter, and top with grilled fish or chicken.

Health dividend: All leafy vegetables teem with beta-carotene, an antioxidant that shields healthy cells from genetic damage, but spinach and chard also come loaded with two others: lutein and zeaxanthin. No one knows exactly why these antioxidants are

standouts, but one recent study found that lutein is five times more likely than beta-carotene to be absorbed into the bloodstream. It makes a difference. Researchers at the University of Utah Medical School have found that people who eat lots of lutein-rich foods run a low risk of developing colon cancer. Diets also high in zeaxanthin have been linked to lower risk of cancer of the esophagus.

romaine lettuce & endive

For a special side dish, says Moore, cut romaine leaves crosswise into thin strips. Then, in a bit of butter, sauté fresh peas until tender, add the romaine, and toss until warm. As for endive (even the Chez Panisse crew can't agree on whether to pronounce it ENdive or onDEEVE), "it's one of our favorites," says Moore. Curly endive, also called frisée, is great wilted with a hot vinaigrette. Or slice Belgian endive leaves lengthwise, steam for several minutes until translucent, brush with olive oil, and grill for a few minutes.

Health dividend: Both these greens deliver generous doses of folic acid, the B vitamin that has been found to prevent some birth defects. Now it appears folic-acid-rich foods fight cancer too. A recent Dutch study linked diets high in folic acid to lower risk of lung cancer. The vitamin also seems to guard against colorectal cancer, say Harvard University researchers. In their findings, women getting an adequate dose were less likely to develop the disease than those running low.

arugula & watercress

Arugula has long been loved in Italy, where it's often found growing wild. Chopped and simmered in tomato sauce, arugula can give pasta a subtle sizzle. The mild pepperiness of watercress is so delicious that Chez Panisse chefs often serve it alone or with a light vinaigrette. It's also tasty in potato salad. And

Scientists are finding substances in leafy vegetables that can block cancer at almost every step of the way.

Chard, Spinach, and Escarole Pasta

SERVES 4
PREPARATION: 15 MINUTES
COOKING: 20 MINUTES

1 bunch chard (about 1 pound)
2 pounds spinach
1 large head escarole, kale, or radicchio
2 large red onions
3 or 4 cloves garlic
1/4 cup olive oil, divided
1 bay leaf
1 tablespoon chopped fresh thyme
1 cup red wine
1 pound linguine
1/2 cup defatted chicken stock or water
2 tablespoons capers*
Salt and pepper to taste

1. Stem chard and spinach, if necessary. Remove core from escarole, and separate leaves. Wash greens, and cut into thin shreds. Peel and coarsely chop onions. Peel and mince garlic.
2. In a large pot over high heat, boil 3 quarts water for pasta.
3. Heat a heavy casserole over medium-high heat. Add half the olive oil and the onions, bay leaf, and thyme; cook, covered, until onions are tender, about 5 minutes. Uncover, and continue cooking about 5 minutes more, or until onions are very brown, just short of burning. Add red wine, and stir to loosen browned bits in pan; cover, turn heat to low, and simmer 3 to 4 minutes.
4. Put linguine on to cook. Uncover onions, and add garlic. After about 1 minute, add greens and stock. Cook 5 minutes, add capers, and season to taste with salt and pepper.
5. When pasta is done (12 minutes), drain, and add to casserole with greens. Pour on remaining olive oil; toss well.

* Use large salt-packed capers, rinsed and coarsely chopped, or brine-packed ones, left whole if they are small.

Per serving: Calories 427 (22% from fat), Fat 12 g (1 g saturated), Protein 18 g, Carbohydrate 65 g, Fiber 13 g, Cholesterol 0 mg, Iron 13 mg, Sodium 539 mg, Calcium 354 mg

Watercress Salad with Belgian Endive and Apple

SERVES 4
PREPARATION: 15 MINUTES
COOKING: 20 MINUTES

3 bunches watercress (about 2 pounds)
2 heads Belgian endive
1 apple
Juice of 1 lemon
1 tablespoon champagne vinegar
2 tablespoons Dijon mustard
Salt and pepper to taste
4 tablespoons olive oil

1. Wash watercress well, and discard any large stems. Dry cress, and put in refrigerator. Remove any damaged outer leaves from heads of endive. Quarter them, and cut away core. Cut quarters lengthwise into long strips.
2. Peel and quarter apple. Cut out core, slice quarters thinly, and cut slices into matchsticks.
3. In a salad bowl, whisk together lemon juice, vinegar, mustard, salt, and pepper. Let stand a few minutes, then whisk in olive oil. Add watercress, endive, and apple to bowl and toss thoroughly to coat with vinaigrette. Taste and adjust seasonings.

Per serving: Calories 209 (55% from fat), Fat 14 g (2 g saturated), Protein 7 g, Carbohydrate 21 g, Fiber 6 g, Cholesterol 0 mg, Iron 1 mg, Sodium 142 mg, Calcium 307 mg

Recipes adapted from Chez Panisse Vegetables *(Harper-Collins, 1996) by Alice Waters and the cooks of* Chez Panisse.

if you're serving fish, try this easy sauce: Quickly plunge one or two cups of watercress into boiling water, then purée them in a blender with one or two tablespoons of flavorful olive oil. Serve with salmon, tuna, or swordfish.

Health dividend: Arugula and watercress are rich in substances called indoles, which nudge the body to produce enzymes that disarm potential carcinogens. New findings suggest indoles may also put the brakes on existing cancer cells. Studying breast cancer,

Collard greens are rich in calcium, a mineral that's not only good for your bones but can shield you from colon cancer.

University of California researchers found that indoles prevent tumor cells from multiplying and may also kill malignant cells. Other findings suggest indoles help boost immune defenses.

collards & turnips

Collards are a favorite in the South, where they're often boiled until tender, up to 30 minutes, then served with a splash of lemon. Turnip greens boil up the same way but are more versatile. For a savory salad, mix chopped and wilted turnip greens, white beans, rosemary, and olive oil. Or let turnips take a star turn. "One of the things I love to do is take young turnips with the greens attached, split them down the middle, and boil or steam them until tender," says Moore. "The combination of the bulb's mellow taste with the spicier flavor of the greens is great."

Health dividend: Think calcium, and you picture a glass of milk. But these greens are full of the bone builder. What's calcium got to do with cancer? At the University of Wisconsin, scientists found that women whose meals were well-stocked with the mineral were about half as likely to develop colon cancer as those whose meals delivered little.

kale & bok choy

Bok choy turns up most often in Chinese stir-fries. But the leaves make a great salad, sliced thin, tossed with minced shallots, olive oil, and white wine vinegar, then topped with cilantro. Of all the varieties of kale, the favorite at Chez Panisse is dinosaur kale—the same prehistoric plants Cannard grows. I took Moore's advice and stripped the leaves from the stems, boiled them for 5 to 10 minutes, then quickly sautéed the drained leaves with some garlic slices in a splash of olive oil. One forkful, and I was right back in that misty Sonoma field.

Health dividend: Both kale and bok choy are brimming with isothiocyanates, the same substances that give broccoli its glowing reputation. Like indoles, they appear to block carcinogens and squelch malignancies. Researchers recently found that Chinese men with measurable isothiocyanate levels in their bodies cut their risk of lung cancer by 40 percent. ✳

Peter Jaret is a contributing Health *editor.*

THE FOOD THAT'S GOOD FOR THE EYES

There's another reason to swerve around the drive-through and head to the farmers' market. A diet high in antioxidants and other nutrients like omega-3 fatty acids may protect against eye diseases, including cataracts, glaucoma, and macular degeneration, which is the leading cause of blindness. A recent study in the *Journal of the American College of Nutrition* reported that people who regularly ate spinach, eggs, and broccoli decreased their risk of cataracts up to 20 percent and macular degeneration up to 40 percent.

Found in abundance in plant-based foods, antioxidants fight free-radical damage. Free radicals create oxidative stress, the harmful condition which has been linked to numerous degenerative diseases.

So what are the superfoods for the eyes? Stuart Richer, Ph.D., chief of optometry at the Department of Veterans Affairs Medical Center in North Chicago, ticks off a list that resembles a Japanese menu. Eat five to nine helpings daily of sulfur-filled garlic, onions, or egg whites; carotenoid-rich kale, spinach, broccoli, or collard greens; and vitamin C-packed oranges, grapefruit, or strawberries. In addition, foods containing bioflavonoids (grapes, berries, green tea), vitamin E (nuts, leafy green vegetables), and omega-3 fatty acids (cold-water fish like salmon, mackerel, and tuna) may also protect your peepers.

FOUND:
Protein Prevents Bone Loss

Make Grandma a tuna sandwich to go with her cottage cheese: A new study suggests that protein may help stave off bone loss in the elderly. Researchers examining more than 600 participants in the Framingham Osteoporosis Study found that the 70- to 90-year-old men and women with the highest daily protein intake—equivalent to either a 9-ounce steak or a cup of tuna salad—lost significantly less bone over a four-year period than those men and women who consumed half as much protein. This confirms several other large studies on the positive link between protein and bones.

t o m a t o e s
even better than we thought

Scientists in Scotland have added yet another reason to celebrate the tomato. Most of us already knew that the succulent veggie comes packed with phytochemicals and antioxidants. Now it turns out that the yellow juice around the seeds contains potent anti-clotting agents.

These agents may prove more effective than aspirin at reducing the risk of harmful blood clots by keeping overactive platelets from clumping together along artery walls.

A N O T H E R   R E A S O N
to love beans

You already eat bananas and drink orange juice to get your fill of potassium. So it may surprise you to learn that eating beans—black, pinto, great northern, and others—is another delicious way to up your intake of this mineral that can help keep blood pressure in check and benefit your bones to boot. A cup of cooked beans contains as many as 950 milligrams of potassium—more than a quarter of your recommended daily allowance.

HEALTH BUZZ

THUMBS UP

MSG
It may be time to rethink your fear of lo mein. A new study suggests that MSG allergies may not really exist.

avocados
Good news for guacamole-lovers. Experts say the tasty fruit contains chemicals that might fight liver damage.

salmonella
Sure, this bug can flatten you with food poisoning. But it turns out it can be harnessed to stall tumor growth.

THUMBS DOWN

cell phones
There's no consensus that they cause cancer. Yet there's evidence they can interfere with medical equipment.

ginko biloba
The extract has been touted to treat tinnitus. But a new study found it did little to quiet the din in people's ears.

cubicles
Wish your office mates would pipe down? A study indicates even mild disturbances can increase stress.

40 percent of cancers: preventable by diet?

The American Institute for Cancer Research estimates that 30 to 40 percent of cancers are directly linked to poor eating and exercising habits. But you may be able to reduce your risk if you log on to the group's Web site (www.aicr.org). It provides reliable research updates, recipes, and free publications explaining what you can do to change your destiny.

bananas:
100 calories of
pure fun

The low-carb diet gurus say bananas can make you fat.
But read on before you give them up for good.

BY JENNA McCARTHY

Bananas are like movie stars: We adore them, but there's a lot we don't know about them. Although they come in hundreds of varieties, for example, most of us are only familiar with the supermarket staple known as the cavendish. Only hard-core afficionados know that each yellow fellow is called a finger and that the bunches stacked in the produce aisle are clusters. (Bunches, truth be told, are giant groupings of clusters that can weigh more than Calista Flockhart wearing combat boots.) And while we're forever referring to the enigmatic edibles simply as fruit, the banana plant is actually the world's largest herb, and each finger is a berry.

Despite their mysterious ways, bananas are the most popular "fruit" in the nation. The average American puts away more than 28 pounds a year. Compare that to the 19 pounds of apples and 15 pounds of watermelon a typical citizen consumes, and it's clear we've gone bananas.

It's not hard to see why: Beyond the brilliantly designed, biodegradable packaging and impressive nutritional profile, bananas rank up there with some pretty decadent confections on the taste-and-texture scale. They're also cheap, portable, and plentiful, and while we're primarily a peel-and-eat culture, the sweet meat is gobbled around the globe in everything from hearty stews to vegetable curry.

Thanks to all their potassium, bananas may help you lower your risk of high blood pressure.

These days, however, not everyone is on the banana bandwagon. A few big-name diet gurus have raised concerns that snacking on a tasty finger is the nutritional equivalent of scarfing down a slice of Wonder Bread.

In his best-selling *New Diet Revolution* (Avon, 1997), Robert Atkins (of all-protein, nothing-but-protein fame) barely deigns to mention the fructose-rich fruit. With about 27 grams of carbohydrate, one medium banana contains more carbs than Atkins recommends that most dieters eat in an entire day.

Pick up *The Zone* (HarperCollins, 1995), another celebrity-endorsed diet book, and you'll find bananas alongside white bread, baked potatoes, and carrots in author Barry Sears's long list of unfavorable carbohydrates. Sears's apparent anti-banana stance is rooted in the glycemic index (GI), a measure of a food's effect on the release of insulin (which Sears terms the fat-storage hormone). The higher a food's GI, the more rapidly glucose enters the bloodstream and the more insulin the body releases. Sears maintains that foods jammed with carbohydrates and carrying a high glycemic rating, force the pancreas into insulin overdrive—a message, according to the book, that tells your body to store fat and keep it stored.

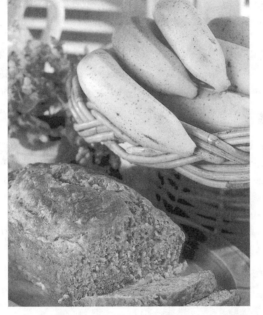

Yet many experts dispute this assertion. "It's absolutely not true that bananas promote fat storage," says Terri Brownlee, nutrition director at Duke University's Diet and Fitness Center. "Insulin is the package through which calories are stored. But this is a normal metabolic process, not one that sends the body into distress."

"A calorie is a calorie is a calorie," says Gerald M. Reaven, a professor at the Stanford School of Medicine and author of *Syndrome X: Overcoming the Silent Killer That Can Give You a Heart Attack* (Simon & Schuster, 2000). "If you want to lose weight, you have to eat less and move more. It's the law of thermodynamics—and it's not going to go away just because someone writes a book." Reaven and others point out that although the glycemic index may be accurate, one major flaw is that the numbers are based on eating one food at a time, something most of us rarely do.

And some experts even question how the diet gurus come up with their numbers. Thomas Wolever, professor of nutritional sciences at the University of Toronto and coauthor of *The Glucose Revolution* (Marlowe & Co., 1998), doesn't even classify bananas as a high GI food, instead grouping them with most other fruit in a more favorable category. (GI ratings for hundreds of foods can be found in Wolever's book or at www.glycemicindex.com.)

While the connection between the glycemic index and weight loss is contentious, there's evidence that foods with a high GI may pose a health risk for some. Low GI meals help diabetics control their blood sugar levels, says Wolever. What's more, studies conducted at Harvard University's School of Public Health found that diets with a low GI are associated with a reduced risk of developing Type 2 diabetes and heart disease.

"We're not saying that high GI foods are poisonous or that you have to cut these foods out of your diet altogether," says Wolever. "The glycemic index is just a tool to help you make the best possible food choices."

There's plenty of evidence that bananas are a wise choice. Weighing in at a lean 100 calories and packing less than one gram of fat, bananas are potassium powerhouses. Numerous studies indicate that this nutrient helps strengthen your bones and lowers risk of high blood pressure and stroke. A single banana contains more than 10 percent of the recommended daily allowance.

Besides all that potassium, bananas contain birth-defect-fighting folate, a B vitamin crucial for anyone who is pregnant or of childbearing age. In addition, they're rich in magnesium, a mineral that helps bones absorb calcium, another boon to lifelong health. Bananas are such an easily digested source of energy, athletes often peel into nature's power bar before a race.

There's really no reason for the nation to stop loving its favorite fruit. Wolever and other nutrition experts advocate a diet that's 50 to 60 percent carbohydrates and that emphasizes a mix of whole grains, vegetables, and fruits—a mix that can certainly include bananas.

According to the U.S. Department of Agriculture (USDA), the average American downs only 1½ daily servings of fruit. (The agency's Food Guide Pyramid recommends two to four.)

"People think it's tough to get that many servings," says Brownlee. "But eat a large banana and you've got two. That's pretty good." So slice one onto your cereal. Stick one in the freezer for a homemade icy treat. Bake a few in a batch of bread. The only way a banana can hurt you is if you slip on the peel. ✳

a tasty banana sorbet you can make in a flash

Bananas do not easily inspire culinary greatness. Sure, we've all whipped up a smoothie or baked a loaf of banana bread. But what else can you do with them? Author Susan Quick has plenty of suggestions —150 of them, in fact. Her recent cookbook, *Go Bananas!* (Broadway Books, 2000), is rich in recipes for exotic curries, deliciously different pancakes, and lots of great dessert ideas. This banana-pear sorbet, adapted from the book, is creamy smooth, packed with fruit flavor, and fat-free.

2 (16-ounce) cans sliced or halved pears in heavy syrup
2 ripe bananas, frozen
2 tablespoons fresh lime juice
2 tablespoons dark rum

1. Freeze the unopened cans of pears until solid, at least 18 hours. Submerge the frozen cans in hot water for one minute. Open them, and slide out the contents onto a cutting board. Using a very sharp knife, slice into 1-inch-thick slices, then into large chunks.
2. Place the chunks in the bowl of a food processor. Slice the bananas, and add to the processor along with the lime juice and rum. Process, pulsing on and off until smooth.
3. Serve immediately, or transfer to a storage container and freeze until ready to serve. Serves 6.

Per serving: Calories 194 (0% from fat), Fat 0 g (0 g saturated), Protein 1 g, Carbohydrate 48 g, Fiber 3 g, Cholesterol 0 mg, Iron 0 mg, Sodium 8 mg, Calcium 10 mg

Q+A

5 servings of fruits and veggies a day: easier than you may think

What, exactly, counts as a serving of a fruit or vegetable?

Probably less than you think. It's really not so hard to eat the recommended five to nine helpings of fruits and veggies each day. That's because the official serving sizes outlined by the U.S. Department of Agriculture are quite small.

Here's how you can keep track. Just about any medium-sized whole fruit equals one serving, as does six ounces of juice. So a breakfast banana and OJ get you off to a good start. If you prefer your fruit cooked or canned, you need only half a cup to make a serving; if you like to snack on raisins and other dried fruit, you need just a quarter cup.

A lunchtime salad made from a cup of raw greens gives you another serving; if it also includes a half-cup of garbanzo beans or other legumes, you've got one more. For dinner, a half cup of a cooked vegetable—such as broccoli—adds a serving, as does a baked potato.

broccoli: eat the whole thing

Are broccoli stems as nutritious as the tops?

Pretty close. The flowery tops do contain more of the anticancer compound sulphoraphane and over seven times more vitamin A (beta-carotene). But both the stalks and the flowers are jam-packed with vitamin C, folate, and fiber—giving you plenty of good reasons to savor those stalks. And using the whole vegetable will also make you feel virtuous.

After trimming off the bottom, just peel off the tough outer layer with a paring knife or vegetable peeler. Julienne the stalk or cut it into small round "pennies" to ensure that it cooks in the same time frame as the tops. Eaten raw, these pennies also make a great crunchy snack.

APPLES: THEY REALLY CAN KEEP THE DOCTOR AWAY

It's a good thing that apples are no longer forbidden fruit. Especially since these shiny, juicy devils are chock-full of nutrients that can keep your heart healthy. That's the finding of a new study by Dianne Hyson, a nutrition researcher at the University of California at Davis. She asked 25 people to gobble down two apples or drink 12 ounces of unsweetened juice every day for 12 weeks.

When Hyson measured the participants' cholesterol levels afterward, she found that the fruit had significantly limited the breakdown of bad cholesterol in the blood. That reduction is important because once the cholesterol deteriorates, it's likely to cause plaque buildup that can clog arteries and lead to heart disease.

Hyson suspects that the protection can be traced to flavonoids, potent antioxidants that apples supply in particular abundance. "To get these benefits, people in the study didn't really have to change anything about their diets," says Hyson. "They just added a little juice or a couple of apples. That's not too hard for most people to do."

berry good news

The word on blueberries just keeps getting better. A recent study indicates that the tasty little beauties, already known to contain potent antioxidants, are packed with yet another disease-fighting powerhouse: resveratrol. U.S. Department of Agriculture chemist Agnes Rimando has found that the berries are brimming with this phytochemical, which is famously found in grapes and wine and has been linked in lab tests and other studies to reduced rates of heart disease and cancer. Rimando also found lesser amounts of resveratrol in cranberries and huckleberries.

perfect smoothies on demand

It's impossible to blend a smoothie without ripe bananas. Fortunately, perfection is always possible—if you have frozen fruit ready to roll. When spots begin to appear, just peel the bananas, wrap them tightly in plastic wrap, and stow them in the freezer. They'll last a few weeks that way.

how vegetables protect you from cancer

Just how do vegetables protect you from cancer? In some cases, they trigger your body's own defenses, a new study suggests. Researchers at Johns Hopkins University Bloomberg School of Public Health found that mice unable to produce a particular protein were more prone to developing stomach cancer than were normal mice. And mice that lacked the protein had higher cancer rates even if they were given a chemical known to be protective against cancer.

This protein, called nrf2, spurs cells to produce enzymes that detoxify cancer-causing substances. And the best way to stimulate the production of nrf2 in your body is to eat your vegetables, says Thomas W. Kensler, Ph.D., who directed the study. "We know that the chemicals in certain plants—particularly cruciferous vegetables like broccoli, cauliflower, and Brussels sprouts—activate nrf2 production," he says. Green leafy vegetables also contain these helpful chemicals.

Increasing production of nrf2 is important whether you're man or mouse, Kensler believes. "We're beginning to understand that if we can elevate the level of these detoxifying enzymes, we can enhance the resistance to carcinogens in animals and, we believe, people."

oats

for weight loss, low cholesterol, and better blood pressure

Help yourself to the world's best breakfast cereal.

BY LAURA FRASER

As a kid, each time I faced a bowl of gray, gummy, lump-strewn oatmeal, I wondered why the three bears weren't grateful to Goldilocks for dipping into their porridge. It wasn't until I was a grown-up that I had the pleasure of cozying up to a breakfast of nutty, steamy specialty oats topped with dried cherries, brown sugar, and warm milk. That's when I realized those bears were on to something.

It's hardly news that oatmeal is good for you: Oats were a mainstay of Scottish and Irish diets for centuries, and the legendary strength of at least one Celtic god is credited to his inexhaustible appetite for porridge. But only recently have scientists begun to understand how oatmeal delivers the goods. Treat yourself to a big bowl every day, and in addition to spooning up plenty of disease-fighting antioxidants, you'll likely see your blood pressure and cholesterol levels drop, protect yourself from some of the ill effects of high-fat foods—and want to eat less the rest of the day too.

Oats are stars, even among whole grains. They're loaded with higher levels of protein, calcium, magnesium, potassium, iron, zinc, and vitamin E than either wheat or corn.

What gives oatmeal its oomph? First, it's made of whole, unrefined grain, which has proved its worth in study after study. The more whole grains you eat, the less vulnerable you are to diabetes, heart disease, and some cancers.

But even among whole grains, oats are stars. They're loaded with higher levels of protein, calcium, magnesium, potassium, iron, zinc, and vitamin E than either wheat or corn. And while all whole grains contain antioxidants, "Oats have hundreds, including some that are unique," says Joanne Slavin, a professor of nutrition at the University of Minnesota. "Together, these antioxidants are as strong and protective as the ones you'd find in most fruits and vegetables."

What really sets oats (and barley) apart is that they contain more soluble fiber than any other grain. Most fiber plows through the body intact, but soluble fiber dissolves to form a viscous fluid that slows things down; food is digested, the stomach emptied, and nutrients absorbed at a more leisurely pace. "Soluble fiber makes it harder to move the meal downstream quickly," says Joseph M. Keenan, a University of Minnesota physician who studies the health effects of oats.

Fiber is also the secret to oats' cholesterol-lowering powers. As it moseys through the small intestine, a soluble fiber called beta-glucan prevents cholesterol-rich bile acids from being reabsorbed into the body. Always on the lookout for cholesterol, the liver then pulls more out of the blood. In their research, Keenan and others have found that a generous bowl of oatmeal every day can reduce LDL cholesterol (the kind you don't want) by an average of 12 percent while leaving HDL cholesterol (the good kind) unchanged.

Soluble fiber can help lower blood pressure too. In a study of 60 hypertensive people, Keenan reported that after 12 weeks, the subjects who ate oatmeal twice a day improved their readings, and half of them were able to go off blood pressure medicine entirely. Keenan suggests that it's the soluble fiber doing yet another good deed: By slowing the rise of insulin in the blood, it keeps blood vessels from constricting. Other studies have shown that oats also keep blood vessels relaxed after high-fat meals, when they usually constrict.

Oatmeal is enjoying a comeback now that food-lovers have discovered nutty-flavored Irish, or steel-cut, oats.

Don't expect to calm your cardiovascular system with an occasional oatmeal cookie, however. Experts agree that to lower cholesterol, you have to eat at least $1^1/2$ cups of cooked oats a day. To lower their blood pressure, Keenan's subjects ate the equivalent of 3 cups of cooked oats a day. Keenan cautions that people at serious risk of heart disease from high cholesterol should not rely solely on oats to lower their numbers.

If you want to reduce your calorie intake, though, you can rely on oats; true to folk wisdom, oatmeal sticks to your ribs. Because oats take a long time to digest, they keep you feeling full longer. In one study, participants ate a 350-calorie breakfast of either oatmeal or sugary cornflakes. Come lunchtime, the porridge group ate about a third fewer calories than did the fiber-free cornflake group. That explains why I can ski a full day on an oatmeal breakfast and not on a meal of cold cereal. It also means that oatmeal makes an excellent breakfast if you're trying to lose a few pounds.

Pancakes: another way to get your oats

Not everyone takes to oatmeal, even with brown sugar on top. But don't let that keep you away from a grain that's good for your heart. These richly textured pancakes, adapted from Deborah Madison's *Vegetarian Cooking for Everyone* (Broadway Books, 1997), will help you work oats into your breakfast repertoire. Top them with fresh fruit, applesauce, nonfat yogurt—or that caloric classic, maple syrup.

$1^1/2$ cups rolled oats*
2 cups low-fat buttermilk
2 eggs
1 teaspoon vanilla extract
2 tablespoons brown sugar or maple syrup
3 tablespoons canola oil
$1/2$ teaspoon salt
$1/2$ cup flour
$1/4$ teaspoon grated nutmeg
$1/2$ teaspoon baking soda

I. In a large bowl, stir together oats and buttermilk; let stand 20 minutes. Beat eggs with vanilla, sugar, and oil, then stir in soaked oats. Combine remaining ingredients, and add to oat mixture.
2. For each pancake, drop $1/4$ cup batter onto a heated griddle, and cook over medium-low heat until tops are covered with holes. Flip and cook other side. Because of the moisture in this batter, the pancakes need to cook slowly, but turn them only once. Makes 14 (4-inch) pancakes.

* To use steel-cut oats, combine the oats and buttermilk, then let the mixture soak overnight in the fridge. The next morning, proceed with the recipe.

Per pancake: Calories 109 (39% from fat), Fat 5 g (I g saturated), Protein 4 g, Carbohydrate 13 g, Fiber I g, Cholesterol 33 mg, Iron I mg, Sodium 175 mg, Calcium 49 mg

The idea of eating oats may raise some people's eyebrows (in 1755 Samuel Johnson defined oats as "a grain which in England is fed to horses, but in Scotland seems to support a people"), but oats have come a long way since the days they were used mainly as animal feed. Once they're hulled—at which point they're called groats—they can take a number of forms.

Americans are most familiar with old-fashioned, quick-cooking, and instant oats, all of which are made by steaming, roasting, and rolling groats to varying degrees. But for first-class texture and taste, you might want to make the leap to steel-cut oats, which are whole groats cut into pinhead-sized pieces.

McCann's Irish Oatmeal, at about $2.50 a pound, is the most popular; natural food stores sell steel-cut oats in bulk for less than half that price. Steel-cut oats must simmer for about 30 minutes—compared with 5 or 10 minutes for rolled oats—but they don't have to be watched the whole time. Just toss them into boiling water, stir a little, turn down the heat, and go read the paper. During the last 10 minutes, give the oats an occasional stir with a wooden spoon

for oats on the run

Many snack bars, muffins, and other items claiming to be endowed with heart-healthy oats contain little whole grain and lots of calories. Read the label—you'll do best with products that give you at least 2 grams of fiber, as do many granola bars made by Barbara's and Health Valley.

(the Scots traditionally use a stick called a spurtle and stir only clockwise, for good luck). Sautéing the oats in a little butter before cooking makes them extra nutty; adding a little milk to the cooking water improves the creamy texture and flavor. Once they're done, the possibilities for enhancement are endless. A dash of milk and brown sugar, a sprinkling of any number of dried fruits and nuts, and you'll start the day in paradise.

As you sprinkle and pour, be grateful you're savoring your oats at this moment in time. The Celts had strict laws regarding the embellishment of oatmeal: A workingman's children were limited to buttermilk or water; the families of chieftains rated butter. Only the sons of kings were allowed to drizzle honey on their porridge. Fortunately, there's nothing to keep us 21st-century common folk from eating like royalty every morning. ✳

....

the truth
ABOUT FOLIC ACID

It's popping up on some folic acid supplements—and the Food and Drug Administration is riled. The claim reads: ".8 mg of folic acid in a dietary supplement is more effective at reducing the risk of neural tube defects than a lower amount of foods in common form." The agency's beef? "Common form" only refers to unfortified items. Scientists say foods to which the vitamin's been added (like cereals and pasta) are what's really responsible for the recent improvements in folic-acid blood levels.

How to Build Your Own Food Pyramid,
courtesy of the USDA

If the food pyramid was based on your eating habits instead of the ideal diet from the U.S. Department of Agriculture (USDA), what would it look like? Check out www.usda.gov/cnpp. Click on the link under the "Healthy Eating Index," register and list your latest meals. In return, you'll get a no-holds-barred analysis of your diet, including a personalized pyramid. If it's a little lopsided, don't despair: You can record up to 20 days' worth of foods, so you have opportunity to build a solid structure.

more GOOD NEWS about fiber

WHILE THE EXPERTS GO BACK AND FORTH over whether fiber protects against colon cancer, some Italian researchers report that it does seem to lower the risk of oral cancers. They examined the diets of some 2,800 hospital patients and found that those who consistently ate the most fiber-rich fruits, vegetables, and whole grain cereals were about half as likely to be diagnosed with cancers of the mouth, throat, and esophagus as those who ate the least.

Organic: what it really means

Don't throw up your hands if you don't know the difference between products labeled "organic" and "100% organic." Though the U.S. Department of Agriculture just implemented its national standards, the word is still slow in getting out on what the many newly defined terms actually mean. To learn more, check out *A Practical Guide to Understanding Organic*, a helpful pamphlet produced by Stonyfield Farm. It's available online at www.stonyfield.com.

5 WAYS TO SNEAK MORE NUTRITION INTO YOUR FAMILY'S DIET

A small change can be a big plus to your diet if it's the right one, says Marjorie Fitch-Hilgenberg, Ph.D., a University of Arkansas assistant nutrition professor. When Fitch-Hilgenberg replaced the standard iceberg lettuce in hamburgers, tacos, and subs with fresh spinach, she was adding jolts of vitamins A and C, folic acid, and other nutrients to meals of the more than 200 subjects in her recent study. And all were none the wiser. While the researchers work with fast-food chains to test-market the spinach switch, you can try these painless ways to sneak more nutrition into your (and your loved ones') favorite foods.

Don't spare that spinach. Toss fresh leaf spinach into salad mixes, sandwiches, and anything else you can think of. "I always put spinach into my lasagna to get more vegetables into the family meal," says Fitch-Hilgenberg.

Build a better oatmeal. For a morning calcium boost, cook instant oatmeal with skim (or soy) milk instead of water.

De-ice your smoothies. Use frozen bananas instead of crushed ice for a nutritious twist to your favorite smoothie.

Mix your cereals. If you're stuck on sweet breakfast cereals, try blending your favorites with better-for-you brands: Mix Honey Nut Cheerios with Grape-Nuts, for instance, or try Cap'n Crunch with a bit of bran.

Modify your muffins. Toss high-fiber, nutrient-dense dried fruits like apricots into your batter; substitute half the all-purpose flour with soy flour.

Cereal Fiber Scores Again

Another reason to eat your Wheaties: The latest word is that eating more cereal fiber—the kind found in whole wheat bread, cereal, pasta, rice, and oats—may help you avoid one type of stomach cancer. Researchers looked at three large-scale Swedish studies and found that participants who consumed the most cereal fiber had a 70 percent lower risk of developing the cancer than those who ate the least.

food designed
just for women

There's a new women's movement, and it's heading to a supermarket near you. Are these new products—supposedly packed with ingredients beneficial to women—really nutritious?

BY DOMENICA MARCHETTI

As a kid, I could always tell which of my parents had made the morning oatmeal. Dad's was strictly utilitarian, cooked with water and topped with a miserly dash of brown sugar. But Mom used milk (sometimes even cream), lots of brown sugar and cinnamon, and maybe a touch of vanilla or maple syrup. The result was sweet, creamy, and soothing—just the sort of comfort food women crave.

So it was my mother's version that came to mind when I tasted my initial rich, cinnamony spoonful of Quaker Oats' new instant oatmeal, Nutrition for Women. The first gender-specific oatmeal (after my mom's, anyway), not only do its texture and flavor play to a female audience, but each packet is specially fortified with calcium, soy protein, iron, folic acid, and vitamins A, B, D, and E—all nutrients of particular importance to women. These ingredients, along with herbs purported to help women better cope with menopausal symptoms, are showing up in all kinds of female-focused foods, from yogurts to juices to cold cereals and even breads.

This is only the beginning, says Bob Messenger,

an observer of the food and beverage industry for the past 25 years. "This is a trend with very long legs," says Messenger, publisher of *Food Trends Newsletter*. "Every single category in the supermarket is a candidate for re-engineering to meet the emerging demands of women consumers."

But aside from the more exotic herbs, such as dong quai (a hot-flash fighter), women can obtain most of the nutrients featured in these new customized foods by stocking their kitchen cupboards and fridges with basic, gender-neutral fare such as legumes, milk, leafy greens, fruit, and tofu, to name a few. So that begs the question: Do you really need cereals of your own to keep menstrual cramps and brittle bones at bay?

"Part of me says this is the quick-fix mentality," says Nancy Clark, R.D., author of *Nancy Clark's Sports Nutrition Guidebook*, Second Edition (Human Kinetics, 1996). "People who dieted or ate badly their whole lives are now looking for nutritional Band-Aids. That same part of me says just eat food responsibly. You may not get the same benefit out of an energy bar that you will from eating a wholesome meal."

That's because nutritionally enhanced processed foods typically don't contain the full complement of nutrients found in whole foods. "I think it's

Do you really need cereals of your own to keep menstrual cramps and brittle bones at bay? Or will gender-neutral foods—like fruit and legumes—work just as well?

wonderful when a product makes people focus more on what they can do to improve their health," says Liz Applegate, R.D., a nutrition faculty member at the University of California at Davis. "But I don't recommend that women center their diet on these functional foods. The best foods out there are what Mother Nature put together. She did a wonderful job with soybeans, oranges, tomatoes. Let's not forget that."

It's also possible to get too much of a good thing. Say you take a multivitamin, wash it down with a glass of calcium-enriched orange juice, and follow that with a heaping bowl of a female-friendly cereal with milk. That's a lot of calcium, an overload of which (more than 2,500 milligrams per day) can interfere with the absorption of iron and zinc. It's more effective to spread your calcium intake out throughout the day,

rather than ingesting it in giant doses. "We could end up seeing new imbalances that we were never aware of before—changes in the immune system, elevated cholesterol levels, possibly anemia," Clark says.

But the fact is, most women do need help meeting their nutritional quotas. Despite general improvements in the American diet, fewer than half of women age 20 or older currently get the recommended dietary allowances for iron, calcium, folic acid, and vitamins B-6, A, and E. "Women today are busier than ever because they've got so much going on in their lives," says Cathy Kapica, R.D., director of nutrition education at Quaker Oats. "They need the nutrients. Let's make it easy."

Tori Stuart, president of the year-old company Zoe Foods, is working to do just that by filling in some

girlfriend groceries, rated

There's good news and bad news when it comes to foods for women. The good: A lot of the products have nutrients sorely lacking in many women's diets, such as folic acid for a healthy heart (and baby); calcium for strong bones and teeth; iron for energy; and soy and flaxseed for hormonal balance, heart and breast health, and reduced cancer risk. The bad: Not all offer amounts large enough to matter, and some have lots of added fat and sugar. Here's a sampling (taste rating: 1=barely edible, 5=couldn't put it down):

Quaker Oatmeal Nutrition for Women

Nutrition profile: Higher calcium and slightly more folic acid and iron than the brand's gender-neutral instant. The single gram of soy is insignificant.

Taste rating: 3. Flavors are very sweet.

Viactiv Energy Fruit Smoothie

Nutrition profile: Beats calcium-added orange juice for folic acid and B vitamins but has 40 more calories per glass; offers 30% of the recommended daily allowance for calcium.

Taste rating: 3.5. Nice thickness; slightly sweet citrus flavor.

Clif Bar Luna Bar

Nutrition profile: Great source of soy protein (9g); 100% of

recommended levels of folic acid and B vitamins, plus 35% of iron and calcium daily quotas.

Taste rating: 4.5. Nearly as indulgent as a candy bar but has an aftertaste.

General Mills Harmony Cereal

Nutrition profile: Calcium (60% of RDA) is the big sell. Good source of folic acid and iron; has less sugar than Kellogg's Smart Start.

Taste rating: 4. Crunchy, slightly sweet, tasty. Makes a nice snack.

Stonyfield Farm YoSelf Organic Yogurt

Nutrition profile: Six live active cultures are a big plus for digestive health; a fiber called inulin aids in the absorption of calcium (20% of the RDA).

Taste rating: 5. Thick and just sweet enough, with authentic fruit flavors.

French Meadow Bakery Woman's Bread

Nutrition profile: Expensive, but its sky-high fiber content (10g per serving), soy isoflavones (80mg), and hearty helping of flaxseed justify the price.

Taste rating: 4.5. Nutty, sourdough-like flavor—filling, but not too dense.

Women can obtain most of the nutrients they need
by stocking their cupboards and fridges with such basic fare as legumes, milk, leafy greens, fruit, and tofu.

gaps. She saw her mother, who was frustrated by hot flashes and other menopausal symptoms, resort to making her own granola with flaxseed and soy protein, two foods that seemed to help.

"My mother had never set foot in a health-food store, yet here she was, making her own granola," Stuart says. "That was a signal to me." Thus was born Zoe Foods' Flax & Soy Granola. "We're touching a note with women," she says.

And reaching out to their taste buds. Decadent-sounding flavors give women the impression that they're indulging without actually indulging, which is why Stonyfield Farm YoSelf, a high-calcium yogurt, comes in chocolate and crème caramel as well as fruit flavors. On first try, a s'mores-flavored Luna bar seemed to be worth far more than the 180 calories listed on the label. There was a definite aftertaste—from all the added nutrients, maybe—but I didn't mind it so much. It made me feel virtuous, not unlike when I remember to take my multivitamin in the morning or floss my teeth before bed.

The next looming question, of course, is: What about men? Several nutrition experts assured me that men could eat any of these women-targeted foods without developing breasts or a crush on Russell Crowe. But will men soon have special products of their own? Women do 70 percent of the grocery shopping in the United States and are typically more concerned with health issues than men, so they're the natural first targets for gender-specific products, Messenger says. Whether we'll soon see male-centric foods on grocery-store shelves is something most food manufacturers won't talk about. One exception, however, is French Meadow Bakery, creator of Woman's Bread (enhanced with heart-healthy flaxseed, soy, and folic acid). The company says that it is currently developing a bread for men, which will be geared to their overall health needs.

One thing is certain, though, Messenger says: Gender-centric, functional foods are here to stay. "Anything that can absorb nutrients can become a nutritionally enhanced food."

Think of all the possibilities: for him, testosterone-laced burgers; for her, estrogen-infused pasta. In such a brave new world, can six-packs of Viagra-enhanced beer be far behind?

Domenica Marchetti is a nutrition, health, and food writer based in Alexandria, Virginia.

Q+A
soy milk: long on protein, short on calcium
I've recently switched from dairy to soy milk. Am I missing out on any nutrients?

If your concern is calcium, you're better off with cow's milk. You'd have to drink three times as much of the soy beverage to match the calcium supply in regular milk. It also has vitamins D and B-12, which aren't in soy.

So why the hype over soy milk? Like dairy milk, it is a great source of protein. And while both kinds have fat (unless you buy the fat-free versions), soy milk's fat is the "healthy" unsaturated kind that improves cholesterol and lowers the risk of heart disease. And because soy is made from beans, it's a good source of fiber and isoflavones, plant estrogens that help ward off osteoporosis, heart disease, and cancer.

If you're lactose intolerant, vegan, or have a history of heart disease or high cholesterol, enjoy your soy. Just choose the enriched version, along with a daily calcium supplement, and don't skimp on nutrient-rich greens.

TEST YOURSELF

What do you really know about food allergies?

FOOD ALLERGIES can cause itchy hives or even anaphylactic shock. How potent can a peanut be?

1. If you're allergic to soy, it's safe to eat food cooked in soybean oil.
   True or False?

2. Artificial flavors cause the majority of food allergies.
   True or False?

3. Which of these can cause an allergic reaction?
   - a) "Natural" cosmetics
   - b) Entering a fish restaurant
   - c) Eating egg whites
   - d) Any of the above

4. Kissing someone who has eaten peanuts can provoke an allergic response.
   True or False?

ANSWERS

1. True. Your body reacts to certain proteins in soybeans, peanuts, and sunflower seeds, and most of the oils sold in the United States are highly refined (as opposed to cold-pressed), so they contain no trace of them.

2. False. Ninety percent are linked to milk, eggs, wheat, peanuts, soy, tree nuts, fish, and shellfish.

3. D. Any of the above. Some beauty products contain enough milk or nut extract to bring on hives. Believe it or not, the tiny proteins released into the air by frying and steaming seafood can also trigger allergic reactions. And most people with egg allergies actually respond to the whites, not the yolks.

4. True. If you're sensitive to goobers, as little as one-eightieth of a peanut can cause an allergic reaction.

when food safety concerns turn into OBSESSION

It's all you hear these days. Everyone's talking food: pure, unadulterated, organic, farm-raised, free-range, genetically unaltered food. Where to buy the best bean curd. Why the fish at the local market is unsafe. Why you should ask for soy milk in your latte. For those folks who still relish the occasional bologna sandwich, this chat takes on an obsessive tinge. And according to Steven Bratman, M.D., the obsession even has its own name: orthorexia nervosa.

Bratman, a physician and self-professed recovering health nut, wrote *Health Food Junkies* (Bantam Doubleday Dell, 2000), a treatise on the symptoms and treatment of this food-quality obsession. According to Bratman, an orthorexic's diet is often too restrictive and might be low in protein, vitamins, minerals, and fat. An orthorexic may suffer the same limitations as an anorexic—a fear of living life fully and a propensity to substitute regimen for experience.

Though not classified as an official psychological disorder, orthorexia showcases the dangers of taking anything to extremes—even concern about your health. For more information, visit www.orthorexia.com.

GO FISH

six sensational ways to reap the benefits of salmon

It's delicious, nutritious, and easy to prepare. But best of all, salmon is good for your heart.

RECIPES BY ROBIN VIETTA-MILLER

"What can I get you?" the clerk asks. I'm standing in the seafood market near my home, a bright place with slick tile floors and gurgling aquariums full of restless lobsters and crabs. A briny scent, like that of the ocean on a cold day, tweaks my nose. Inside tidy glass cases are glistening fish steaks and fillets laid out in trays on ice. The fish looks perfect—bone-white halibut, dusky red tuna, blond sea bass—and placing my order ought to be easy. But no. I dither, I debate, then say what I said the last time I was in: "Two-thirds of a pound of salmon, please."

I love salmon. Never mind that it's every cardiologist's darling, rich in the fish oils that help to keep hearts beating steadily and to stave off the ultimate misfortune known as sudden cardiac death. Or that the oils seem to repel depression. Salmon is just plain delicious, easy to cook, and no less versatile than chicken or beef.

HOW TO COOK *perfect grilled salmon*

Salmon on the grill is one of life's joys—except when it sticks. To avoid that mishap, scour the rack with a wire brush, wipe off any grit with a rag, then preheat the rack over medium-hot coals (just fading from orange to gray).

1. Using tongs, grasp a clean paper towel that's been folded, then soaked with 2 tablespoons of vegetable oil; wipe the hot grill to remove as much lingering grime as possible.
2. With a pastry brush dipped in oil, lightly coat both sides of the fish. The oil variety isn't crucial; use whatever kind the recipe you're following calls for.
3. Place the fish near but not directly over the coals' hottest spot. Wait 2 to 3 minutes, then with a spatula, lift the fish and rotate it a quarter turn; cook 2 minutes more. Turn the fish over and cook 3 to 5 minutes more.
4. Check for doneness by using a knife or fork to peek inside the salmon's thickest part. When the flesh is nearly but not entirely opaque, remove the fish to a warm platter. It will cook through on its way to the table.

Doubt that last claim? Then try these recipes. Grilled salmon steaks with cilantro pesto and teriyaki-glazed fillets are ideal fare on a warm summer evening. But keep on exploring. Salmon is also terrific baked; simmered in a chowder; cooked gently and then nestled in a Caesar salad; or rubbed with chili and roasted.

To find the best salmon, pick a seafood seller you trust. Atlantic salmon, always farmed, tends to be mild and rich. Pacific (wild) salmon can be strong or mild, fatty or lean, depending on the variety and where it was caught.

Salmon Chowder

SERVES 4
PREPARATION: 10 MINUTES
COOKING: 15 MINUTES

2 teaspoons olive oil
2 leeks, rinsed well, ends trimmed and chopped
2 cloves garlic, minced
2 bay leaves
1 teaspoon dried tarragon
1/2 teaspoon salt
1/2 teaspoon freshly ground black pepper
6 small red potatoes (about 1/2 pound total), cut into
    1-inch cubes
2 1/2 cups nonfat reduced-sodium chicken broth
1 pound salmon fillet, skinned and cut into 1-inch cubes
1/2 cup fat-free half-and-half
4 teaspoons minced fresh chives (optional)

1. Heat oil in a large stockpot over medium-high heat. Add leeks and garlic, and sauté 3 minutes, stirring, until tender. Add bay leaves, tarragon, salt, and pepper; stir to coat. Add potatoes and chicken broth, and bring mixture to a boil. Reduce heat to medium-low and simmer 8 minutes. Add salmon and simmer 2 minutes, or until fish is cooked through and potatoes are fork-tender.
2. Remove from heat, remove bay leaves, and stir in half-and-half. Ladle chowder into bowls, and top with chives.

Per serving: Calories 304 (29% from fat), Fat 10 g (1 g saturated), Protein 26 g, Carbohydrate 27 g, Fiber 3 g, Cholesterol 61 mg, Iron 3 mg, Sodium 666 mg, Calcium 62 mg

Baked Salmon with Potatoes, Onions, and Fennel

SERVES 4
PREPARATION: 10 MINUTES
COOKING: 45 MINUTES

Olive oil-flavored cooking spray
2 Yukon gold potatoes (about 1 pound total), peeled, halved,
    and thinly sliced
Salt and freshly ground black pepper to taste
1 yellow onion, halved and thinly sliced (about 2 cups)
1 fennel bulb, ends and stalks trimmed, bulb halved and thinly
    sliced (about 2 cups)
1 tablespoon sugar
1 teaspoon dried thyme
2 tablespoons drained capers
4 (5-ounce) salmon fillets
4 tablespoons crumbled feta cheese
3 tablespoons seasoned dry breadcrumbs
1/4 cup vermouth, dry white wine, or chicken broth

1. Preheat oven to 400°.
2. Spray an 11 x 7-inch baking pan with cooking spray. Arrange potato slices in 4 slightly overlapping rows in the bottom of prepared pan. Sprinkle with salt and pepper. Bake 10 minutes.
3. In a large bowl, combine onion, fennel, sugar, and thyme. Toss to combine. Arrange onion and fennel mixture over potatoes. Sprinkle the top with capers. Bake 15 minutes.
4. Reduce oven temperature to 350°.
5. Arrange salmon fillets on top of vegetables.
6. In a small bowl, combine feta, breadcrumbs, and vermouth. Toss gently to combine. Sprinkle mixture over salmon and vegetables. Bake, uncovered, 20 minutes, or until fish is fork-tender.

Per serving: Calories 379 (26% from fat), Fat 11 g (4 g saturated), Protein 30 g, Carbohydrate 41 g, Fiber 5 g, Cholesterol 75 mg, Iron 2 mg, Sodium 563 mg, Calcium 147 mg

the facts

Nutrition facts are given to help healthy individuals select daily meals that are low in calories, saturated fat, cholesterol, and sodium. Recipes are tested for taste, appeal, timing, ease of preparation, and presentation.

Teriyaki-Glazed Salmon with Noodles

SERVES 4
PREPARATION: 5 MINUTES
COOKING: 15 MINUTES

Cooking spray

2 tablespoons water

1/4 cup packed light brown sugar

2 tablespoons rice vinegar

2 tablespoons reduced-sodium soy sauce

1/2 teaspoon ground dried ginger

1/2 teaspoon garlic powder

4 (5-ounce) salmon fillets

8 ounces uncooked vermicelli or somen noodles

2 teaspoons dark sesame oil

1/4 cup chopped fresh scallions

1. Preheat oven to 400°.*
2. Coat a shallow roasting pan with cooking spray. Set aside.
3. To prepare teriyaki glaze, in a shallow dish, whisk together water, brown sugar, vinegar, soy sauce, ginger, and garlic.
4. Add salmon, and turn to coat. (Salmon can marinate, covered, in the refrigerator up to 1 hour.)
5. Transfer salmon to prepared roasting pan, and pour teriyaki mixture over it. Roast 15 minutes or until fork-tender.
6. Cook noodles in a medium-sized pot of rapidly boiling water according to package directions. Drain and transfer to a large bowl. Add sesame oil, and toss to coat.
7. Transfer noodles to four individual plates, and top each portion with a salmon fillet. Spoon any teriyaki glaze remaining in pan over salmon, and sprinkle chopped scallions on top.

* Salmon may also be grilled or broiled 3 minutes per side until fork-tender.

Per serving: Calories 451 (20% from fat), Fat 10 g (1 g saturated), Protein 28 g, Carbohydrate 62 g, Fiber 2 g, Cholesterol 61 mg, Iron 3 mg, Sodium 325 mg, Calcium 30 mg

Creamy Salmon Caesar Salad with Sourdough Croutons

SERVES 4
PREPARATION: 15 MINUTES
COOKING: 10 MINUTES

2 cups cubed sourdough bread

Olive oil-flavored cooking spray

1 pound salmon fillet

1/2 cup fat-free sour cream

1/4 cup nonfat reduced-sodium chicken broth

3 tablespoons grated Parmesan cheese, divided

2 tablespoons fresh lemon juice

2 cloves garlic, sliced

2 anchovy fillets (optional)

2 teaspoons Dijon mustard

2 teaspoons Worcestershire sauce

1/8 teaspoon freshly ground black pepper

8 cups torn romaine lettuce, rinsed well and patted dry

1. Preheat oven to 400°.
2. To prepare croutons, arrange sourdough cubes on a large baking sheet. Spray cubes with cooking spray. Bake 10 minutes until golden brown. Set aside.
3. Place salmon in a shallow, microwave-safe baking dish.* Cover dish with plastic wrap, and microwave on HIGH for 3 minutes or until fish is fork-tender, rotating dish halfway through cooking.
4. Transfer salmon to a cutting board, and using two forks, break up fish into 2-inch pieces. Discard skin, and set salmon pieces aside.
5. In a blender combine sour cream, chicken broth, 2 tablespoons Parmesan, lemon juice, garlic, anchovies, mustard, Worcestershire sauce, and pepper. Purée until smooth.
6. Place lettuce in a large bowl, and add salmon and croutons. Drizzle dressing over top of salad, and gently toss to coat. Transfer mixture to 4 individual serving bowls, and sprinkle remaining Parmesan over top.

* You may poach salmon, if desired: Place salmon in a large saucepan, and add water to cover. Set pan over high heat. Bring to a boil; immediately remove from heat. Let stand 10 minutes; drain. Use as directed.

Per serving: Calories 307 (28% from fat), Fat 9 g (2 g saturated), Protein 32 g, Carbohydrate 24 g, Fiber 3 g, Cholesterol 65 mg, Iron 3 mg, Sodium 443 mg, Calcium 177 mg

Chili-Rubbed Salmon with Gazpacho–Black Bean Salsa

SERVES 4
PREPARATION: 10 MINUTES
COOKING: 15 MINUTES

Chili-Rubbed Salmon

Cooking spray

2 tablespoons fresh lemon juice

1 tablespoon sugar

3 teaspoons chili powder

2 teaspoons finely grated lemon zest

1 teaspoon ground cumin

$^1/_2$ teaspoon salt

$^1/_8$ teaspoon freshly ground black pepper

4 (5-ounce) salmon fillets

Gazpacho–Black Bean Salsa

1 cup tomato juice

2 large tomatoes, seeded and diced

1 green bell pepper, seeded and diced

1 small cucumber, peeled, seeded, and diced

$^1/_4$ cup diced red onion

$^1/_4$ cup canned black beans, rinsed and drained

2 tablespoons fresh lemon juice

2 tablespoons chopped fresh parsley

1. Preheat oven to 400°.*
2. Coat a baking sheet with cooking spray, and set aside.
3. In a shallow dish, combine lemon juice, sugar, chili powder, lemon zest, cumin, salt, and black pepper. Mix with a fork, or whisk until blended. Add salmon fillets, and turn to coat. Transfer salmon to prepared baking sheet, and roast 15 minutes until fork-tender.
4. Combine all salsa ingredients in a medium-sized bowl. Toss to combine. Cover and refrigerate until ready to serve.
5. Serve salmon with salsa on top and alongside.

* Salmon may also be grilled or broiled, 3 minutes per side until fork-tender.

Per serving: Calories 237 (29% from fat), Fat 8 g (1 g saturated), Protein 25 g, Carbohydrate 17 g, Fiber 4 g, Cholesterol 60 mg, Iron 3 mg, Sodium 583 mg, Calcium 52 mg

Grilled Salmon Steaks with Cilantro Pesto and Cumin-Dusted Toasts

SERVES 4
PREPARATION: 10 MINUTES
COOKING: 7 MINUTES

Cilantro Pesto

2 cups fresh cilantro leaves

4 tablespoons fresh lime juice

2 tablespoons water

2 tablespoons grated Parmesan cheese

2 cloves garlic, sliced

1 teaspoon sugar

$^1/_4$ teaspoon salt

$^1/_4$ teaspoon freshly ground black pepper

Grilled Salmon and Cumin-Dusted Toasts

4 (5-ounce) salmon steaks, about 1 inch thick

Salt and freshly ground black pepper to taste

Olive oil-flavored cooking spray

1 baguette, sliced crosswise into 1-inch-thick rounds

1 bunch fresh asparagus (about $^1/_2$ pound), woody ends trimmed

1 teaspoon ground cumin, or more to taste

1. Preheat grill.*
2. To prepare pesto, in a blender combine cilantro, lime juice, water, Parmesan cheese, garlic, sugar, salt, and pepper. Purée until smooth. Set aside.
3. Season both sides of salmon with salt and pepper to taste. Spray baguette rounds and asparagus with cooking spray. Sprinkle both sides of bread slices with cumin, and salt to taste. Place salmon on hot grill, and arrange bread and asparagus around the outside, where the grill is not as hot. Grill salmon, bread, and asparagus 5 to 7 minutes; turn fish and bread halfway through cooking, and turn asparagus frequently, until fish is fork-tender, bread is golden brown, and asparagus is crisp-tender.

* Salmon may be broiled, 5 inches from heat source, 5 minutes per side, until fork-tender. To prepare bread and asparagus: Place bread slices and asparagus on a baking sheet. Roast in a 400° oven 10 minutes, until bread is golden and asparagus is crisp-tender.

Per serving: Calories 356 (25% from fat), Fat 10 g (2 g saturated), Protein 30 g, Carbohydrate 37 g, Fiber 3 g, Cholesterol 63 mg, Iron 4 mg, Sodium 595 mg, Calcium 142 mg

the wine–lover's
GUIDE
to risk-free
drinking

*If good wine is a necessity of life for you, here's how
to enjoy the benefits and skip the risks.*

BY DOROTHY FOLTZ-GRAY

've always loved wine. Even as a kid I relished the occasion of champagne—December 31, the sip my grandmother offered before I bent into the cold dark to shout "Happy New Year." I also liked the communion sips I took at church, the solemn nod into the silver chalice, the illicit burn right there in front of everyone. Never mind that my first adult wine was syrupy Spañada. In spite of its sweetness, it made a simple meal a celebration, turned an ordinary evening exotic.

Over the years my wine drinking has become something else as well, a second food passion that isn't about taste alone. Pinot Grigio, Sangiovese, Chianti: The sensuality begins before the cork's out, in the rolling names, the inquisitive stroll through the wine store. But then I open a bottle, a Syrah, say, and enter a dark, lush wood. Or an oaky Chardonnay, full of sun and blue sky. Will the next white wine I sample be silky and sweet or hard-edged and tart?

Once in a while, though, I worry that I love wine too much. Alcoholism trails through both sides of my family, and the tales of disappearances, of sudden angers, of lost opportunities I heard as a child all revealed a face of alcohol I never want to see in my life. That family history makes me wonder: Doesn't my drinking habit clash with my commitment to daily exercise and a veggie-filled diet?

So I've done some digging. I can't say I've been shocked to find that wine's been linked to good health—the French paradox is still a hot topic. But I have been thrilled to discover that the findings have deepened and apply to me especially, a woman who's turned the corner into midlife. Far from harming me, my habit is actually shielding me from the one illness likely to shorten my time on the planet.

"Several hundred studies since the early '90s show that moderate alcohol intake reduces the risk of heart disease," says R. Curtis Ellison, a professor of medicine

> A healthy drinker's motto:
> Find the sweet spot where wine, good
> food, and companionship merge.

women and wine: a health scorecard

All pleasures have risk trade-offs, whether you're skiing, sunbathing, traveling overseas, or just strolling in your neighborhood. Here's a research update on risks and benefits for wine-lovers.

Heart disease: Studies over the past decade provide convincing evidence that moderate drinkers run a 30 to 40 percent lower risk of heart disease than do teetotalers. Still up in the air: whether wine beats beer and spirits.

Breast cancer: Most studies show that breast cancer risk rises about 10 percent with each drink you down per day. But when Curtis Ellison of Boston University examined data on women in the Framingham Heart Study, he found no increased risk among moderate drinkers compared with nondrinkers. Still, if your family history suggests you're at risk for breast cancer, it safest to limit your drinks to several a week.

Other cancers: Several studies link alcoholic beverages with added risk for cancers of the mouth, throat, and esophagus. However, a recent Danish study found that moderate wine drinkers had half the cancer risk of nondrinkers, while those who drank beer or spirits had triple the risk. A study issued in 2000 showed that wine drinkers were less likely to develop colorectal cancer than were imbibers of beer or mixed drinks.

Fertility: Put away the corkscrew if you're trying to get pregnant. Researchers in Denmark discovered that moderate drinkers were 66 percent less likely to conceive than women who didn't drink.

Weight: Moderate wine drinking has been linked to both weight gain and loss—you get 100 calories per five-ounce glass, but scientists can't say if those calories matter.

Bone strength: Overindulging can weaken bones, but a 2000 study of 7,600 French women age 75 and older found that those who drank moderately actually added bone mass.

Mental acuity: Long-term heavy drinking can cause brain damage and dementia, but in France researchers found that compared with nondrinkers, moderate drinkers ran a 75 percent lower risk for Alzheimer's disease and an 80 percent lower risk for dementia. In the Honolulu-Asia Aging Study, elderly men who had imbibed a drink a day during middle age performed better than nondrinkers or heavy drinkers on tests involving concentration, memory, and language.

Digestive complaints: Though wine, beer, and spirits can ignite flare-ups in heartburn sufferers, alcoholic beverages appear to kill bacteria that trigger food poisoning and ulcers.

and public health at Boston University School of Medicine. What's clear from the latest papers is that alcohol—when used moderately—raises good cholesterol and lowers the bad, staves off heart attacks and strokes, and may even lower blood pressure slightly. And evidence is mounting that polyphenols, antioxidant compounds plentiful in red wines, can amplify these benefits.

I love hearing such news, but it doesn't completely erase my worries. My husband and I drink wine almost every night, a practice that makes us rarities where we live, in the buckle of America's Bible Belt. So I sometimes get a little self-conscious. Isn't a daily dose overdoing it?

> Savoring wine slowly with meals is the best way to claim its health benefits.

Actually, no, experts say. Wine seems to work its magic when you imbibe slowly and steadily throughout the week, much as folks do in comparatively heart-healthy countries like France. Once wine's compounds have begun circulating in your blood, they mingle with sticky little disks called platelets, preventing the sudden clots that can plug an artery and trigger a heart attack or stroke. But that effect lasts just 24 to 36 hours.

As a matter of fact, Ellison says, what appears healthiest for a wine-lover like me is to drink moderately every day. How much is okay? Down more than three drinks daily, experts say, and you're flirting with heart failure, liver disease, and cancer.

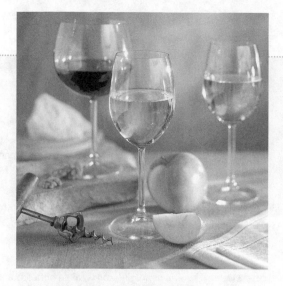

eight wines you'll love

Ann Littlefield doesn't just enjoy the fruit of the vine, she uncorks bottles by the score as a senior wine merchant for www.wine.com, an online retailer. She's been an oenophile for 30 years, since taking a course in wine appreciation as a student in Europe, but there's nothing snooty about the business to her. "Wine is for every day," she says. "I love to cook and share meals with friends, and wine is just part of the camaraderie." Here are some of her current favorites, all available for between $10 and $17 a bottle from the Web site above.

- Beaucanon 1997 Napa Valley Reserve Chardonnay
  Excellent with chicken or light pasta dishes.
- Dry Creek 1998 Sonoma Chardonnay
  Great with salmon and hearty seafood dishes or pasta with mushrooms.
- Ballentine Vineyards 1996 Napa Valley "Libero" Zinfandel
  Goes well with pizza, spaghetti, and lots of everyday dishes.
- Buena Vista 1997 Carneros Cabernet Sauvignon
  Complements roasted meats—even chicken—or tomatoey pastas or full-flavored New Mexican dishes.
- Chateau La Fleur 1997 "Clemence" Graves (France)
  Delicious with most foods, from vegetable frittatas to chicken or pork stew.
- d'Arenberg 1998 McLaren Vale "Footbolt" Shiraz (Australia)
  Perfect with hearty dishes such as veal ragu or osso buco.
- Tuatara Bay 1999 Marlborough Sauvignon Blanc (New Zealand)
  Ideal with crab, smoked trout, or any light seafood.
- Wagner Vineyards 1998 Finger Lakes Semi-dry Riesling (New York)
  Just right with Asian dishes and Indian curries.

At the same time, health agencies say a woman can enjoy up to one glass a day—but no more. (Men get two.)

Yet I admit that sometimes one glass feels like too little—is too little. We have friends over for dinner, and when their glasses are empty I offer to refill them. But the point is never the drinking. It's not a frat party we're throwing. We're sharing a meal, recharging our souls as we might during a hike or a spell in a health club sauna.

And that ultimately is the key, say experts who have hammered out healthy drinking guidelines. The way you drink can be as important as how much. Almost instinctively, my friends and I have found the sweet spot where wine, good food, and companionship merge. No one's tippling behind the potted plant or staggering out to her car. It also happens that savoring wine with meals is the best way to claim its health benefits, says Ellison. It's after a meal that fats circulate, upping the blood's tendency to clot. That's when wine's protection kicks in.

But am I really a healthy drinker? If, as Ellison says, staying well means keeping your weight down, exercising, not smoking—and granting yourself some wine every day—then I suppose I am. I drink the way I eat: moderately but with enthusiasm.

Do I push away a celebratory hunk of rib eye or gooey chocolate cake? Do I staunchly refuse that second glass of Zinfandel, mindful as I am of my family history? Sure, but not always. I'm not interested in eating and drinking by rote, taking their measure like medicine. After all, wine's not medicine. It's part of a well-set table, a finished day, a happy reunion—sometimes more, sometimes less. And like most things, it's something I love not alone but as a piece of something bigger I'm building: a good life. ✳

Dorothy Foltz-Gray is a contributing Health *editor.*

HOW TO GET THE "RECOMMENDED DAILY ALLOWANCE" FOR EVERY NUTRIENT

Nutrition experts love to scrutinize what we eat. For years they've been poring over research and analyzing our diets to determine if we're getting enough—or too much—of key nutrients. Their latest dispatch revises the guidelines for some 14 vitamins and minerals. But be patient if you're waiting for the new recommended dietary allowance (RDA) figures to appear on nutrition labels. It likely will be a few years before the proposals are translated into practice. Here are highlights of the recommendations.
Vitamin A: Experts dropped the daily requirement slightly to 700 micrograms (mcg) for women and 900 mcg for men. And for the first time they set an upper limit, declaring that a long-term daily dose of more than 3,000 mcg (or 10,000 IU) may cause irreversible liver damage and birth defects. The scientists also reported that certain A-rich foods provide the body with only about half as much of the vitamin as previously thought.

Still, it's not hard to get your fill, says Robert Russell, a professor of medicine and nutrition at Tufts University who led the panel: "If you choose right, you can do it easily with one serving a day, like half a cup of carrots." Other good sources include fish, dairy products, and red, orange, and dark green veggies such as broccoli, spinach, and sweet potatoes.
Iron: Postmenopausal women likely get more than they need, so their RDA fell from 10 to 8 milligrams (mg). Premenopausal women, however, require a little more, so the experts raised the RDA from 15 to 18 mg. Also, they instituted an upper safety limit of 45 mg.
Other nutrients: Zinc's RDA was bumped down to 8 mg for women and 11 mg for men. The mineral is thought to fight infection and prevent reproductive and vision problems. The panel also suggested specific doses for chromium: 25 mcg for women and 35 mcg for men.

Three Yummy Nuts
that can help prevent a stroke

WHILE THE JURY IS STILL out on whether vitamin E supplements can ward off heart disease, recent research suggests that a diet packed with the nutrient can protect women from a stroke. Researchers at the University of Minnesota tracked 35,000 postmenopausal women and found that those who often ate foods high in vitamin E were 60 percent less likely to die from stroke than those who rarely did. It's easy to get your fill by munching on almonds, hazelnuts, or peanuts. A handful gives you a decent dose with hardly any saturated fat.

getting to know your freezer

Sure, you've lived together for years. But how much do you really know about your freezer? Take this quiz.

• Which can be stored longer: ground beef or fresh shrimp?

• How long will frozen food last if there's a power outage?

• Is it OK to store ice cream in the freezer door?

If you answered "fresh shrimp," "two days, if the freezer's full," and "no way!," consider yourself freezer-savvy. If your score was less than perfect, don't worry. Head to the National Frozen Food Association's new Web site, www.easyhomemeals.com, to learn more. They've also got tips on microwave usage and germ-proofing your kitchen.

the truth about garlic

Do the health benefits of this potent herb live up to its reputation?
Get the facts behind the hype about garlic's impact on your health.

BY CATHERINE GUTHRIE

Here's a familiar story. An herbal supplement with disease-fighting properties rooted in the ancient East gains newfound popularity in America, is buoyed by a nationwide marketing campaign, and becomes widely accepted as a potent recipe for good health. Then, after years of immense commercial success, the herb comes under increased scrutiny, and research indicates that the purported health benefits aren't all the supplement makers claim. Consumers are left wondering what the truth is.

That's what has happened with garlic. Medical use of the herb dates back to Hippocrates, who prescribed it for everything from heart trouble to uterine tumors. In ancient China, people used it to cure respiratory infections, and athletes at the first Olympic games popped garlic cloves to build physical endurance.

In the more recent past, garlic's main claim has been as a cholesterol buster. Larry King promotes it on the radio, while colorful bottles of supplements proclaim their cardio cures from drugstore shelves: "Clinically proven to lower cholesterol." "Promotes healthy circulation." "Supports a healthy cardiovascular system." Each assertion is a promising lure for the 60 million Americans with heart disease—and together these claims

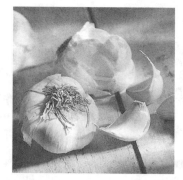

have helped make garlic one of the best-selling herbal supplements in the United States. In 2000, American consumers spent more than $61 million on the stuff.

But there's a problem: Comprehensive new research debunks garlic's lipid-lowering notoriety. In three separate studies, researchers showed that there is no proof that the herb offers long-term cholesterol-lowering help. New evidence, though, suggests that garlic may offer other health benefits. Where does this leave folks who are concerned about protecting their health the rational way?

To help you sort out the claims, here's a hype-free assessment of garlic's powers.

Garlic vs. High Cholesterol

Some scientists still believe that garlic's wealth of antioxidants prevents bad cholesterol from damaging artery walls. The thinking is that antioxidants break the chain of events that lead to artery-hardening, or atherosclerosis. To test this theory, among some of the herb's other health claims, the Agency for Healthcare Research and Quality convened an expert panel in fall 2000 to analyze existing research.

When it came to garlic and cholesterol, the group discovered a troubling trend. Of the 36 papers that charted garlic's effect on lowering cholesterol, the studies in which volunteers experienced the most dramatic improvements lasted three months or less.

Curious, the panel took a closer look at eight studies that lasted six months

Some scientists still believe garlic offers long-term cholesterol-lowering effects. But new research shows the benefits are temporary.

Despite doubts about garlic's cholesterol-lowering potential, there is evidence that garlic might help prevent blood clots, heart attack, stroke, and some forms of cancer.

or more. The result? Initially garlic caused a dip in "bad" cholesterol levels, but over the long haul, it fared no better than placebos at keeping arteries clear. That was the first comparison of short- versus long-term benefits, according to David Schardt, a panel member and nutritionist at the Center for Science in the Public Interest in Washington, D.C. It also marked the beginning of the end of the herb's cholesterol-lowering career.

Garlic's reputation suffered another blow when Germany's Commission E, one of the most respected councils for evaluating the safety and efficacy of herbal remedies, dropped cholesterol lowering from the authorized claims that can be made about garlic.

Again in fall 2000, garlic suffered its third strike in less than a year. Researchers at the University of Exeter in England published an analysis of 13 garlic and cholesterol studies in the *Annals of Internal Medicine.* Results from the six most reliable studies found no relationship whatsoever between garlic and cholesterol. In the end, the authors admitted that the use of garlic to treat high cholesterol was "of questionable value."

The bottom line on garlic and cholesterol? Garlic may trigger an initial drop in LDL levels, but don't expect any long-term benefits. The short-lived improvement is not a viable alternative to a low-fat diet or prescription cholesterol-lowering medication. (See "The All-Natural Way to Reduce Cholesterol" on page 238 to read about the fight against high cholesterol.)

Heart Attack and Stroke Prevention

Despite discouraging news about garlic and cholesterol, researchers remain hopeful that the herb offers other substantial health benefits. In fact, studies show garlic may reduce the risk of heart attack or stroke. The Agency for Healthcare Research and Quality's garlic panel examined 10 trials that looked specifically at the herb's ability to stop potentially dangerous blood clots from forming. All but one of these trials showed that garlic indeed offered some protection.

Where does garlic get its clot-busting powers? Recently, scientists identified a substance in the herb called Ajoene that lubricates platelets in the blood.

pushing garlic's powers

Most at-home cooks have figured out their personal favorite techniques for peeling and using garlic to perfect the taste of a dish. But there are still a few tricks to preparing the herb to enhance its health benefits.

Garlic's compounds are particularly volatile. Like an expensive Merlot, its fickle personality shifts depending on age, storage, handling, and preparation. Raw garlic will exhibit different properties than cloves cooked in last night's stir-fry. Only when garlic cloves are sliced, diced, mashed, or broken in some way do they release those powerful enzymes that combine to make the antioxidants responsible for its purported health benefits.

It takes time for garlic's disease fighters to arm themselves. One new study shows that the sulfur compounds in the herb need 10 minutes to kick in once a clove is crushed. So, the next time you use garlic, keep this in mind and be sure to plan accordingly. Chop a few cloves first, then either gather the meal's remaining ingredients or simply sit back and sip a glass of Chardonnay.

The more slippery platelets become, the less likely they are to clump together and form a clot, the first step to a heart attack or stroke.

While early evidence continues to support garlic's reputation as a blood thinner, more research is needed before experts can draw firm conclusions about the herb's role in preventing heart attack and stroke.

Cancer-Fighting Potential

Health experts are perhaps most encouraged about garlic's potential cancer-fighting capabilities.

The evidence is still under debate, but researchers are pinning their hope on a sulfur compound called allicin, which is the active ingredient in garlic. Garlic-supplement users will no doubt recognize allicin as the ingredient highlighted on product labels. The reason for allicin's high profile: When you chew garlic, it breaks down into antioxidants, which are known for their cancer-fighting abilities. These antioxidants neutralize reactive molecules in the blood (known as free radicals), which can damage a cell's DNA and trigger cancer. Scientists believe these compounds play a crucial role in cancer prevention, and they are continuing to research the possibilities.

One significant study occurred in fall 2000 at the University of North Carolina (UNC) in Chapel Hill, where scientists gathered garlic and cancer research from around the world, including China, Italy, Sweden, and the Netherlands. Overall, they found that garlic- lovers (those who regularly ate six or more cloves a week) showed a 30 percent lower risk of colorectal cancer and a 50 percent lower risk of stomach cancer compared to those who shunned the herb. To a lesser extent, garlic appeared to aid in protection against prostate, laryngeal, bladder, and breast cancers.

Carmia Borek, Ph.D., professor of community health at Tufts University School of Medicine in Boston, is one of the optimistic researchers. She says there is strong evidence that garlic not only prevents cancer but also slows the growth of tumors. In particular, she says, studies have indicated that people who eat a significant amount of garlic have a reduced risk of colon and stomach cancer. In other studies, animals that had certain tumors were given aged garlic extract (AGE). The results? The garlic seemed to inhibit the growth of some of those tumors. Although she emphasizes that further study is needed, Borek says that garlic "appears to attack different stages of cancer—from initiation to promotion."

So why aren't docs doling out the herb like candy on Halloween? One problem is in isolating garlic's effect, Borek explains. For many study participants who stayed cancer-free, the herb was just one component of a diet rich in fruits and vegetables. Her hope is that future studies will clarify and validate the herb's status as a cancer-fighter.

This research could be enough to put garlic back in the health experts' good graces. But more studies are needed to determine how much of the herb you should swallow and which form works best. Borek, though, is a believer in the herb's potency. "I'd recommend adding garlic in any form" to your diet, she says.

Supplement or the Real Thing?

Although many of garlic's health benefits are still being sorted out, it is already a part of many people's health regimens. If you are committed to taking the herb, fresh is best: Garlic in its natural state is the most potent and complete version of the herb. As long as your self-esteem and loved ones can handle the occasional awkward side effects (such as bad breath or residual body odor), regularly consuming six or more cloves a week—the amount used in the UNC-Chapel Hill study—may help protect you from cancer.

If you are someone who is ultrasensitive to the herb, though—it gives you gas, heartburn, or even a rash—you may want to skip the fresh stuff and consider taking a supplement instead. Herbal experts aren't certain which form of supplement is superior: powdered garlic or age. Unfortunately, the composition of powdered garlic supplements isn't standardized, so it's hard to determine what you get in one brand compared with another. If you decide to take powdered garlic anyway, look for one containing 5,000 micrograms of allicin a day. Thanks to a special coating, powdered garlic is odorless at the onset, but it may leave a lingering scent. To ward off unpleasant garlic-flavored burps, swallow the capsules before bedtime.

On the other side of the lab, cancer researchers swear by AGE. The rationale is that garlic's antioxidants multiply as the herb ages, increasing its potential cancer-fighting properties. One of its most significant perks is that AGE is odorless. A daily dose of 1,200 to 1,600 milligrams of AGE, sold in health food stores under the brand name Kyolic, should be plenty. However, avoid garlic supplements altogether if you already take a daily anticoagulant, such as aspirin or warfarin (Coumadin).

Whether or not the new evidence boasting garlic as a cancer and clot preventer holds up or goes the way of its cholesterol-lowering abilities, no one can say. If nothing else, though, garlic—at least in its natural state—can't hurt you and may be a delicious way to preserve your health. ✳

Catherine Guthrie is a freelance health and medical writer whose work has been published in Self *and* Yoga Journal, *and on* WebMD.

Is our food safe?

What you need to know before your next trip to the grocery store

The foods we eat are treated with pesticides, hormones, or antibiotics. How do you know what's safe and what isn't? Here's the middle ground where you can enjoy healthy food without worrying.

BY BILL GOTTLIEB

What could be simpler than stopping at the market for a few basic items: a quart of milk, some chicken breasts, salad greens, and a bag of chips? Zip over to the express lane, and with luck, you'll be out in a few minutes. But no sooner have you grabbed a basket and headed down the aisle than questions start to clutch at your mind like thorny weeds.

Should you buy milk from a dairy whose cows were treated with hormones? Should you shell out for a free-range chicken that wasn't fed antibiotics and for organic greens that haven't been near pesticides? What if they're tainted

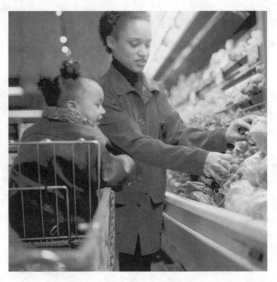

with dangerous microbes? And there's the chip dilemma: Most packaged foods now include ingredients from genetically modified crops. Should you skip them? It's hard enough keeping an eye on your fat and calorie intake, but all these other concerns can turn a quick food run into a marathon.

Fortunately, help is at hand. We talked to dozens of medical researchers, government officials, consumer advocates, and industry scientists about the safety of the food you eat every day. Not surprisingly, the experts don't all see eye to eye, and the attitudes range from carefree to cautionary. Yet between the extremes lies a middle ground with a range of reasonable choices. Want to enjoy healthy food without becoming a fanatic? Here's what you need to know before your next trip to the supermarket.

Hormones in Milk and Meat

To boost milk output, many American dairy cows are regularly dosed with a synthetic hormone called recombinant bovine growth hormone, which is produced by genetically altered yeast cells. Meanwhile, at least 75 percent of beef cattle are given sex hormones to spur them to grow extra muscle, producing leaner, more tender meat. Tests of meat and milk sold in U.S. supermarkets reveal minuscule residues of these or related compounds.

Is there really any danger?

Most scientists say the hormones pose no health risk. The milk of hormone-treated cows shows slightly increased levels of a compound called insulin-like growth factor 1. Studies of lab animals show that this compound, which regulates cell growth, may at high levels make the animals more prone to breast, prostate, and colon cancers. In addition, milk from treated cows may show slightly increased levels of thyroid hormone enzymes, which some critics say could result in the disruption of thyroid function in humans. Treated cows' milk has also been shown to have an unusual mix of fatty acids, which may raise the risk of heart disease in milk drinkers. But to date, no one has found that people who drink milk from hormone-dosed cows are any more likely to develop these illnesses.

As for beef, American cattle are routinely given one or more natural or synthetic sex hormones. The government sets rules for their use, requiring tests for residues and prohibiting the sale of meat with amounts that exceed set levels, which generally fall in the range that occurs naturally in the animals. Still, enforcement could be much more stringent, and some worry that doses of one often-used hormone—estradiol—may be reaching consumers. Estradiol, a type of estrogen, can play a role in the growth of breast and uterine cancers. Still, there's no evidence that women who regularly eat beef run any extra risk for those diseases.

What you can do

If you'd rather drink milk produced without hormones, look for brands that say so on the label. New federal rules specify that dairy products and meat from hormone-treated animals cannot be labeled "organic," so be cautious and shop for organic brands.

Pesticides on Produce

About 95 percent of all the fruits and vegetables grown in this country are at some stage treated with insecticides or fungicides. Surveys regularly find residues on produce in markets that exceed Environmental Protection Agency (EPA) limits.

Is there really any danger?

For adults, probably not; but for children, possibly. The safety of pesticide residues used to be gauged by research on adults, and few alarms were raised. But a five-year study by the National Academy of Sciences (NAS), published in 1993, showed that although the entire population is exposed to these residues, fetuses, infants, and children run the greatest chance of harm.

Young children are exposed to higher doses than adults because they have smaller bodies and, pound for pound, eat more than their parents do. They also tend to eat the same foods over and over, including more items that contain pesticide residues, like fruit juices. Also, their bodies aren't as efficient at eliminating chemicals. Because their brains are still developing, these realities put them at heightened risk.

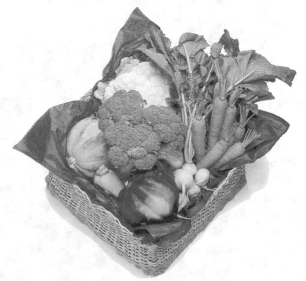

Residue of insecticides, often found on supermarket produce, can pose a health hazard to children.

Many of the commonly used pesticides are organophosphates, which kill insects by destroying their nervous systems. NAS found that they also harm the brains of young rodents—resulting in impaired reflexes, delayed learning, and shortened attention spans. Young children, if overexposed to these pesticides, may be affected in the same way. Farm workers and others who work in close contact with pesticides are at a greater risk for developing a host of health problems, including higher rates of cancer and miscarriages. In 1996, the U.S. Congress unanimously passed a bill to review the risk of pesticides to children; so far the EPA has limited the use of two common organophosphates: methyl-parathion and chlorpyrifos. But it may be years before the agency has an opportunity to review all 600 pesticides licensed for use on foods in the United States.

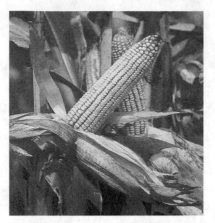

There is no evidence so far that genetically modified crops pose any risk to humans.

What you can do
To play it safe, remember to thoroughly wash fruits and vegetables under running water. To be extra cautious, always peel fruits and vegetables with removable skins. And, if your budget allows, buy organic produce or foods available at a farmer's market, which typically have lower pesticide residues.

Genetically Modified Foods

Some 70 percent of all packaged foods now contain certain ingredients—vegetable oils, mainly—produced using biotech methods that allow scientists to splice genetic codes from one species into another. For example, one new variety of corn approved only for animal feed contains bacteria genes that make the plants toxic to insects, ideally permitting farmers to cut back on pesticides. But it has raised worries about risks to people who eat the meat or corn kernels.

Is there really any danger?
There's no evidence that anyone is being harmed by the genetically modified (GM) foods that are on the market. However, the method is so new and the possibilities for tinkering so vast that it's impossible to declare all present and future biotech ingredients risk-free.

Scientists have for centuries tampered with the genetic makeup of plants and animals, of course, by crossbreeding or by propagating seeds from plants that by mutation developed new traits—sweeter apples, say, or crisper greens.

But the new technique is very different. To create one of these so-called GM crops, scientists trick special viruses called "promoters" into taking up a snippet of DNA from one species, and then attaching it to DNA in cells from another. The modified cells are then grown into plants that have new DNA and new traits. Some people worry that the promoters could infect other plants or animals or develop into harmful new viruses, but so far there's no evidence this has happened.

It is possible, however, to endow a crop with an unwanted trait. Steve Taylor, Ph.D., head of the University of Nebraska's food science and technology department, tested a new soybean whose protein content had been boosted by the addition of a Brazil nut gene. His studies suggested the modified beans could cause severe reactions in people allergic to the nuts.

Taylor, like most food scientists, takes such findings in stride, noting that after the tests, production of the soybean was stopped. But many people fear that safety testing is inadequate and government rules too lax to keep a public health crisis from someday breaking out.

What you can do
Unless you've been actively avoiding them, you probably already eat GM foods and are not in grave danger of harm. If you prefer not to eat them, start by cutting back on processed foods. Beyond that, shop for 100 percent organic products. Federal rules require them to be free of GM ingredients.

Antibiotics in Meat

Pigs, chickens, cows—virtually all farm animals—are routinely fed small doses of antibiotics, which make them mature faster, for reasons no one fully under-stands. The practice has been a boon to farmers, but now it appears to be promoting the development of drug-resistant bacteria.

Is there really any danger?

Your chances of being felled by a resistant bug are very low, but they should not be discounted. Say you acci-dentally undercook some chicken or ground beef and come down with intestinal distress that lasts several days. It's uncomfortable, but you recover and carry on. Now suppose the bacteria were antibiotic-resistant. That won't matter if, like most people, you're simply waiting out your symptoms. But if you're a person with a weak immune system—you're

under 5 years old or over 65, have a chronic disease, or are undergoing chemotherapy—you might not survive, even if you seek medical treatment. "We have patients dying because some of the antibiotics we have are not working," says Stuart Levy, Ph.D., professor of molecular biology and microbiology at Tufts University in Boston, and author of *The Antibiotic Paradox: How Miracle Drugs Are Destroying the Miracle* (Perseus Press, 1992).

Consider the drugs called fluoroquinolones, used to treat infections of the foodborne microbe *Campylobacter jejuni.* They're also given to poultry to treat respiratory tract disease. A study by researchers from the Minnesota Department of Public Health in Minneapolis found that 14 percent of chickens sold

clean up your act

Following three rules can dramatically cut your risk of getting sick from a foodborne contaminant.

Keep it hot. Cooking is the best way to destroy disease-causing organisms. Use an instant-read food thermometer to make sure you cook all meats thoroughly, following these guidelines:

> **Beef, lamb, and veal:** 145° (rare), 170° (well-done)
> **Chicken and turkey:** 165°
> **Ground meat:** 160° (medium), 170° to 180° (well-done)
> **Pork:** 160° to 170° (reheat ham to 140°)
> **Casseroles and egg dishes:** 160°
> **Leftovers, reheated:** 165°

Keep it cold. Refrigerate perishables as soon as you get them home. Keeping food cold slows or stops the growth of bacteria and viruses. Set the refrigerator at 40°. Never let perishables stay at room temperature longer than two hours—unless, of course, they're whole fruits that need be stowed in the fridge only after they've been cut or peeled.

Defrost meat in the refrigerator, not on the counter. For safe, rapid defrosting, place the meat in a sealed plastic bag and surround the bag with cool water; the meat will defrost in about 30 minutes.

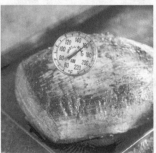

Cook meat thoroughly to minimize the potentially hazardous effects of antibiotics and foodborne microbes.

At picnics, keep meats and other perishables in a closed ice chest in the shade, with cold packs on top of the food. Put out only small amounts of food at a time and, when possible, surround the food with ice.

Keep it clean. The cleaner things are, the less likely you are to get a foodborne illness. Using hot, soapy water, wash and rinse every surface, cutting board, plate, and utensil (including your hands) that touches food before and after each use. This will help eliminate cross-contamination, when a pathogen is moved from one object to another. For example, if you use a knife to cut up raw chicken, don't rinse the knife and then use it to cut open a watermelon. This could infect the watermelon with pathogens from the chicken.

Proper hand washing would eliminate half of all foodborne infections. Be sure to wash your whole hands, not just the palms. And take your time. Most people just give their hands a quick rinse. To be supersafe, scrub continuously through two full choruses of the happy birthday song, about 20 seconds.

Most people don't realize their "stomach flu" is from something they ate, usually microbes on foods such as undercooked beef or eggs, mishandled dairy products, or produce tainted by animal waste.

in the state's markets carried fluoroquinolone-resistant campylobacter. What's more, many Minnesotans were being infected, and doctors frequently couldn't treat them with fluoroquinolones.

Though the Food and Drug Administration has on occasion ordered farmers to stop using drugs too similar to those in wide medical use, experts believe the resistance problem is growing.

What you can do

First, make sure you're doing what you can in the kitchen to cut your chances of falling victim to a foodborne illness. (See "Clean Up Your Act" at left.) Second, take antibiotics only when you really need them. (Many cold sufferers talk their doctors into prescribing the drugs, a gambit that always fails since colds are caused not by bacteria but viruses, which carry on unfazed.) Levy has found that people on antibiotics are more prone to foodborne infections, since the drugs kill off the benign bugs in their digestive tracts, giving resistant ones a perfect competitor-free environment.

Foodborne Microbes

At least 80 million Americans suffer a foodborne illness each year, according to the Centers for Disease Control and Prevention. "But I believe that figure is low," says Philip Tierno, M.D., director of microbiology and diagnostic immunology at New York University Medical Center in Manhattan. "My estimate is 135 million people, or about half the population of the United States." Most don't even realize their gut-wrenching "stomach

People on antibiotics are more vulnerable to foodborne infections because the drugs kill off both bad and good bugs in their digestive tracts.

flu" is from something they ate, usually microbes on foods such as undercooked ground beef or eggs, mishandled dairy products, or produce tainted by animal waste.

Is there really any danger?

Most sufferers recover completely in several days and without seeing a doctor, but some aren't so lucky. One in every thousand people who has an identified infection by the common foodborne bacterium *Campylobacter jejuni* (usually carried by poultry) will develop Guillain-Barre syndrome, a chronic disease that slowly paralyzes the body from the legs up.

Every year, 1,000 or more pregnant women will have a spontaneous abortion after eating a food contaminated with the bacteria *Listeria monocytogenes* (which tend to hang out in soft cheeses like Brie, pâtés, rolled and jellied pork, and even hot dogs). Two to 3 percent of those infected with the foodborne microbes salmonella, campylobacter, shigella, or clostridium (which are largely associated with eggs) will get Reiter's syndrome, a fast-developing or "reactive" arthritis of the feet and legs that can become chronic.

Each year an estimated 9,000 of those with a foodborne illness will die from it—typically the very young or old, those with chronic conditions, such as heart disease and diabetes, or others with immune systems crippled by AIDS, hepatitis C, chemotherapy, or immune-suppressing drugs.

What you can do

Outbreaks that make the headlines can usually be traced back to restaurants, but the vast majority of foodborne infections start at home, where they're easy to prevent.

If you don't do anything else, remember these simple rules: Keep it hot. Or keep it cold. And always keep it clean. ✳

Bill Gottlieb is the author of Alternative Cures *(Rodale, 2000).*

Changing the way America eats

From the classroom to the kitchen, the lab to the garden, these seven women are spreading a simple, welcome message:

You don't have to sacrifice good flavor for good health.

BY PETER JARET

PHOTOGRAPHY BY SUSAN SALINGER

Americans are fed up with being told what we should and should not eat, the pollsters tell us. We're tired of being force-fed foods we don't like just because they're good for us.

Thanks to the seven women that we celebrate here, though, a healthy diet has never looked more appealing. Each of these women is helping change the way we eat for the better. And you won't find a stern-faced finger-wagger among them.

We began our search for nutrition's most influential women with three criteria in mind. First, we looked for innovators with bold new ideas about what constitutes a healthy diet. Second, we wanted crusaders, women who aren't afraid to swim against the current. Most important, we searched for people with a passion for good food.

The women we honor here are all that and more. Not only are they deeply committed to food that's both good for you and delicious, but also they're smart, funny, and opinionated—just the sort of people you'd love to sit down to dinner with.

Rena Wing:
Diets Do Work

We've all heard the gloomy reports that diets don't work. Even people who manage to lose weight, the naysayers tell us, will most likely gain it back.

Rena Wing, Ph.D., a professor of psychiatry and a behavioral scientist at both the University of Pittsburgh and Brown University, doesn't buy those discouraging words. As one of the first few researchers to explore behavioral approaches to dieting in scientifically controlled studies, Wing knows better. "Maintaining weight loss is difficult for everyone, but it's not impossible. Some people do lose weight and successfully keep it off," Wing says. "We think what they've learned can

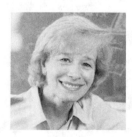

teach us a lot about successful weight loss."

To counter the prevailing pessimism with a dash of hope, Wing helped create the National Weight Control Registry, which compiles the stories—and strategies—of

Eat less. Exercise more. That's the real magic bullet when it comes to losing weight. It may not be easy, but we know it works.—Rena Wing

successful dieters from around the country. The registry serves as a research tool, enabling scientists to learn what works and what doesn't. It has reinforced the crucial message that losing a moderate amount of weight can help reduce the risk of heart disease or diabetes, and it offers inspiration to thousands of people struggling with their weight. The registry shows that, despite all the diets of the moment, a simple formula often works best. Those who succeed—that is, those who maintain their weight loss over time—report exercising regularly and following a diet that's lower in calories and fat.

"Fad diets get all the publicity," Wing says. "But we've found that very few people who succeed in losing weight do so with approaches such as high-protein regimens or very low-calorie diets. Almost all of them succeed by combining moderately low-calorie diets with lots of exercise."

> **A change** most Americans should make is to eat more foods from plants—fruits, vegetables, grains, nuts, and oils like olive, peanut, and canola.—Penny Kris-Etherton

increasing the risk of heart disease.

Thankfully, Kris-Etherton's research highlights a delicious alternative. A diet rich in monounsaturated fats lowers total cholesterol without dragging HDL levels down, and it keeps triglycerides from climbing.

That's great news for food-lovers, of course. No more trying to strike every ounce of fat from the menu. No more nonfat foods with all the flavor of sawdust. Instead, as Kris-Etherton has shown us, we can once again enjoy moderate amounts of healthy fats like olive oil and canola. "For too long, dietary advice was all about saying no to this and no to that," she says. "We're showing that, with foods like nuts, olives, and avocados, you can say yes."

Penny Kris-Etherton:
Fat Is Not the Enemy

Many of us have welcomed a host of once-banished foods back into our kitchens, all because of the pioneering research of Penny Kris-Etherton, Ph.D., R.D., a professor and researcher in the department of nutrition at Pennsylvania State University. "For years the official message was to cut back on all fat," Kris-Etherton says. "But in our studies we've helped to show that diets very low in total fat may not be 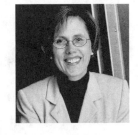 as healthy as diets that include some good fat. On the other hand, a diet with generous amounts of foods rich in unsaturated fats, like peanuts, olive oil, or avocados, turns out to be a healthier choice, as long as you don't overdo the calories."

Here's why: While very low-fat diets do lower total cholesterol, they also lower high-density lipoprotein, or HDL, the so-called good cholesterol that helps keep the harmful low-density lipoprotein (LDL) from collecting in blood vessels. What's more, very low-fat diets raise levels of triglycerides, or fat particles in the blood,

Wendy Rickard and Fran McManus:
Farm Fresh Is Best

In an age in which some chefs are treated like rock stars, Wendy Rickard and Fran McManus want local farmers to share the spotlight. "Even the superstar chefs out there will tell you that behind every great chef is a great farmer," McManus says. "Small, local farmers produce the freshest, most flavorful produce you can find. And they help keep local communities economically diverse and vibrant."

To give farmers more recognition, McManus and Rickard are writing a series of books that includes collections of recipes and essays, as well as listings of local farmers and restaurants that feature their produce. The first, *Eating Fresh From the Organic Garden State* (Northeast Organic Farming Association, 1997), focuses on New Jersey. A similar guide to the San Francisco area is *Cooking Fresh from the Bay Area* (Eating Fresh Publications, 2000). Now the two crusaders are working on the third book, which will focus on the mid-Atlantic region.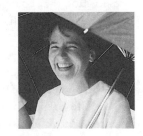

Support your local farmers. Shape your menu around what's in season, and you'll help yourself to the freshest, healthiest, most flavorful food around.—Fran McManus

McManus and Rickard aren't alone in emphasizing the importance of small farms. Nor are they the only advocates for the health and environmental benefits of organic farming. But they are the first to bring these issues together in the form of regionally focused books that help people support their local growers. And they remind us that great food, good health, strong communities, and a robust environment are all woven from the same cloth.

"We're trying to help people learn about what's going on in their own backyards—the small farmers who are growing the best foods, and the restaurants that support them," says Rickard. "Sure, there are environmental and economic reasons to support local farmers, but we also want to give people another reason to buy locally grown produce: because it's simply delicious."

culinary pleasures and the health benefits of traditional cuisines. Working with Oldways' founder, Dun Gifford, Baer-Sinnott played a leading role in developing the group's familiar Mediterranean Diet pyramid—featuring olive oils, legumes, fruits, grains, nuts, and vegetables—which many experts say is a healthier guide than the U.S. Department of Agriculture's food pyramid. Since then, Baer-Sinnott has helped create pyramids based on Asian, Latin American, and vegetarian cuisines. Under her watch,

The lesson of the world's great traditional cuisines—from the Mediterranean to Asia—is that healthy food can be rich, varied, and truly satisfying.—Sara Baer-Sinnott

Oldways helped promote the idea that unsaturated fats are healthy. The federal government, spurred in part by the group's work, changed its official advice to include moderate amounts of healthy fats.

That success hasn't meant complacency for Baer-Sinnott. Now she is focusing on Oldways' newest effort: bringing together researchers, dietitians, and food experts to promote the health benefits of antioxidants, those disease-fighting substances abundant in fruits and vegetables.

Sara Baer-Sinnott:
Learn from the Past

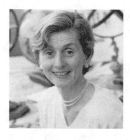

Sara Baer-Sinnott remembers standing in a taverna on the island of Crete, watching a crowd of more than 100 nutrition scientists, chefs, and food experts singing, dancing, even smashing plates on the floor in the finest Greek tradition. "That moment, more than any other, seemed to capture the essence of what we're about at Oldways Preservation & Exchange Trust: combining a deep love of food traditions with the latest scientific research," Baer-Sinnott says.

Over the past nine years, the 47-year-old executive vice president of Oldways, a nonprofit organization, has coordinated more than two dozen conferences around the world. They have brought leading nutrition researchers together with food experts to explore the

Bonnie Liebman:
Expose the Bad, Celebrate the Good

For 24 years, Bonnie Liebman has been one of this country's most diligent nutrition watchdogs, exposing unhealthy food wherever it's served. As the director of nutrition for the Center for Science in the Public Interest (CSPI), an outspoken consumer group, Liebman helped uncover the truth about movie-theater popcorn, warning that a large bucket popped in coconut oil

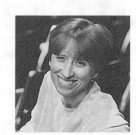

can contain as many as 77 grams of fat (most of it saturated)—and that's without butter. When she and her investigative team sampled the entrées being served in many of America's most popular restaurants, the news was just as scary. Some versions of beef-and-cheese nachos contain as much fat as seven glazed doughnuts, she warned. An order of fettuccine Alfredo at certain Italian restaurants is laden with as much fat as three pints of ice cream.

One of Liebman's proudest moments came when she noticed that a character in one of Tom Clancy's novels calls fettuccine Alfredo a "heart attack on a plate." "I was thrilled," Liebman says. "Those are exactly the words we used to describe the fat-laden pastas served up in many Italian restaurants. I figure if we've made it into a Tom Clancy book, we must be reaching a few people."

More than a few, it turns out. CSPI's *Nutrition Action Healthletter*, for which Liebman is a contributing editor, has a devoted audience of more than 800,000 subscribers. Liebman isn't interested only in pointing the finger of blame, though. She's also quick to praise food items that are good for you, like whole grain breakfast cereals and convenient frozen vegetables.

To eat a healthy diet, learn to resist messages that are constantly urging us to eat, eat, eat.—Bonnie Liebman

"If I didn't love good food, I wouldn't be in this business. I enjoy cooking. I love to eat. That's really what motivates me to point out to people exactly what they're being served." Her latest target: meals served up in food courts, such as those in airports and shopping malls. "Of course, what we're finding is what we see almost everywhere. What used to be an adult-size serving of French fries is now the kid-size helping. And the adult size is so big that it packs almost a half day's worth of calories."

We know what a healthy diet consists of. It means eating less fat in the form of meat, dairy, and processed food. It means eating more plant foods and consuming fewer calories than most Americans now eat.—Marion Nestle

Marion Nestle:
Spreading the Good-Nutrition Gospel

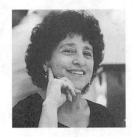

If anyone deserves the title of America's Nutritionist, it's Marion Nestle, Ph.D., chair of the department of nutrition and food studies at New York University (NYU). In 1986, after earning a master's degree in public health nutrition, Nestle went to Washington, D.C., to help put together the Surgeon General's Report on Nutrition and Health—a landmark document that alerted many Americans for the first time to the dangers of saturated fat. She has continued to play a leading role in steering the nation's official nutrition advice, speaking out on everything from vitamin supplements (mostly a waste of money) to hospital food (appallingly unhealthy).

From her post at NYU, Nestle is training a new generation of nutritionists and food-lovers. Since taking over the department in 1988, she has turned it into a vibrant center for the study of the culinary, cultural, and health aspects of food. She has also helped make food studies a recognized academic discipline that can go a long way toward changing the kind of food we eat in restaurants and at home. "We're turning out chefs who know more about food as it relates to culture and society, food writers who know about nutrition, and scholars who are interested in both the culinary and cultural aspects of food," Nestle says.

Now she is writing again, finishing a new book called *Food Politics* (due out in 2002), which exposes how food manufacturers have tried to lobby and influence federal nutrition policy. Nestle is also working on a book about the politics of food safety and biotechnology.✳

Peter Jaret is a contributing Health *editor.*

the 10 top
diet supplements that work

The supplement craze may have stalled in the face of negative press and questionable test results. But the fact is, some natural compounds do work.

BY TIMOTHY GOWER

Throughout the 1990s, the dietary-supplement industry took off running almost as dramatically as dot-coms. Each year during the last decade, sales of all-natural medicinal herbs and other health boosters spiked ever higher.

But America's love affair with these supplements is beginning to show signs of strain. According to industry journals, the overall growth rate of supplement sales has hit a plateau, and sales of such superstar herbs as ginseng and ginkgo biloba have plummeted. Consumer enthusiasm for these products may be waning because watchdog groups have found serious problems with the ingredients in some supplement brands. But the public's passion may have fizzled for a much more basic reason: They have doubts about whether or not dietary supplements actually work.

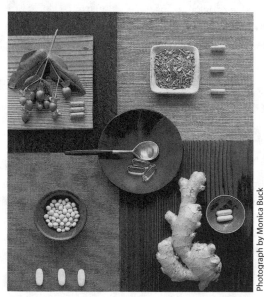

Photograph by Monica Buck

These pills, powders, and other potions aren't closely monitored by the Food and Drug Administration, so companies can sell them whether or not there's proof they live up to their hype. Research suggests that many might not.

That's no reason to dismiss all supplements, though. We've reviewed the research, explored the claims, and sifted through the side effects to come up with this list of 10 natural compounds that offer real benefits. In this group, you'll find supplements that may help prevent or treat major causes of pain, such as osteoporosis, arthritis, and migraines—and even help combat such serious killers as heart disease. We've also developed a confidence scale, so you can see at a glance exactly how strong the proof is behind each pill. That said, you still need to play it safe: Always talk to your physician before taking any supplement.

confidence ratings

🌿 Has shown promise in early clinical trials, but needs more study to verify its safety and efficacy.

🌿 🌿 Has undergone serious scrutiny, yet many doctors in this country remain skeptical.

🌿 🌿 🌿 Has an accepted role in mainstream medicine.

calcium

Rating: 🌿 🌿 🌿

The claim: Calcium builds stronger bones and helps prevent osteoporosis, which can lead to crippling fractures.

The evidence: Scientists know that calcium is critical for healthy bones; the recommended daily intake is 1,000 milligrams (mg), 1,200 mg for women over 50. A study in *The New England Journal of Medicine* found that taking 1,000 mg of supplemental calcium a day slowed bone loss in post-menopausal women by 43 percent.

The caveat: Exceeding the recommended daily intake could block the absorption of other minerals.

evening-primrose oil

Rating: 🌿

The claim: Herbalists recommend supplements made from this plant for many inflammatory conditions, especially rheumatoid arthritis.

The evidence: Evening-primrose oil contains several essential fatty acids, including gammalinolenic acid, or GLA. In a few small studies, some people with rheumatoid arthritis who took supplements containing GLA had less joint pain, swelling, and stiffness. Evening-primrose oil probably can't replace anti-inflammatory drugs, which are standard therapy for rheumatoid arthritis. But some arthritis sufferers who use the herb are able to reduce their drug dosage.

The caveats: Evening-primrose oil appears to be nontoxic, but the safety of using it for extended periods has not been studied. Side effects include nausea and headaches.

five supplements to avoid

Some dietary supplements have no proven value; others may be harmful. For either of these reasons—and sometimes both—these potions are best left on the shelf.

Bee pollen. There is no proof that these exotic-sounding pills increase physical vigor and energy, as is often claimed.

Bilberry. Extract of these berries supposedly improves night vision. But in a pair of studies published in the late 1990s, the men who took these supplements remained in the dark.

Ephedra. A review in *The New England Journal of Medicine* in 2000 found that this herb, widely used for losing weight and increasing energy, raises the risk of heart attacks and strokes. (To learn more, see "Ephedra: Dieter's Miracle . . .or Menace" on page 77.)

Kelp. There's no scientific evidence to support the use of seaweed-based pills and powders. And because of their potentially high iodine content, they could cause thyroid problems.

Shark cartilage. A book called *Sharks Don't Get Cancer* (Avery, 1992) promoted these supplements as a miracle cure. But sharks *do* get cancer, and there's no evidence that these pills fight the disease.

feverfew

Rating: 🌿

The claim: Prevents migraine headaches, which afflict about 28 million Americans (75 percent of whom are women).

The evidence: British researchers have found that migraine sufferers who took a daily capsule containing the equivalent of two feverfew leaves (roughly 80 mg per capsule) had 24 percent fewer attacks than patients given a placebo. Several other small studies have found similar benefits. Lab research suggests that chemicals in feverfew thwart production of hormonelike molecules called prostaglandins, believed to be a factor in many migraine attacks.

The most promising supplements may relieve pain as well as fight serious diseases.

The caveats: Larger studies would clarify feverfew's role in treating migraines. It doesn't appear to diminish the duration of attacks. Quitting this herb may cause rebound headaches, as well as nervousness, insomnia, and other symptoms. Feverfew may also interact with drugs used to prevent blood clotting and with iron supplements.

fish oil

Rating: 🌿 🌿

The claim: It reduces the risk of heart disease and eases symptoms related to some forms of arthritis and depression.

The evidence: One study found that people who eat fish at least once a week are half as likely to suffer sudden cardiac death. Fish oil appears to prevent blood clots and, at doses up to 6 grams (g) per day, may also reduce levels of triglycerides, blood fats associated with an increased risk of heart disease. A few small studies suggest that taking fish-oil pills may allow patients with rheumatoid arthritis to decrease drug dosage. Preliminary research hints that the supplements may also help control bipolar disorder (manic depression).

The caveats: There's little evidence that taking these supplements offers benefits you wouldn't get from eating salmon or other fatty varieties of fish a few times a week. People who take blood-thinning drugs shouldn't use fish-oil pills.

folic acid

Rating: 🌿 🌿 🌿

The claim: Taken before and during pregnancy, this B vitamin prevents birth defects that can result in diseases of the skull and spine, such as spina bifida.

The evidence: Two large studies published in the early 1990s found that women who took folic-acid supplements were up to 72 percent less likely to have babies with neural tube defects. Based on these studies, the U.S. Public Health Service recommends that

women who may become pregnant should consume 400 micrograms of folic acid a day—preferably from foods such as chickpeas, spinach, and oranges but by supplement if necessary. Some evidence suggests that folic acid and other B vitamins could also reduce the risk of heart disease, but more study is needed.

The caveat: Very high doses of folic acid may mask a vitamin B-12 deficiency (see "Are You Running Low on B-12?" on page 288).

ginger

Rating: 🌿

The claim: This spice is often taken in supplement form to prevent motion sickness and relieve nausea, particularly among pregnant women.

The evidence: A study published in 2001 found that 90 percent of expectant mothers who took four 250-mg capsules of ginger experienced less nausea and vomiting than pregnant women who took placebos. At least two studies suggest that taking ginger will reduce the risk of seasickness. In one, ginger was more effective than Dramamine.

The caveats: Other studies suggest that ginger may not prevent nausea and vomiting related to surgery and anesthesia. High doses might interfere with blood-thinning drugs such as warfarin, as well as medications that control blood sugar in diabetics. Some experts also question ginger's effect on fetal development.

glucosamine & chondroitin

Rating: 🌿 🌿

The claim: These natural compounds (which are sometimes combined in one pill) are said to ease joint pain and stiffness caused by osteoarthritis, the most common form of arthritis.

The evidence: A scientific review for the National Institutes of Health (NIH) analyzed 15 studies involving glucosamine and chondroitin—taken separately or together, in various dosages (there's no consensus on dosage yet). Although the NIH panel said some of the studies were flawed, the overall evidence suggests that these natural joint-pain relievers likely provide modest relief for osteoarthritis pain. A large NIH study is under way and is expected to wrap up in 2004.

The caveat: An arthritis sufferer may need to take glucosamine and/or chondroitin for several months before feeling any benefit.

multivitamins

Rating: 🌿 🌿 🌿

The claim: These pills safeguard health by providing the recommended daily dose of vitamins and minerals.

The evidence: Although a few surveys have found that people who pop multivitamins are no healthier than non-users, some preliminary studies have detected lower rates of colon cancer among women who use multivitamins. An ongoing study of more than 15,000 physicians should shed more light on the benefits of multivitamins, but its results won't be known for several years. There's no question, however, that taking a multivitamin each day increases blood levels of nutrients believed to fight various illnesses, including cancer and heart disease.

The caveats: Many multivitamins sold today are blended with herbs and other nonessential compounds that have not been well-studied and, therefore, could be dangerous. Ignore label buzzwords such as "time-release" and "chelated," which are meaningless.

niacin

Rating: 🌿 🌿 🌿

The claim: This B vitamin lowers cholesterol and other risk factors for heart disease.

The evidence: In a 1994 study, high doses of niacin (up to 4.5 g per day—more than 200 times the recommended daily intake) lowered LDL cholesterol (the "bad" kind) by 23 percent after six months, but the prescription drug Lovastatin fared much better.

Niacin, however, boosted HDL cholesterol (the "good" kind) more than four times higher than did lovastatin.

The caveats: Therapeutic doses of niacin can cause liver damage, which is why anyone taking these supplements must be monitored by a doctor. There is also some evidence that niacin may raise blood levels of an amino acid called homocystine, which could actually increase heart-disease risk. A variety of health conditions, including diabetes, gout, and glaucoma, may be worsened by the use of this supplement, so check with your physician. Side effects include flushing, tingling, or a sensation of warmth that usually stop with continued use.

saint-john's-wort

Rating: 🌿 🌿

The claim: Although it has many purported uses, Saint-John's-wort is best known as an herbal antidepressant.

The evidence: Two separate scientific reviews have determined that Saint-John's-wort (typical dosage: 900 mg per day) seems to improve mood in people with mild to moderate depression. An NIH-sponsored study scheduled for completion in 2002 should show if it's as effective as prescription antidepressants.

The caveats: Saint-John's-wort does not appear to be effective in treating major depression, according to a widely publicized study in *The Journal of the American Medical Association*. Saint-John's-wort may interfere with a long list of medications, including drugs used to thin blood, treat HIV, and prevent transplant rejections. ✳

Contributing editor Timothy Gower is the author (with Robert S. DiPaola, M.D.) of A Doctor's Guide to Herbs and Supplements *(Henry Holt and Company, 2001).*

Are you running low on
B-12?

A new study suggests that people of all ages
are missing out on this essential vitamin.
Here's how to be sure you're getting enough.

BY BILL GOTTLIEB

There are certain things in life you can't go wrong with: jumper cables in the trunk, a little black dress in the closet. A traditional, balanced diet used to be on this list of things, too, until a recent study found that it doesn't deliver on all of its promises. It turns out that even if you're eating the right amounts of produce, grains, and animal foods, you may still be missing out on a vital nutrient that can give you the energy of Mia Hamm and the clarity of Cokie Roberts: vitamin B-12.

A recent study from Tufts University in Boston uncovered the surprising fact that 40 percent of young, otherwise healthy women and men have low enough levels of vitamin B-12 to threaten good health. And that was even when their diets contained three times the recommended daily intake.

Before this news, B-12 deficiency wasn't something to worry about—especially if you ate beef, chicken, or fish—until age 50 or older. (After 50, lower levels of stomach acids can block absorption.) But this study suggests that even seemingly healthy people under 50 need to rethink their "everything's OK" approach to B-12.

The study, led by Katherine Tucker, Ph.D., of the U.S. Department of Agriculture Human Nutrition Research Center at Tufts, tested B-12 blood levels in 3,000 adults. "The correlation was lower than expected between vitamin B-12 levels in the blood and age," Tucker says. "Low blood levels were prevalent in the entire population, among all adults, in both women and men." The study was based on individuals' self-reported dietary intakes, rather than monitored diets, so more research is needed. But the results are startling: Of the participants, 39 percent had levels at or below the borderline, 17 percent had low levels, and 9 percent had levels that were low enough to be considered clinical deficiencies.

"This study is a real eye-opener," says Jeff Hampl, Ph.D., R.D., a spokesman for the American Dietetic Association and professor of nutrition at Arizona State University. "Based on this evidence, dietitians should be concerned about ensuring that everyone gets enough B-12—not just senior citizens."

Fortunately, you can prevent low levels if you know where to look. And it's not to the red meat, chicken, and fish that nutrition scientists have long touted as being good sources of B-12. In the study, people had low levels of the vitamin even if they included these foods in their diets. "The knowledge that B-12 is not

A vitamin B-12 deficiency can leave
you tired, forgetful, and depressed. It may
also be linked to heart disease and stroke.

well-absorbed from most protein foods—not just in the elderly but in the entire population—is completely new," Tucker says.

Sub-par levels of B-12 can leave you tired, weak, and eventually even forgetful and depressed. Without enough B-12, oxygen-carrying red blood cells can grow to an abnormal size, a condition called macrocytic anemia. The precious outer coating of nerves, the myelin sheath, can begin to dissolve, and with it vanishes sharp memory, clear thinking, and positive moods. The nerve damage can also cause tingling, numbness, and burning in the hands and feet, along with balance problems. The circulatory system is hit hard too: Low levels of B-12 can cause an increase in homocystine, an amino acid linked to heart disease and stroke.

With the exception of anemia, these health problems don't develop quickly; chronically low B-12 levels can take 10 or more years to produce symptoms. Unfortunately, once a doctor detects a B-12-related problem, the memory loss, nerve damage, or circulatory disease may be irreversible, Tucker says. That's why it's important that you pay attention to B-12 levels now.

No one knows for sure why blood levels of B-12 are so low in the under-50 set, but Tucker has a theory: "The use of antacids and acid-blocking and acid-suppressing drugs to treat heartburn in the general population has skyrocketed: In terms of total sales, they are the number one drug," she says. "B-12 absorption from food depends on the presence of adequate levels of stomach acid—so these acid-suppressing drugs make vitamin B-12 very difficult to absorb from food. Although it remains to be proven, preliminary data suggest that people who take more antacids have lower blood levels of vitamin B-12."

Experts have long known that older people don't absorb B-12 well because they have lower levels of stomach acid and the enzyme pepsin. These factors help digest protein, which is what the B-12 in food is attached to. That's why the government's National Academy of Sciences recommends that everyone over age 50 get B-12 from a nutritional supplement or B-12-fortified cereal products. These sources contain the vitamin in its free form: It's not attached to protein and, therefore, doesn't need acid or pepsin for absorption.

Tucker says that the advice for those over 50 may now be important for people well under that age. In fact, she found that people who took supplements, ate fortified cereal, drank milk, or consumed other dairy products were more likely to have normal levels of the vitamin than people who ate more meat such as beef, chicken, or fish. Scientists don't know why B-12 in dairy is more absorbable than B-12 in meat, though it may be because when meat is cooked, B-12 becomes bound more tightly to the protein.

A few basic steps, though, will help make sure you have enough B-12 in your diet. Tucker recommends any of the following methods to get your fill.

It isn't hard to replenish your supply of B-12: Just add fortified cereal, milk, and vitamin supplements to your diet.

a daily dose of dairy

Though you'll have to polish off several servings to meet your needs, the vitamin B-12 in dairy products is believed to be more absorbable than that in meat. In a recent Tufts University study, people with the third-highest intake of B-12 were getting 8.2 micrograms of the vitamin a day, mostly from dairy foods. Here's where you can find vitamin B-12 in the dairy case.

dairy product	micrograms
1 cup of regular or low-fat (1%) cottage cheese	1.4
8 ounces of low-fat fruit yogurt	1.1
8-ounce glass of milk	0.9
1 ounce of Swiss cheese	0.5
4 ounces of light vanilla ice cream	0.4
4 ounces of frozen yogurt	0.2
1 ounce of Cheddar cheese	0.2
1 ounce of low-fat Cheddar cheese	0.1

should you get tested?

Anyone can ask her doctor for a B-12 test, but if you don't take supplements or don't often eat fortified cereal or dairy products, make the test a priority. You may also want to get tested if you use antacids two or more times a week. Having two or more alcoholic drinks a day can also cut absorption levels. Latin Americans and African-Americans may have more absorption problems with B-12 than Caucasians or Asian-Americans, according to a study by Ralph Carmel, Ph.D., a professor in the department of medicine at the New York Methodist Hospital in Brooklyn.

If you decide to get tested, Tufts University researcher Katherine Tucker, Ph.D., advises that you make sure your doctor uses the right cutoff for diagnosing a deficiency. Tucker's study used a measurement system that's not as common in most doctor's offices, so the terminology can be confusing.

Borderline B-12 deficiency is 258 picomoles per liter. But most doctors wait until you're clinically deficient and have only 148 picomoles per liter before bringing it up. Tucker advocates concern at a higher level. "If your B-12 level is below borderline, you should take a supplement."Those who score below 258 should have further medical testing for the amino acids homocystine and methylmalonic acid. High levels of either could mean you have some nerve or circulatory symptoms of B-12 deficiency, and you may need treatment with high doses of the nutrient.

Make it a multi. Take a daily multivitamin or other supplement with a minimum of 2.4 micrograms (mcg) of B-12, the recommended dietary allowance (RDA) for women 19 and older. Tucker recommends a supplement with 25 mcg for women over age 50. In the study, the people with the highest B-12 levels took a daily vitamin supplement that included B-12.

Try fortified foods. People in the study with the second-highest levels of the vitamin ate breakfast that consisted of cereal fortified with B-12 at least four times a week. To be safe, Tucker says, you should choose a product that is fortified at 100 percent of the daily value for B-12. Don't simply assume that all fortified cereals have the same levels of a vitamin; for instance, Product 19 qualifies, but Wheaties and Cheerios don't.

Get milk. The people in the study with the third-highest levels of B-12 had an average intake of 8.2 mcg daily, mainly from milk or other dairy products. Getting that amount may mean consuming more dairy than you're used to. An 8-ounce glass of milk, for example, has 0.9 mcg (see "A Daily Dose of Dairy" on page 289 for levels in other dairy products). ✳

Bill Gottlieb is a freelance writer and author of Alternative Cures *(Rodale, 2000).*

Q+A The not-so-real benefits of wheat grass and powdered greens

Are wheat grass and powdered greens as healthy as they're claimed to be? I would love a way to get my five to nine a day without having to eat spinach for lunch!

Fans swear by them, but experts disagree. Most nutritionists will tell you that grasses—whether wheat or barley, juiced or powdered—don't do everything their followers maintain. Despite claims that wheat grass and other greens are wonder cures for everything from headaches to cancer, downing a shot a day won't grant you the immunity from disease that you seek.

Wheat grass does contain the same vitamins, minerals, and phytochemicals found in leafy vegetables—and it's often easier to fit a wheat-grass cocktail into a busy schedule than, say, to steam a bunch of broccoli.

Unfortunately, the quantity of nutrients in this popular green drink is scant. A combination of various greens, such as the souped-up powdered versions you'll find in a health-food store, provides larger amounts and a bigger variety of vitamins and minerals.

Still, no juice or powder can fully replicate the fiber and other benefits of the real thing. So drink up, but don't forget to eat your broccoli too.

Shining a new light on *dining after dark*

Delaying dinner can lead to extra pounds. But the reason why may surprise you.

BY DOMENICA MARCHETTI

As my husband and I sat down to eat dinner one recent evening, I glanced at the clock: 9:35 p.m. A minor miracle, I thought. Rarely on a weeknight do we eat before 10 o'clock.

With two young kids and odd working hours, we often put dinner on the back burner. That is, dinner usually takes place late, after the kids are bathed, read to, tucked in, and asleep.

We are far from alone in our nocturnal dining habit—and it's not just harried parents in search of a peaceful or romantic meal who are delaying dinner. We are joined by professionals who toil late at the office or bring bulging briefcases home, and folks who use their evenings to work out or squeeze in a trip to the grocery store.

Such a schedule has its consequences: bad eating habits, fitful sleep, and weight gain. Experts used to believe that calories eaten close to bedtime piled on pounds because metabolism slows while you sleep, leaving little chance to burn off a meal. But later studies showed that what matters weight-wise is the number of calories you consume and burn each day—when you eat them makes no difference to your metabolism. Since late-night noshing indeed leads to larger waistbands, researchers went looking for the real culprit. The problem, they found, is that people who eat late tend to consume more calories than those who don't.

Blame it, at least in part, on the lighting. A study published in the July 2001 issue of the journal *Personality and Individual Differences* examined the eating behaviors of 151 undergraduates and found that those who stayed up later were more likely to overeat. The probable reason, according to study author Joseph Kasof, Ph.D., a researcher in psychology and social behavior at the University of California at Irvine, is that people are less inhibited in general when lights are low, as every would-be Casanova knows.

"When you're standing in a floodlight, you're very self-conscious," Kasof says. "But when the lights are down low, you're much less self-conscious. And when you're less self-conscious, research shows that you're more at risk for misbehavior." In his studies, Kasof found that even a small difference in lighting can affect how much people are likely to overeat, particularly among dieters. He became interested in the theory after observing his own eating behavior. A vegetarian who admits to being "aesthetically attracted to meat," Kasof noticed that he only strayed from his vegetarian diet in the evening. Now he eats dinner earlier—with the lights turned up.

Low lighting is not the only reason late-night diners may experience weight gain. People who dine late often find they are not hungry in the morning, making them more likely to skip breakfast. They may skimp at lunch too. While this might seem like a benefit for people trying to manage their weight, it's just the opposite.

"Your hunger pattern is determined by your eating pattern," says C. Wayne Callaway, M.D., an endocrinologist and obesity specialist in Washington, D.C. "People who skip a meal or undereat tend to be more hungry following the next meal. If you skip lunch, you're setting yourself up to eat two desserts after dinner."

If the time you spend eating is at the expense of exercise, it's double trouble because you're burning fewer calories and taking in more. There's a simple cure, says Barbara J. Moore, Ph.D., president of Shape Up America!, a nonprofit organization started by former U.S. surgeon general C. Everett Koop. Moore points out that although Europeans eat later, there is a tradition of the paseo, a post-dinner walk through the streets. "Europeans also tend to eat late lunches, snack

less, and consume smaller portions than Americans, which may explain the lack of obesity in countries such as France, Italy, and Spain—despite a tradition of dining late."

For some, however, the problem can't be solved by a simple stroll. There's an extreme form of late-night eating, known as night-eating syndrome, in which those afflicted eat nothing or very little during the day and consume about 40 percent of their daily calories after their last meal, often waking up in the middle of the night to eat.

The disorder was first identified in 1955 by Albert Stunkard, M.D., a professor of psychiatry at the University of Pennsylvania. Unlike binge eating (which Stunkard is also credited with identifying), night-eating syndrome remains virtually unknown to the public, even though it is fairly widespread. Stunkard, who has just been awarded a grant from the National Institutes of Health to study the disorder and its treatment, estimates that as much as 5 percent of the country's population may suffer from it.

The syndrome tends to be precipitated by stress, Stunkard says. But it's not like other stress-related disorders: "Even when the stress goes away, once this thing gets started it tends to become chronic," he says. "I know patients who have had it for 30 years."

Besides contributing to obesity, the disorder may be related to depression and sleep problems as well. Stunkard has noticed that the late-night snacks tend to be very high in carbohydrates, which raise the level of the sedative-like brain chemical seratonin, thus helping people get back to sleep. He believes chronic night-eaters are simply self-medicating. Whether depression or insomnia leads to the eating disorder, or overeating precipitates mood problems and sleeplessness is not clear. These problems are evidently connected, though, and can escalate into a debilitating illness.

> *When the moon hits your eye, put down that pizza pie—or you may put on some extra pounds. Research shows the dimmer the light, the more you tend to eat. That's why eating late can be hazardous to your weight.*

Curb late-night binges with small, healthy meals throughout the day and a light dinner before you go to bed.

There is no reason to believe a lopsided eating schedule will lead to night-eating syndrome, Stunkard says. However, the habits associated with late-night eating—lack of exercise and consumption of additional calories—can contribute to weight gain or an increased risk of obesity.

For many of us, eating earlier is just impossible. So what can be done to minimize the consequences of a late-night eating schedule? Try these steps.

Don't skip breakfast or lunch. "The best way to reduce overeating at night is to eat adequately during the day," Callaway says.

Choose easy to digest foods. Try vegetables, fruits, and small amounts of starches, advises Terri Brownlee, nutrition director at the Duke University Diet & Fitness Center.

Watch portion sizes and calories. "This will ensure that your total calorie intake for the day is not out of line," Brownlee says.

Eat at least half your calories by early afternoon. Replace three large meals with four smaller ones every four hours.

Go for a walk after you eat if at all possible, Moore says.

And let's not forget Kasof's advice: Skip the romantic candlelit dinner—and turn up the lights. ✳

Domenica Marchetti is a Virginia-based nutrition, health, and food writer.

Q+A
love the pizza, hate the heartburn

I love pizza, but every time I eat it, I get heartburn. Do I need to be under a doctor's care?

Heartburn, also called acid reflux, is extremely common. The American College of Gastroenterology estimates that more than 60 million Americans suffer from it, and 50 percent of pregnant women experience it in the latter stages of pregnancy. The pain you feel comes when the valve that separates the esophagus from the stomach weakens and allows stomach juices to creep up. Most people who get a little heartburn after eating certain foods can just chew a couple of Maalox, and it's no big deal. There are also other terrific over-the-counter remedies like Tagamet and Zantac.

But for some people, it can be a serious problem that must be dealt with. Occasionally, cancer of the larynx or esophagus may develop if there's been a very long history of severe reflux. This doesn't happen very often, but over time, if left untreated, reflux does raise the risk of this type of cancer.

Before you reach for medicines, there are some simple things you can do to cut down on the problem. First of all, don't eat or drink anything other than water after 7 p.m. This will give your stomach time to empty its contents before you go to bed. Second, avoid cigarettes and alcohol because they relax the lower esophageal valve, making it easier for stomach acids to climb up. Third, sleep on two pillows; the gravity will help keep the stomach contents down where they belong. And finally, stay away from the foods that you know trigger the pain. (Here's a tip: If you have a problem with reflux and you're on your way out of a restaurant, don't grab a chocolate-covered mint. The chocolate and mint together not only relax the valve, but also increase acid secretions.) For most people, doing these things will help.

How do you know if you actually have a more serious problem? There are a couple of signs: a lump in the throat, as if something is stuck there, or chest pain that doesn't go away. If symptoms persist after three weeks of consistent use of over-the-counter remedies, you should see a doctor.

warmth in winter
simple comfort foods

RECIPES BY KAREN A. LEVIN

W ish I had time for just one more bowl of chili," said the legendary western scout Kit Carson on his deathbed, and who would quarrel with his hankering? Chili is classic comfort food, the kind of dish that makes you feel cozy and warm and happy to be home. Equally comforting is a batch of lean meat, fish, or poultry browned until fragrant, then simmered to succulence in a luxurious sauce. Think piping hot chicken and onions stewed in white wine, garlicky pork loin with tender sweet potatoes, or lamb shanks and white beans braised in red wine and beef broth.

Hold on a minute, you say—what's braised? It's the term for food that's been slow-cooked in a small amount of liquid in a tightly closed pot, traditionally in the oven instead of on the stove top. Granted, slow is a dirty word in many kitchens these days. But slow cooking doesn't mean slow to prepare or slow to reach the table.

For starters, these recipes are dead easy. In most cases, you simply brown some meat and cut a few vegetables. The ingredients all go together in a casserole or Dutch oven that you then pop in the oven and ignore for long enough to scan a magazine or go for a brisk stroll.

And here's the trick: You can make most of these superbly light dishes hours or days ahead. In fact, they're even better after a night's rest in the fridge. Warm the pot over a low flame or heat separate portions in the microwave. Add some sliced bread or boiled potatoes, and your dinner's ready in minutes. Now, that's true comfort food.

Braised Red Snapper

SERVES 6
PREPARATION: 30 MINUTES
BRAISING: 25 MINUTES

1/4 cup all-purpose flour

2 teaspoons Old Bay seasoning

1 whole red snapper or striped bass (3 to 4 pounds), scaled, head and tail removed

1/4 cup olive oil

3/4 cup chopped shallots or sweet onion

3 cloves garlic, minced

2 cups dry white wine or vermouth

2 sprigs tarragon or Italian parsley, plus 2 tablespoons chopped tarragon or parsley

2 sprigs thyme

1 teaspoon coriander seeds

1 teaspoon whole peppercorns

1/2 teaspoon salt

1 tablespoon butter

I. Preheat oven to 350°. Combine flour and Old Bay seasoning in a shallow dish or pieplate. Dredge both sides of fish in flour mixture, patting to coat. Discard excess flour mixture.

2. Over medium heat, warm a large, deep ovenproof skillet or roasting pan big enough to hold fish. Add olive oil; when it's hot, add fish. Cook 5 minutes per side or until deep golden brown. Carefully transfer fish to a platter; set aside.

3. Pour off oil. Add shallots and garlic to skillet; cook 30 seconds. Add wine, herb sprigs, coriander, peppercorns, and salt; bring to a simmer, scraping browned bits from bottom of skillet.

4. Return fish to skillet. Cover with lid or heavy-duty foil; braise in oven 25 minutes or until fish is opaque throughout.

5. Carefully transfer fish to a serving platter. Strain pan juices; return to skillet. Bring to a boil; remove from heat. Stir in butter until melted; spoon juices over fish. Garnish with chopped tarragon or parsley.

Per serving: Calories: 236 (27% from fat), Fat 7 g (2 g saturated), Protein 21 g, Carbohydrate 8 g, Fiber 0 g, Cholesterol 96 mg, Iron 2 mg, Sodium 421 mg, Calcium 40 mg

Coq au Vin

SERVES 4
PREPARATION: 15 MINUTES
BRAISING: 40 MINUTES

$^1/_4$ cup all-purpose flour
2 teaspoons paprika
2 teaspoons dried thyme
$^1/_2$ teaspoon salt
$^1/_2$ teaspoon freshly ground black pepper
4 chicken breast halves, bone in, skin on
1 tablespoon olive or vegetable oil
12 cipollini onions, medium shallots, or large pearl onions, peeled
1 pound button mushrooms, halved if large
1 pound baby carrots
1 cup white wine
1 cup low-sodium chicken broth
2 tablespoons chopped fresh thyme (optional)

1. Preheat oven to 350°. Combine flour, paprika, thyme, salt, and pepper in a plastic or paper bag. Rinse chicken in cold water; shake off excess water. Add chicken to flour mixture, 1 or 2 pieces at a time, shaking to coat. Reserve mixture remaining in bag.
2. Heat a 5-quart Dutch oven or ovenproof covered casserole over medium heat until hot. Add oil; when it's hot, add chicken, meaty side down, and cook 4 minutes or until golden brown. Turn; continue to cook 3 minutes. Transfer chicken to a plate; set aside.
3. Add onions, mushrooms, and carrots to the Dutch oven; cook 1 minute, stirring often. Add reserved flour mixture; mix well. Add wine and broth; bring to a boil. Set chicken over vegetables, and cover; braise in oven about 40 minutes or until chicken is cooked through.
4. With a slotted spoon, transfer chicken and vegetables to a serving platter; tent with foil, and keep warm. Boil pan juices in Dutch oven over high heat until reduced to 1$^1/_2$ cups, about 8 minutes. Serve chicken and

vegetables with pan juices. Garnish with chopped fresh thyme, if desired.

Per serving: Calories: 401 (29% from fat), Fat 13 g (3 g saturated), Protein 35 g, Carbohydrate 27 g, Fiber 4 g, Cholesterol 82 mg, Iron 5 mg, Sodium 510 mg, Calcium 73 mg

Osso Buco with Butternut Squash

SERVES 4
PREPARATION: 20 MINUTES
BRAISING: 1$^1/_2$ HOURS

$^1/_4$ cup all-purpose flour
$^3/_4$ teaspoon freshly ground black pepper
$^1/_2$ teaspoon salt
4 meaty veal shanks (about 2 pounds), trimmed well and cut 1$^1/_2$ inches thick
1 tablespoon olive oil
1 medium onion, chopped
5 cloves plus 1 clove garlic, minced
1 cup fat-free beef broth
$^1/_2$ cup dry white wine or vermouth
1 tablespoon dried herbes de Provence or fines herbes
1 butternut squash (about 1$^1/_4$ pounds)
8 ounces uncooked no-yolk broad egg noodles
$^1/_4$ cup chopped parsley
1 teaspoon finely grated lemon peel

1. Preheat oven to 350°. Combine flour, pepper, and salt in a plastic or paper bag. Add veal; shake to coat. Reserve remaining flour in bag. Heat a 5-quart Dutch oven or large ovenproof covered casserole over medium heat. Add oil; when hot, add veal. Brown well on all sides, about 10 minutes.
2. Transfer veal to a plate; set aside. Add onion and 5 cloves minced garlic to Dutch oven. Cook 5 minutes, stirring frequently. Add reserved flour mixture; cook 1 minute. Add beef broth, wine, and herbs; bring to a boil. Return veal to Dutch oven. Cover; braise in oven 50 minutes.
3. Meanwhile, peel squash; discard seeds and membrane. Cut squash into $^3/_4$-inch chunks. Stir into veal mixture; return to oven, and continue to braise until veal is fork tender, about 40 minutes longer.
4. Cook noodles according to package directions. Combine parsley, lemon peel, and remaining clove minced garlic; mix well. Spoon veal mixture over

drained noodles; top with parsley mixture.

Per serving: Calories: 576 (14% from fat), Fat 9 g (2 g saturated), Protein 49 g, Carbohydrate 64 g, Fiber 7 g, Cholesterol 143 mg, Iron 4 mg, Sodium 596 mg, Calcium 140 mg ✄

Pork Loin with Sweet Potatoes and Garlic

SERVES 6
PREPARATION: 30 MINUTES
BRAISING: 55 MINUTES

1 tablespoon all-purpose flour
2 teaspoons paprika
2 teaspoons dried sage
1 teaspoon dry mustard
1 teaspoon salt, divided
$^1/_2$ teaspoon freshly ground black pepper
$^1/_4$ teaspoon cinnamon
1 well-trimmed center-cut boneless pork loin roast
    (2 to 2$^1/_4$ pounds)
2 tablespoons vegetable oil
1 (14$^1/_2$-ounce) can low-sodium chicken broth
3 pounds sweet potatoes, peeled and cut into 2-inch chunks
1 head garlic, cloves separated but not peeled

1. Preheat oven to 350°. Combine flour, paprika, sage, mustard, $^1/_2$ teaspoon salt, pepper, and cinnamon in a pieplate or shallow dish; mix well. Dredge roast in flour mixture, patting to coat. Discard any remaining flour mixture.
2. Heat a 5-quart Dutch oven over medium heat. Add oil; when it's hot, add roast. Cook, turning as needed, until browned on all sides, about 10 minutes. Transfer roast to a plate; set aside. Pour off drippings from Dutch oven. Add broth; bring to a boil, scraping up browned bits on bottom. Add sweet potatoes and unpeeled garlic cloves. Place roast on sweet potatoes. Cover; braise in oven 50 to 55 minutes or until internal temperature of meat reaches 150°. Transfer pork to carving board; tent with foil, and let stand 5 minutes. (Its internal temperature will rise to 155°. Do not overcook or pork loin will be tough.) Transfer sweet potatoes to a medium saucepan with a slotted spoon; add remaining $^1/_2$ teaspoon salt. Mash with a potato masher; cover and keep warm over low heat. Transfer garlic cloves to a small plate; set aside.

3. Cook pan juices in Dutch oven over high heat 5 minutes. Squeeze cooked garlic from skins; mash into a paste. Stir garlic paste into pan juices; heat through. Carve meat into slices; arrange on plates with sweet potatoes. Spoon juices over pork and sweet potatoes.

Per serving: Calories: 477 (34% from fat), Fat 18 g (6 g saturated), Protein 36 g, Carbohydrate 42 g, Fiber 3 g, Cholesterol 93 mg, Iron 3 mg, Sodium 504 mg, Calcium 83 mg ✄

Minestrone

SERVES 6
PREPARATION: 15 MINUTES
BRAISING: 35 MINUTES

1 ounce pancetta or 2 slices bacon, diced
1$^1/_2$ cups thinly sliced leeks (white and light green parts only)
1 cup thinly sliced carrots
5 cloves garlic, coarsely chopped
1 (28-ounce) can Italian seasoned diced tomatoes or Italian plum tomatoes, coarsely chopped, juice reserved
1 (14$^1/_2$-ounce) can fat-free beef broth
1 cup water
2 ounces ($^1/_2$ cup) uncooked ditalini or small shell pasta
2 teaspoons dried basil
1 teaspoon dried oregano
$^1/_4$ teaspoon red chili pepper flakes (optional)
1 (16-ounce) can cannellini or great northern beans, rinsed and drained
1 cup frozen baby peas, thawed
$^1/_4$ cup grated (or 1 ounce shaved) Parmigiano-Reggiano or Pecorino Romano cheese
1 tablespoon basil- or rosemary-infused olive oil, such as Consorzio brand
2 tablespoons chopped fresh basil or Italian parsley

1. Preheat oven to 350°. In a 5-quart Dutch oven or ovenproof covered casserole, cook pancetta over medium heat until it starts to brown, about 3 minutes. Add leeks, carrots, and garlic; cook 3 minutes, stirring occasionally.
2. Stir in tomatoes with juice, broth, water, pasta, dried basil and oregano, and pepper flakes; bring to a full boil. Cover; braise in oven 35 minutes or until vegetables are tender. Stir in beans and peas; cover and let stand 5 minutes. Ladle into bowls; top with cheese. Drizzle $^1/_2$ teaspoon oil over each serving;

garnish with fresh basil.

Per serving: Calories: 261 (30% from fat), Fat 9 g (3 g saturated),

Protein 11 g, Carbohydrate 33 g, Fiber 7 g, Cholesterol 8 mg,

Iron 3 mg, Sodium 564 mg, Calcium 132 mg

Chipotle Chili Con Carne

SERVES 6
PREPARATION: 15 MINUTES
BRAISING: 50 MINUTES

1 pound lean boneless pork shoulder or beef chuck, cut into
   $^1/_2$-inch cubes

1$^1/_2$ tablespoons chili powder

1$^1/_2$ tablespoons ground cumin

$^1/_4$ teaspoon salt

2 teaspoons vegetable oil

1 large onion, chopped

4 cloves garlic, minced

1 (10-ounce) can tomatoes with green chiles, undrained

1 cup beer (not dark)

1 to 2 tablespoons pureed chipotle chiles in adobo sauce*

2 teaspoons dried oregano, preferably Mexican

1 (16-ounce) can pinto or black beans, rinsed and drained

1 (15-ounce) can 50%-less-salt black beans, rinsed and drained

$^1/_2$ cup coarsely chopped cilantro

Optional garnishes: light sour cream, diced avocado, and tomato

I. Preheat oven to 350°. Toss meat with chili powder, cumin, and salt; set aside. Heat a 4- to 5-quart Dutch oven over medium heat. Add oil; when it's hot, add onion and garlic, and cook 5 minutes, stirring occasionally. Add seasoned meat; continue to cook 5 minutes, stirring occasionally.

2. Stir in tomatoes, beer, chipotle chiles, and oregano; bring to a boil. Cover; braise in oven 50 minutes or until meat is fork tender. Stir in beans and cilantro; cover and let stand 5 minutes. Ladle into bowls; garnish as desired.

* Find cans of chipotle chiles in the ethnic section of the supermarket. Purée in a blender or food processor. Refrigerate unused purée up to 1 week, or freeze up to 3 months.

Per serving: Calories: 282 (26% from fat), Fat 8 g (2 g saturated),

Protein 23 g, Carbohydrate 28 g, Fiber 9 g, Cholesterol 51 mg,

Iron 2 mg, Sodium 682 mg, Calcium 82 mg

Wine-Braised Lamb Shanks with White Beans

SERVES 4
PREPARATION: 30 MINUTES
BRAISING: 1 HOUR, 15 MINUTES

3 tablespoons all-purpose flour

$^3/_4$ teaspoon freshly ground black pepper

4 small, well-trimmed lamb shanks (about 4 pounds)

2 tablespoons olive oil

1 medium onion, chopped

4 cloves garlic, minced

1 cup fat-free beef broth

1 cup dry red wine, such as merlot

1 teaspoons dried rosemary, crushed

1 pound baby carrots

1 (19-ounce) can cannellini beans, rinsed and drained

Rosemary sprigs (optional)

I. Preheat oven to 350°. Combine flour and pepper in a plastic or paper bag. Add lamb shanks (in batches if necessary); shake to coat well. Reserve any remaining flour in bag.

2. Heat a 5-quart Dutch oven or ovenproof covered casserole over medium heat. Add oil; when hot, add lamb shanks (in batches if necessary). Brown the shanks on all sides, about 10 minutes. Transfer shanks to a plate. Pour off all but 1 teaspoon drippings from Dutch oven. Add onion and garlic; cook 4 minutes, stirring occasionally. Sprinkle reserved flour mixture over vegetables; cook and stir 1 minute. Add broth, wine, and dried rosemary; bring to a boil, scraping up any browned bits from bottom of Dutch oven. Return lamb shanks to Dutch oven. Cover; braise in oven 45 minutes. Stir in carrots; cover and continue to braise 30 minutes or until lamb is fork tender.

3. Remove from oven, and transfer lamb shanks and carrots to a serving platter. Tent with foil; keep warm. Spoon off and discard fat from pan juices. Boil pan juices in Dutch oven over high heat until thickened, about 3 minutes; stir in beans, and heat through. Spoon bean mixture over shanks and carrots; garnish with rosemary sprigs, if desired.

Per serving: Calories: 551 (38% from fat), Fat 23 g (9 g saturated),

Protein 37 g, Carbohydrate 38 g, Fiber 8 g, Cholesterol 109 mg,

Iron 4 mg, Sodium 462 mg, Calcium 72 mg

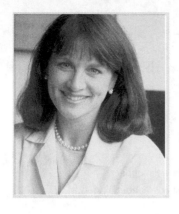

Good Question
about Food and Nutrition

by Nancy Snyderman

Is There a Link Between Wheat and Headaches?

I get a lot of migraine headaches, and I've heard that wheat could be causing them. Should I stop eating it?

I know how eager most headache sufferers are for a cure—especially people who get migraines, three-quarters of whom are women. But the truth is, wheat doesn't cause headaches in otherwise healthy people. It's a problem only for the relative few—about 1 in 200—who suffer from gluten intolerance, known as celiac disease, a condition in which the body cannot process a protein that's found in wheat, rye, and barley.

When a sufferer eats one of these foods, her immune system unleashes an antibody that damages the small intestine, causing diarrhea, cramping, and other stomach distress. (In fact, celiac disease is often misdiagnosed as irritable bowel syndrome or Crohn's disease.) But gluten intolerance can also lead to a confusingly wide array of symptoms, including anemia, skin rashes, and neurological problems. A recent study adds headaches to the list.

If you suspect you have celiac disease, a simple blood test can screen for it. It's hard to self-diagnose, since so many foods contain wheat that it's very difficult to eliminate from your diet. And you don't want to go wheat-free unless you really have to, since whole grain foods that contain gluten are critical to healthy eating.

Assuming you don't have celiac disease, I advise you to keep a daily diary, noting all the facts that could be relevant to headaches. Your diet is key (chocolate, red wine, and some cheeses are classic triggers), but also write down where you were in your menstrual cycle and whether you were particularly tired or stressed when you had a headache. Many people eventually discover some direct links and can take steps to avoid them.

Can You Outgrow a Peanut Allergy?

I've been allergic to peanuts since I was a kid, but I recently heard that you can outgrow the allergy. Is it safe for me to try peanut butter again?

Nowadays, a PB&J is practically a lethal weapon: Many schools are considered "peanut-free zones" because of the growing number of kids with peanut allergies.

If you've been allergic before, **don't eat nuts again without medical supervision**—no matter how much you want a Reese's Cup.

Whether you become less sensitive to peanuts with age, though, is a matter of debate. A recent study offers hope: In it, researchers at Johns Hopkins University gave a group of adults who were allergic to peanuts as children small amounts to sample, with doctors on standby in case any problems occurred. These folks had low levels of a blood marker for peanut allergy (peanut-specific IgE) and had not had a reaction within a year. More than half the adults passed the peanut challenge without a glitch and were pronounced allergy-free.

If I had been allergic to peanuts as a child, though,

I would never risk eating them as an adult, especially without medical supervision. No matter how much you might want a Reese's Peanut Butter Cup, it's not worth it. Your throat could swell, you could get hives, you could even stop breathing. But if you've got a craving and you want to find out whether you can eat peanuts—or any food to which you have been allergic in the past—do it the safest way: Take the "peanut challenge" at a doctor's office. There, if you have a reaction after eating a couple of nuts, you can get a shot of adrenaline quickly. I would not rely solely on a blood test; it's better to trust experience. But trying this at home would be like playing Russian roulette with your health—and your life.

New and Improved Eggs

I've noticed a new brand of eggs at the grocery store that's supposed to contain extra omega-3 fatty acids. Are the new eggs healthier than regular eggs?

Omega-3 fatty acids, typically found in cold-water fish such as salmon, are good for you for a number of reasons: Studies show that they may contribute to heart health, help ease the symptoms of rheumatoid arthritis, and even combat psychiatric disorders such as manic depression. It's natural, then, for food manufacturers to look for ways to boost the omega-3s in their products. Egg producers do that by feeding hens flaxseed or algae (good vegetarian sources of omega-3s). The results look and taste the same as regular eggs, but can contain as much omega-3 fat as a 4-ounce serving of tuna (the amount of omega-3 acid found in eggs varies; check the labels for specific information). Can eating omelettes made from these eggs make a real difference, healthwise?

According to a University of Nebraska study, it can. Researchers fed participants on a low-fat diet a dozen of the omega eggs per week and found that the eggs reduced their triglyceride levels 14 percent compared with people who ate the same number of regular eggs. While I certainly think that is interesting, I probably wouldn't go out of my way to buy these eggs unless I had a pre-existing cholesterol or triglyceride problem. Instead, I'd just eat my salmon—and stick with my regular eggs.

Cholesterol Drugs Hold Promise in Battle Against Alzheimer's

I heard that cholesterol-lowering drugs can prevent Alzheimer's disease. Is that true?

Recently, fascinating evidence surfaced out of a study conducted at Loyola University. Researchers found that patients who used statin drugs (such as Zocor or Lipitor) to lower their cholesterol had a 30 to 40 percent decreased risk of dementia, of which Alzheimer's is the most common form. The study brings up two questions. One, do these statin drugs work in ways that doctors haven't figured out yet, such as changing brain chemistry and stopping Alzheimer's? And, two, could there be a link between heart disease and dementia?

Statin drugs may turn out to be sort of like Rogaine, which was originally intended to help hypertension and then was found to cause hair to grow.

Unfortunately, physicians don't yet know what causes Alzheimer's, and it's often misdiagnosed or under-diagnosed. And they really don't know how to treat it because there's not one perfect drug. But I think this may be one of those cases where a medication intended for one particular medical problem is found to have benefits in other far-reaching areas. Statin drugs may turn out to be sort of like Rogaine, which was originally intended to help hypertension and then was found to cause hair to grow.

I suspect that there's a link with statins and Alzheimer's, although there's still no clear evidence. The possibility of a connection opens the door for new research, and several studies are in the works. So should people start taking these cholesterol-lowering drugs to ward off dementia? I would say the answer is, right now, no.

Nancy Snyderman, M.D., is a medical correspondent for ABC News and author of *Guide to Good Health for Women Over Forty* (Harvest Book, 1996).

the power
of food

Calories are more than pesky numbers that build bulging thighs—they are units of energy. Instead of figuring out how many minutes you need to spend on the treadmill to burn off a Pop Tart binge, consider what those calories could do if used for power. The calories in a piece of cherry cheesecake, for example, could light a 60-watt bulb for an hour and a half. Look below for more on the power of food.

• A bagel with cream cheese (540 calories) would power an electric tooth brush for 52 hours and 20 minutes or give you the energy to brush your teeth for 3 hours and 23 minutes.

• A powerbar (230 calories) would run a 34-horsepower motorcycle going 40 mph for 0.4 miles or give you the energy to cycle 6.25 miles at 10 mph.

• A Big Mac (590 calories) would keep a vacuum cleaner going for 98 minutes or give you the energy to clean your house for 88 minutes.

• One cup of Ben & Jerry's Chubby Hubby (350 calories) would operate a riding mower for 89 seconds or give you the energy to push a power mower for 69 minutes.

• Six handfuls of pretzels (600 calories) would operate a radio for 4 hours or give you the energy to sing for 90 minutes.

chapter 7

stress
management

a woman's guide to energy, confidence, and calm

how to make your
temperament
suit your
LIFE

**If you're chronically anxious and stressed,
the first step to feeling better may be understanding
the disposition you were born with.**

BY JANE MEREDITH ADAMS

JOYCE H. is a pale blonde with a round face who, before moving to Manhattan, was the kind of confident Midwesterner who believed that hard work and talent would see her through.

But a few months after arriving in the city, vowing to make it there so she could make it anywhere, Joyce (whose name has been changed) was a nervous wreck. Plagued by headaches, muscle tension, and constant despair, the young actress asked around for a good psychiatrist. Then, dragging herself up Park Avenue, she settled into the office of Alexander Thomas and pleaded for help.

Thomas, a genial man now in his late 80s, ran through the list of questions any psychiatrist would ask a patient suffering from anxiety and depression. Nothing in Joyce's story popped out: no family history of mood disorders; no deep, dark secrets or unresolved traumas. At this point, another therapist might have turned to a Freudian analysis of Joyce's relationship with her parents, discussed breathing exercises and other behavioral techniques to control her stress, or pulled out a prescription pad and ordered up some Valium or antidepressants.

But Thomas isn't just any therapist. Along with his wife and collaborator, psychiatrist Stella Chess, he's a leader in the study of temperament: the behavioral and emotional characteristics we're born with that help shape how we relate to the world. For more than four decades, Thomas and Chess have been teasing out the various traits that make up temperament—such as our innate curiosity, our wariness of strangers, our need for physical activity, even our sensitivity to noise and nasty smells. They've also looked at how these traits interact with our environments: the families we're born into, the schools we attend, the society we inhabit. Since the 1950s, the couple and their followers have helped to revolutionize our understanding of kids and ways to rear them so they are confident and resilient.

Now, in the twilight of their distinguished careers, Thomas and Chess have turned their attention to the largely overlooked role that temperament

> Accepting yourself
> as you really are may be the
> key to mental health.

Choosing a job or creating a family that doesn't match your temperament could lead to depression and anxiety.

plays in the psychology of adults. They have a theory: Some so-called mood disorders, including who knows how many cases of depression and anxiety, have a basis in temperament—or more specifically, in how well our adult temperament meshes with the jobs we choose, the people we encounter, and the families we create. If you're lucky enough to find yourself in a good fit with your environment, Thomas says, then you're probably pretty content. (This assumes, of course, that you don't have some other biological or emotional vulnerability to depression or anxiety.) But if you're stuck in a situation that's a poor temperament fit—if, for example, your natural intensity puts you at odds with your low-key coworkers or insecure mate—you may be unhappy indeed.

A mismatch doesn't necessarily mean you need to quit the job or dump the guy, say Thomas and Chess, authors of *Goodness of Fit: Clinical Applications from Infancy Through Adult Life* (Brunner/Mazel, 1999). In many cases, you can change the situation, or your own response to it, to make a more comfortable fit. At other times simply accepting yourself as you really are may be the key to mental health.

Take Joyce, for example. Her downward spiral began when she got a job on a television sitcom, her first major acting role. She was nervous but confident, and in the second week she improvised, waving her hand and raising her voice in a way she thought her character would. She'd always been praised for putting her personal stamp on a role. But the star of the show, an egotist named Bob, said her changes were stupid and demanded that she stick to the script. When she did, the director blasted her performance as shallow and dull. "It gets worse every week," Joyce told Thomas, referring to her performance and the director's criticism. She was so demoralized she was thinking of giving up on acting, her lifelong

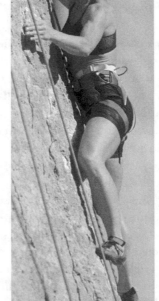

dream. Of course, that possibility made her more depressed.

Yet Joyce's finding a new career didn't strike Thomas as the answer. Her temperament—she approached new situations eagerly and threw herself into them in inventive ways; she was exuberant (although not at the moment) and slightly intense—seemed just right for an actress. The problem was that around Bob, who by nature seemed dour and resistant to change, she was stifled. Thomas had an idea. Before the next show, he suggested, Joyce should practice in private how she'd perform the role if she had her druthers. Then she should forge ahead boldly, not during rehearsal as in the past, but when the cameras were rolling—too late for Bob to stop her. Joyce was aghast.

"I'll be fired," she objected.

If you don't take the chance, you'll end up quitting anyway, Thomas pointed out. And is getting fired from a job that saps the joy from life such a bad thing? Joyce admitted he had a point. She decided to give his plan a shot.

Sure enough, when the taping was finished, Bob exploded. "Fire her!" he demanded. But the director disagreed. "For the first time," he said, "Joyce has given a splendid performance." Ta da!

Here, Chess, who has seen Joyce perform in small yet distinctive roles in Broadway plays and major movies, picks up the story with evident pride. "She became the kind of actress who could always be counted on to make the character interesting."

And she didn't have to pop a single pill to do it. Could Thomas and Chess really be onto something with their "goodness of fit" theory?

Ms. Adventurer

Seeks out new experiences.
Adapts well to change.
Loves to be stimulated.
Hates schedules.
Has energy to burn.

People are born sensitive, but they are not born insecure. They become insecure as a result of experience and environment.

The idea that temperament is important isn't brand-new, at least not as far as babies and pets are concerned. No one asks a Labrador, for example, to herd like a sheepdog or yap like a Chihuahua. Similarly, parents have always observed that their children have very different dispositions from the moment of birth. One baby greets the world calmly and snuggles at her mother's breast; her brother screams like a banshee and thrashes as if he'd really rather go back where he came from.

Indeed, Chess and Thomas are responsible for much of what we know about babies' innate dispositions. In the mid-1950s, they embarked on a landmark study, hoping to solve two of the mysteries of child development: What makes some babies born to the same parents so strikingly dissimilar? Why do some easygoing mothers have "difficult" children, and vice versa?

After observing babies from three months to one year of age, Chess, Thomas, and their colleagues concluded that human temperament breaks down into nine basic traits. The first to emerge, at birth or soon after, are a baby's level of sensitivity to changes in light, sound, taste, and texture, and the intensity of her emotional responses (does she shriek with displeasure or fuss more quietly?). As she gets older, more traits become apparent: the regularity of her bodily functions like eating and sleeping; her ability to adapt to changes in routine; and her level of curiosity or wariness when faced with the unfamiliar. Eventually, as she starts to explore the world, the remaining blanks in her temperament fill in: How energetic and physically active is she? How long is her attention span compared with the average baby's? How easily is she frustrated? And what is her overall mood—sunny and smiley or sad and prone to tears?

Some traits tend to cluster, researchers noted: energy level and emotional intensity, regularity and adaptability, sensitivity and wariness. Some combinations make up classic "types." For example, the "difficult" or "inhibited" child is sensitive, easily overwhelmed, and cautious of strangers; she dislikes changes in routine and reacts intensely by screaming and wailing. The "easy" or "uninhibited" child is at the opposite extreme.

What accounts for differences in temperament? Genetics and biology both play definite roles. Scientists at the University of Minnesota found that identical twins tend to be alike in disposition, whether raised together or apart.

Bolstering this idea, Jerome Kagan, a professor of psychology at Harvard, has done studies showing that certain types of behavior seem to be hardwired. Inhibited babies, those who kick and cry when faced with a new toy or person, have significantly higher brain levels of norepinephrine, a chemical released during arousal, as well as high levels of cortisol, the hormone associated with wariness. Other scientists have found that babies showing greater activity in the left region of their frontal cortex, the part of the brain associated with expressing and controlling emotions, tend to be cheerful and outgoing. Those with more brain wave activity in the right section are more likely to cry when separated from their mothers.

Ms. Sunshine

Needs peace and quiet.
Feels everything deeply.
Is wary of strangers.
Appreciates nuance in language, music, and mood.

Yet another piece of the puzzle may be how efficiently the brain processes dopamine and serotonin, chemical messengers that influence the ability to feel pleasure and pain. Israeli researchers recently reported that infants with a long form of the dopamine receptor gene known as D4DR were more likely to show signs of curiosity and boldness.

In adults, of course, low levels of these substances are associated with anxiety and depression. Does this mean the die is cast at birth? Will the fussy, fearful infant inevitably grow into a cranky, jittery adult?

Not necessarily. This is where Chess and Thomas's "goodness of fit" research comes in. After identifying the basic temperament traits, the psychiatrists began looking at how well the dispositions of the children they were studying seemed to mesh with those of their parents.

The results were astounding. Consistently, they found that well-adjusted children had a good fit with their family environments and troubled children had a poor fit. If, for example, a sensitive, fussy kid had parents who ridiculed her need for quiet and routine, she was more likely to grow up anxious, insecure, depressed, and shy. But if her parents valued sensitivity and learned how to handle her—say, by giving her lots of time to warm up to new people—there was no problem. She learned to manage her fearfulness and grew up happy and secure.

Chess and Thomas didn't stop there. Over the next 40 years, they did several follow-ups with the children in their 1956 New York Longitudinal Study. Subjects who fit well with their parents from the start continued to thrive as long as their home and school environments remained warm and nurturing. Those in a continuously poor fit tended to have all kinds of problems into adulthood.

But the researchers also discovered that a poor-fit subject who suddenly found himself in a more encouraging environment frequently began to flourish. And a good-fit subject, forced into the wrong school or work setting, tended—like Joyce H., the actress—to become anxious and insecure.

Obvious? Maybe to enlightened professionals like career counselors, who depend on the Myers-Briggs test and other temperament tools to match clients to suitable work. But not, apparently, to psychologists used to thinking of adult mood disorders in terms of Oedipal complexes and chemical imbalances. "A lot of psychotherapy has no awareness of the temperament issue," Thomas says.

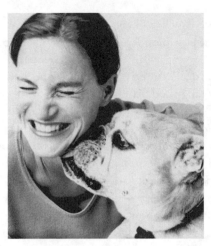

Ms. Too-Easygoing for-Her-Own-Good

Happy just hanging out.
Loves a distraction.
Slow to get riled.
Low-maintenance
to a fault.

One big reason: Adult temperament is more elusive than the kid variety. Most adults are in the normal range of most characteristics, so their temperament is hardly visible, says Sean McDevitt, a psychologist at Arizona Behavioral Health Specialists in Phoenix. "It's the people who are either very, very easygoing or very, very difficult who tend to be noticeable."

Temperament is also more complicated in adults than it is in children. As we grow up, we interact with the people and the events around us. We learn to curb our natural tendencies or gravitate toward situations that suit us, and we lose touch with our underlying temperament traits. What's more, depending on whether we find ourselves in a good or poor fit, innate disposition may express itself in different personality traits. For example, someone who craves regularity, has trouble adjusting to changes in routine, and gets a little nervous around anything new might, in the right circumstances, be superorganized and efficient. In the wrong situation, she might be bossy and demanding. Or anxious and insecure.

Insecurity is an example of a personality trait that we frequently assume is innate but that really results from a poor fit. "People are born sensitive, but they are not born insecure," says Joseph Nowinski, a psychologist at the University of Connecticut Health Center and author of *The Tender Heart: Conquering Your Insecurity* (Fireside, 2001). "They become insecure as a result of experience and environment." This is good news, Nowinski believes. "It means there is much that can be done to heal the insecurity in ourselves."

Similarly, a person may be born sensitive and wary, but not shy, says Elaine N. Aron, who most recently

Many intense people are also high-energy and need regular exercise. Go to the gym and take your anger out on the StairMaster.

wrote *The Highly Sensitive Person in Love* (Broadway Books, 2001). "Shyness develops as one possible adaptation to some of life's situations."

Sensitivity is starting to receive a good deal of attention, in part because of its association with mood disorders and the drugs that treat them. But sensitive types aren't the only ones who feel anxious and insecure when the fit is poor. In their book, Thomas and Chess discuss numerous cases in which a patient's depression or stress vanished once she learned to work with her temperament instead of against it. The key, says Thomas, is to "reach a point of self-awareness" about your innate disposition and needs and to go from there. But where do you start?

Test Yourself

Begin by taking our quiz below, which is similar to the one developed by Chess and Thomas. Other tools include the Myers–Briggs test, the Keirsey Temperament Sorter (found in *Please Understand Me II: Temperament, Character, Intelligence,* by David Keirsey, Prometheus Nemesis Books, 1998), and questionnaires in Aron's and Nowinski's books. On the Internet, see the Big Five Personality Test at www.outofservice.com.

Talk to Other People

Temperament tests are fairly subjective. Get a more complete picture of your disposition by asking your parents, siblings, and friends. You can also gain

what's your type?

ON A SCALE OF 1 TO 6, how do you rate yourself in the following areas compared with others? Traits in which you score either 1 or 6 are the ones most likely to put you at odds with your job or other people.

Activity/Energy Level: Do you fidget and talk really fast? Bounce between a million projects a day? Or do you saunter through errands instead of running them and consider the remote control a form of exercise equipment?
1= a live wire   6= a couch potato

Rhythmicity: Are you the punctual, plan-ahead, highly scheduled type? Or do you keep irregular hours, revel in spontaneity, and hate anything that makes you feel hemmed in?
1= proud to be predictable   6= devil-may-care

Adaptability: Do you find it hard to get revved up in the morning? Become irritated at a sudden change in plans? Or can you go from one thing to another with no discernible downtime?
1= flexible as a noodle   6= stiff as a board

Sensitivity: How quickly do you note changes in noise, temperature, texture, light, language, and other stimuli? How easily are you influenced by other people's moods?
1= utterly oblivious   6= Princess and the Pea

Novelty Seeking: Do you seek out the latest fashions, movies, and music? Or do you shy away from anything new—ideas, people, places, even the daily specials at your favorite restaurant?
1= shock it to me   6= I know what I like

Distractibility: Are you able to tune out noise, problems, other people? Or are you constantly diverted by conversation in the next cubicle or the scene as you walk down the street?
1= always engrossed   6= easily sidetracked

Emotional Intensity: Do you guffaw instead of giggle, make passionate proclamations, fly into rages, and cry over the silliest things? Or are you low-key, soft-spoken, and hard to read?
1= meek and mild   6= living large

Frustration Tolerance: Do you lose patience easily? Tend to give up without a fight? Or do you stick out bad situations long after others bail and refuse to give in?
1= practically Sisyphus   6= quick to move on

Mood: Are you cheerful most of the time, or do little setbacks get you down? Are you an optimist or a pessimist?
1= a ray of sunshine   6= not a happy camper

You're attracted to someone because he's so different from you—now those differences are driving you crazy. Many of these battles trace back to profound differences in disposition.

important clues by looking at photos of yourself as a child or watching home movies, Nowinski says. James Cameron, a temperament expert and executive director of the Preventive Ounce, a nonprofit mental health foundation in Oakland, California, suggests asking your mate or a close friend to assess you, using the same tests you take, then comparing the results.

Take a Hard Look at Your Life

The next step is to examine how your general temperament affects the way you live your life. The best place to start is with a situation where something clearly isn't working, Cameron says. Let's say you're a high-energy, extremely focused, and persistent person who has trouble shifting gears and adapting to change. Now choose a problem: Your new dream job as a manager isn't working out very well, and your mate is unhappy with you, too.

Next, try to analyze how your traits play out in this situation. Some possibilities: You are so focused that you tune out your staff, hurting people's feelings. Your persistence and low adaptability mean that you have a hard time letting go of projects. Your tendency to keep your nose to the grindstone robs you of the simple pleasures of a job well done.

Now look at your troubles on the home front. Perhaps your focus on your job means that you ignore your family. Perhaps you have difficulty switching from work to play, so you unconsciously build in transition time for yourself—dawdling at the train station or arriving home grumpy so everyone leaves you alone. Maybe your persistence means that in

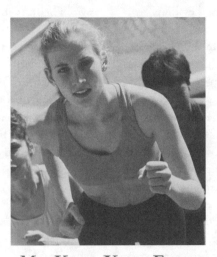

Ms. Keep-Your-Eyes-on-the-Finish-Line

Craves physical activity. Has an intense desire to win. Never loses focus. Persists to the bitter end.

arguments you always want the last word.

Try applying this approach to a number of scenarios. Talking with family and friends and writing in a journal can also help. "The goal," says McDevitt, "is to understand patterns in your life. Then you can do something about them."

Step Outside Yourself

"When you're in a mismatch situation, your temperament will rule you," Cameron says. "You have to learn to manage it. Then you can gain control."

One effective strategy is to practice self-awareness, not just in retrospect, but in the heat of the moment. Say your secretary has missed another deadline, and you're ready to fire her. "Get out of the situation for 10 minutes," Nowinski says. "Go to the bathroom or get a cup of coffee." Or go to the gym and take your anger out on the StairMaster; many intense people are also high-energy and need regular exercise, Cameron says. Remind yourself: "I'm intense, I'm easily frustrated, so I get angry easily."

Shy or insecure types also benefit greatly from learning to step back, Nowinski says. But even an easygoing person might find it useful to develop this skill. Let's say you work in an office with a bunch of prima donnas. You pride yourself on getting along with everyone, but the result is that you tolerate their tirades and take on tasks they disdain. The next time this happens, instead of letting the situation pass unremarked (or letting it stress you out), grab your coat, go for a walk, and think about how you can assert yourself.

Make Concrete Changes

Some bad-fit situations do require that you make real changes in your life. If, for instance, too much hubbub drives you batty, wear earplugs at work, buy a silent dishwasher, ask for a quiet table in the restaurant, and avoid launching a heart-to-heart conversation in a noisy room. Go outdoors instead—nature soothes many temperaments.

Carie Graves, 47, an Olympic gold medal winner in rowing and head rowing coach at the University of Texas at Austin, used to get burned out during the evening, throwing herself into household chores with the same intensity that she puts into her job. "I've learned about setting limits for myself," she says. Now she helps her son with his homework or chats with a friend. She's also stopped dating intensely competitive guys, who make her feel anxious. "Now I tend to be with men who are very nice, loving, and mellow, thank goodness," she says.

Sometimes feeling better requires making tough trade-offs. Margaret Butler of Oskaloosa, Iowa, wound up with a stress-related hernia after her first year as an Episcopal priest. She had been pushing herself hard, ignoring her sensitive nature. "I need lots of renewal time and solitude," she says. So now Butler, 60, builds plenty of downtime into her schedule. "Sometimes I settle for less-than-perfect work. I know if I stayed up another hour I could make the sermon better, but that will color the whole next day with fatigue and irritability."

Remember That Other People Have Temperaments, Too

It's an old story: You're attracted to someone because he's so different from you—bold where you're hesitant, flexible where you're rigid. Now those very differences drive both of you crazy. You blame each other for refusing to change, but the problem may be innate and manageable rather than intentional and destined to irritate you both forever.

Nearly 70 percent of all conflicts between couples—happy ones as well as those destined to split—are unresolvable, Aron notes. She guesses that many of these battles trace back to profound differences in disposition. "Couples in better relationships understand the perpetual problems differently," she says. "They talk about them rather than fighting over them and blaming each other for refusing to change."

How do you get to that point? Begin by suggesting that your mate (or best friend or mom) take a temperament test. Then start a dialogue about what you discover about yourselves—the similarities as well as the differences. Discuss how temperament may contribute to a specific, long-running conflict—say, his tendency to be distant when he comes home from work. Maybe the solution is as simple as realizing you shouldn't take his remoteness personally. Or maybe he'll realize that by taking public transportation, he can have the transition time he needs without making you upset.

But don't feel you must blindly accept a loved one's bad behavior any more than you should expect him to tolerate yours. "Because you know what your temperament is doesn't mean you have license to be that way," Cameron says. "You have to take responsibility for yourself."

It also helps to cultivate a sense of humor. Jane Ericson, a 35-year-old English teacher in suburban Los Angeles, used to feel ashamed of her tendency to be easily hurt by other people's comments. Reading books about sensitive people broke the spell. Once, after she bought her parents an expensive gift certificate, her mother remarked, "Why did you spend that kind of money?"

"I said, 'Can you just say thank you?' " Ericson says. "Before, everything hurt my feelings. Now I can make a joke of it." ✳

Jane Meredith Adams lives in San Francisco.

The key is to reach a point of
self-awareness about your innate disposition and
needs and to go from there.

THE BEST WAY TO STOP WORRYING

CHRONIC FRETTING IS A BAD HABIT that can literally make you sick. But there's an upside: World-class worriers can be great goal setters, says Lucinda Bassett, author of *Life Without Limits* (Harper-Collins, 2001). *Health* asked Bassett how a fretter can turn stressful thinking into an advantage.

Q: What type of worry are we talking about?
A: The kind that robs us of happiness, drains our energy, and creates depression or anxiety.

Q: Is it tough to stop cold turkey?
A: You bet. It takes time to change any bad habit. Try scheduling a "planned worry time" each day for, say, 15 minutes. Set aside until then the concerns that bombard you all day. Then, ask yourself, "Do I need more information, should I take action, or is this fear irrational?"

Q: Can I dwell on my problems then?
A: No! This is a time for constructive thinking, what I call "worry reversal." You use all that energy reserved for worrying to accomplish wonderful things. I've found it takes the same skills to succeed as it does to worry: anticipation, creativity, analytical ability, and imagination.

Q: If I think something bad will happen, what can I do?
A: Say you're anxious about a presentation. Instead of imagining failure, visualize your boss complimenting you on a job well done. This positive anticipation can be exhilarating.

Q: What if I start overanalyzing?
A: It's easy to fall into the trap of asking yourself "Why is this happening to me?" or "Why did he say that?" But train yourself to use this thinking to pursue what you want. When you analyze your goal, think of all the ways you can make it work. Get a pencil and write down 10 different ways you could make your goals come true.

Q: Are you a big worrier?
A: Not anymore. Chronic fear and a severe anxiety disorder plagued me for years. But when I began to focus on what I wanted instead of what I was afraid of, it really changed my life.

....

using the herb
Saint-John's-wort
to heal depression

Want to use herbs to manage your state of mind? Psychiatrists at King-Drew Medical Center in Los Angeles, California, recently reviewed a decade's worth of research on herbs in psychiatric treatment. Studies that pitted Saint-John's-wort against conventional antidepressants suggest it works as well as prescription drugs to combat mild to moderate depression. And 39 out of 40 trials of ginkgo found it helps ease dementia in elderly patients. But experts say brands vary wildly in potency, and the pills can have side effects. So check with a doctor before taking herbs.

How to Complain Effectively

Psychologist Robin Kowalski's study on pet peeves turned up some good news: Complaining can be healthy if done sparingly. Those who gripe selectively get more psychological satisfaction and, not surprisingly, are less likely to alienate friends and coworkers when compared with continual whiners.

More discriminating complainers also tend to target the people who can address their problems, says Kowalski.

Want to take charge of your life? Stop worrying so much?
Sleep soundly and exercise more? Grab a pen and let yourself go.

from anxiety to overweight

How keeping a journal can help solve any problem

BY ELIZABETH BERG

'VE KEPT MANY TYPES OF JOURNALS in my life. The first, a white leatherette diary, was surely designed with a 12-year-old like me in mind: It came with that most alluring of things, a gold key. I lost the key almost immediately and was forced to cut open the latch, then use tape to keep it closed. I backed up this dubious form of security with a stern and unoriginal warning, written boldly across the front cover: KEEP OUT!!!!!!!!!! The exclamation points ended with little circles, yet the gravity of their message must have been clear; I never saw any evidence of a break-in.

But then, why would I? A typical entry would first and foremost record what our family had eaten for dinner. Next might be an analysis of some aspect of my love life. I was very much interested in boys, though at times my fascination was mixed with a delicate nausea. *Todd L. put his* tongue *in Mary Lou's mouth!!!!!!* I chronicled injustices of various teachers, the death of a grandparent, the time I fell into a river and almost drowned.

In high school, I abandoned the write-this-much-every-day diary format for the comparative freedom of lined paper, saving the pages in a black plastic notebook. I am embarrassed by these pages now and have thought more than once about burying them in my backyard. (Seriously. I have the spot all picked out.) I could not stop raging about hypocrisy and all the wrongs done to me, real or imagined. I took issue with people's obsession with the way they looked, even while I agonized over my split ends and lusted after a pair of Weejuns. I longed mightily for a great love and pretended I found it over and over again. *"Oh, Randy,"* one entry begins. *"Oh, Frank,"* goes another. And yet another, I'm afraid, *"Oh, Jim, Jim, Jim!"* I was oblivious to the Vietnam War as well as the bolstering beauty of nature and art. My focus was unrelentingly narrow and narcissistic.

Yet however superficial my first explorations of self, they were also enormously helpful. I was a sensitive girl who took everything much too seriously, and I spent much of my adolescence cocooned in misery.

I saw my journal as a kind of aproned lap I could crawl into, a place where I could speak and not be judged.

I remember sitting alone on the bus after school, hunched over my books and staring straight ahead, my insides aching. I couldn't wait to get home and write myself out of pain. When I settled behind my closed bedroom door, a blank page before me, I felt a rare inner warmth, a wash of comfort that started at the top of my head and slowly worked its way down. I saw my journal as a kind of aproned lap I could crawl into, a place where I could speak and not be judged, even (perhaps especially) by myself. Finally, I could say all that I needed to.

When I had children, I necessarily focused on someone besides myself, and my journal (now a grown-up, black-bound specimen) reflects this new maturity. I wrote about Julie asleep as a newborn, her hands curled into fists so small they made my heart skip. I wrote about Jenny, my second born, dressing herself in a pink tutu and striped T-shirt to go outside and stir mud with her boyfriend—"We're making soup," she said. One winter morning I sat curled up in a chair in the living room and wept while I wrote that I loved staying home with my daughters, but I needed more in my life. Later, I described the rewards and hardships of my work as a nurse; later still, I confided that what I really wanted was to be a writer, to see my words on a printed page—just once.

putting pen to paper

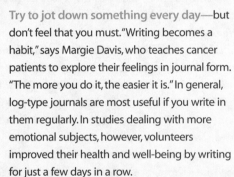

getting ready

Pick a place that's comfortable and private. Many writers find (and it's borne out by the research) that a new setting, free of the usual distractions, can be stimulating—and liberating.

Choose whatever format you find convenient and inspiring: Maybe a pretty diary and special pen, an innocent-looking steno book, or a computer you can secure with a password.

Set a time limit. In most studies, volunteers got enormous benefit from scribbling for a mere 15 or 20 minutes. If you're really busy, 5 or 10 minutes will do just fine.

Try to jot down something every day—but don't feel that you must. "Writing becomes a habit," says Margie Davis, who teaches cancer patients to explore their feelings in journal form. "The more you do it, the easier it is." In general, log-type journals are most useful if you write in them regularly. In studies dealing with more emotional subjects, however, volunteers improved their health and well-being by writing for just a few days in a row.

Get help if you feel emotionally overwhelmed.

Reward yourself when you're done.

sitting down to write

Misspell that word. Dangle that participle. No one, especially your high school English teacher, ever needs to know.

Go deep. Researchers have found that people who delve into important experiences become mentally and physically healthier than people who write about trivial things. Of course, pleasant events are significant, too. The key is to discuss how they make you feel.

Explore the positive along with the negative. Researchers have found that people who do nothing but vent in their journals get no more benefit from the writing process than people who stick to the superficial and mundane.

Safeguard your privacy. If you're worried about a sensitive entry, write it on a separate piece of paper and seal it in an envelope—or even burn it, as one researcher suggests.

staying inspired

When a blank page just stares back at you, try these thought-provoking ideas from *The Way of the Journal* (Sidran Press, 1998), by psychotherapist Kathleen Adams, director of the Center for Journal Therapy in Lakewood, Colorado:

Answer the question "How am I feeling right now?"

Create your ultimate to-do list, one that helps you chart your path through life. Use one or more of these questions as a springboard: Who am I? Why am I here? What do I want?

Make a list of the major emotional turning points in your life. Pick one or two to write about, now or later.

Finish the sentence "I want to explore…."

Write a letter to someone you care about who is no longer in your life. (You don't have to send it.)

Then, when I was 35, I was diagnosed with an incurable lymphoma. First, I turned to my family and friends for comfort. Then I turned to my journal. That is to say, I turned to myself. There are certain kinds of work no one can do for you. And coming to terms with cancer is one of them.

It was in the pages of my journal that I could open up most fully to my fears. *S. says that when he was diagnosed with cancer, the writing in his journal got smaller. I see that mine is getting so, too. I think it has to do with not wanting to use things up. A need to preserve. Translated: A desire to keep living. A hope that if you keep things small, you will keep them longer. But my dreams betray me. Last night I dreamed a doctor told me all would be well so long as she didn't find a mole in a certain place. But she did find one there.*

I wrote about needing to understand that everything is one thing. I planned my funeral. I wrote: *I think in the end, in anyone's end, it'll be the small things that we loved the most. The image of things that mean home and comfort and safety, the cooling pies, the winter boots lined up, the click of the doors locked against the blackness of night. We strive for big things, only to find that what feels best is returning to things that don't try so hard, but simply are.*

It occurs to me now that this sentiment went on to become a theme, or at least a subtheme, in every novel I've written. So an integral part of my work as a fiction writer was born in the pages of my journal.

In the way that one can get used to anything, I got used to having cancer. *Inside the oven, the aroma of gingerbread competes with the bar-b-que sauce smell of the chicken,* I wrote six months after I was diagnosed. *I'll go down to the basement, soon, and fold some laundry. I worked on an article about cancer for a magazine this morning. It's so matter-of-factly in my life now. Another thing about me, like the gray in my hair or my hazel eyes. When I write about it now, it doesn't seize me up, make some inside part of myself grow cold and still. It is no more complex than life, death. The pondering of it now is, for the most part, no more bothersome than those middle-of-the-night reckonings I used to have—those chilling taps on the shoulder that said, "Listen. Everything changes. Everyone dies. You, too." The smell of gingerbread has assumed its*

a journal for what ails you

Women are writers by nature, it seems. We scribble on everything, all the time. E-mails, to-do lists, memos on yellow Post-Its, bills—let's face it, the world as we know it would fall apart without our keyboards, our No. 2 pencils, our trusty Bics.

Why, then, don't more of us keep journals? Lack of time, perhaps. Fear that our scariest secrets will be found out. The ghost of Anne Frank looking askance at our ungainly sentences and trivial plights.

But, in truth, a journal can be nothing more complicated than a pocket-sized notebook in which you record what you eat, when you exercise, or all the little things that drive you crazy. It can be a collection of glorified lists: counted blessings or heartfelt goals.

Research shows that journals make us feel better—mentally and physically. Insomniacs, the panic-prone and depressed, cancer patients, people trying to lose weight—all have been shown to benefit. Students who wrote about painful events for just 20 minutes, four days in a row, boosted their immune function and reduced the number of times they visited a doctor. Asthma and arthritis sufferers who described an intense experience were more likely than other patients to see their symptoms ease. James W. Pennebaker, the University of Texas psychologist who led many of the studies, believes that repressing difficult emotions creates stress. Writing about them defuses their power to harm—and, suggests Joshua Smyth, a researcher at North Dakota State University, helps us learn to cope better in the future.

That said, different types of journals can have different benefits. The following techniques are especially useful, experts say.

• a story book •

When it's helpful
If you're depressed, struggling with a sudden crisis or unresolved tragedy, or living with a chronic ailment.

What it involves
The idea here is to put experiences in context with a beginning, a middle, and an ending, much as you would tell a story. Say a car crash has left you in constant pain. Try writing about the

accident from the moment you woke that morning: how you were feeling, where you were going, what caused the wreck, the ambulance, and so on. Any difficult event—a divorce, a cancer diagnosis, a loved one's death—can be turned into story form. Some therapists advise writing about the same episode several times; the retelling often gives new perspective. Even if a health problem isn't obviously related to a particular event, research suggests you might benefit from writing about a trauma in this way.

Why it works
Pennebaker believes that humans rely on narratives to make sense of our experiences. Once we understand them, they become less stressful. Learning to cast events in a new, more optimistic light—known as reframing—has also been shown to reduce depression.

• a worry book •

When it's helpful
If you suffer from anxiety, stress, insomnia, or related complaints.

What it involves
Draw a line down the center of a page. On the left side, briefly discuss some of the issues that are upsetting you: unpaid bills, an argument with your teenager. On the right, describe steps you've taken to address the problem or solutions you can try. You can also prevent worrying by using this space to plan, organize, and strategize for the future.

Why it works
Agonizing on the page defuses stress and gives you a sense of control over your problems so they're less apt to take over your life—or rob you of sleep. For best results, write a little every day, ideally several hours before bedding down.

• a log book •

When it's helpful
If you want to lose weight, get morefit, spend less money, understand your body's rhythms, or chart your recovery from illness.

What it involves
Simply record relevant information—how many calories you eat at every meal, how far you walk, how you feel after taking a certain pill—in a small notebook. Try to do it every day.

Why it works
Jotting down the minutiae of our lives helps keep us mindful and motivates us to make healthful changes. It also allows us to detect patterns, such as how our sleep and menstrual cycles mesh.

• a memory book •

When it's helpful
If you're becoming absentminded, recovering from a head injury, or have a learning disability or bipolar disorder.

What it involves
This technique, devised by memory researchers at Beth Israel Deaconess Medical Center in Boston, is like your trusty day planner on steroids. Find a good-sized notebook that's still small enough to tote everywhere. Fill it with the usual to-do lists for the day, week, and month; phone numbers; addresses; birthdays; but also medical information, directions, random musings—you name it—organized by tab. Write down hard-to-remember details at least once a day and check the notebook frequently.

Why it works
Researchers have found that this superorganizing strategy improves recall by enhancing a sense of control and reducing stress. What's more, repetition—in this case, scribbling details more than once—has been shown to sharpen the wits.

• a gratitude book •

When it's helpful
If you're inclined to be pessimistic, depressed, stressed-out, or anxious, or if you're in the throes of a major crisis.

What it involves
Popularized by Sarah Ban Breathnach of *Simple Abundance* (Warner Books, 1995) fame, this type of journal simply entails listing a few things every day for which you are thankful.

Why it works
Training yourself to think positively is one of the best ways to improve your emotional health, psychologists say.

• a scrapbook •

When it's helpful
If you have trouble putting feelings into words.

What it involves
The goal is to supplement other journal-writing techniques by including magazine clippings, snapshots, sketches, and cherished mementos that add layers of nuance and meaning to your prose. For example, if you're battling a poor body image, you might attach photos of women who strike you as strong and sexy—and who look something like you.

Why it works
Researchers haven't studied the benefits of scrapbooks per se. But anything that helps you express deep emotion is worth a try.

rightful place in the scheme of things.

I am 51 now, in good health, treating the occasional flare-up successfully. For me, recovery means not that the disease is cured but that it is controlled. The bulldog grip was long ago loosened, and I can breathe freely, be at home inside myself.

It is tempting to say that the most important function my journal ever served was to help me through that difficult period of my life. But that's not true. What's most important about a journal is its ongoingness. A journal is there for everything, from the recording of anguish over split ends to the contemplation of mortality. It is the place to be congruent with your soul because it keeps you in the habit of telling the truth, whatever that truth may be at the moment. A journal chronicles your growth. It teaches you that things change—not only outside you, but inside you. It gives you perspective, and in so doing, it gives you hope. It is a kind of true camera, offering views of yourself that cannot be seen in any other way.

Sometimes, when you reread journal entries, you cherish them. Sometimes you pray no one will ever see them. Sometimes you are acutely embarrassed by their inanity, by their immaturity. But none of that matters. The simple act of recording your life helps you celebrate, conspicuously, consciously, your presence here. ✳

Elizabeth Berg has published a number of books, including Escaping into the Open: The Art of Writing True

HOW TO OVERCOME FEELINGS OF INSECURITY

The term gets thrown around a lot, but few of us know how deeply insecurity affects people and their relationships, says psychologist Joseph Nowinski, author of *The Tender Heart: Conquering Your Insecurity* (Fireside, 2001). *Health* spoke to Nowinski to learn how sensitive souls can find some much-needed confidence.

Q: What is insecurity?
A: Well, it's not a flaw or a mental illness. It's a personality trait that reflects both the temperament a person is born with and life experiences. Unfortunately, people with sensitive natures are far more likely to become insecure. And insecurity ends up making those who fall prey to it approach life defensively.

Q: So are thin-skinned folks doomed?
A: Not at all. People can shake the nagging self-doubt and lack of confidence that breeds insecurity.

Q: Isn't that an awfully tall order?
A: Yes. But if they start by examining their expectations, they'll soon find that many are unrealistic. Then they can work on changing them.

Q: How exactly do you do that?
A: Say you're constantly looking for approval. If you struggle with insecurity, then this impossible expectation is always there. Even in the best relationships—with your lover, family, or coworkers—your actions won't always be applauded. Every day you may have to take an inventory of what's reasonable to expect from people.

Q: It sounds like insecure people demand a lot from the folks in their lives.
A: Often they do. And they're hypercritical of themselves. More secure people can keep criticism in perspective. But to an insecure person, any censure can be devastating. If you learn to hear out someone else's complaint—without getting defensive, retaliating, or fleeing—you'll likely be facing some tough emotions. But I promise you'll feel better in the long run.

Q: Again, how do you do that?
A: Remember these three words: Listen, learn, and compromise. Find out exactly what the other person expects of you. Is it reasonable? Be sure to resist the urge to view a disagreement as a win-lose proposition. Good relationships don't have a winner and a loser.

Why Overeating When You're Stressed is Bad for Your Heart

We all know that mental strain can spell weight gain–just think of how many times you've reached for a pint of Häagen-Dazs when life got a little too hard. Now a study suggests that overeating triggered by stress sends extra pounds straight to your belly—with potentially damaging consequences for your heart.

Researchers at Yale University assembled 59 premenopausal women with varying shapes; some were "apples," with more fat around their waists, while others were "pears," carrying more weight in their hips. They then put the women through nerve-racking tests, such as subtracting large prime numbers and convincing a mock committee that each was the best applicant for a job. They also measured the women's levels of the stress hormone cortisol. It turns out the apple-shaped women secreted more cortisol, did worse on the tests, and reported more day-to-day stress than did the pears.

Study leader Elissa Epel, a psychologist now at the University of California at San Francisco, believes there is a direct relationship between the way these women respond to pressure and their apple shapes. So-called visceral fat is located deep within the torso, packed around the organs; the surfaces of its cells have more receptors for cortisol than do other kinds of fat. When cortisol meets these cells, it can activate an enzyme that causes them to get bigger.

This isn't just a problem when it comes to buying pants. Plumped-up visceral fat cells are more likely to release fat into the bloodstream, where it can clog arteries, hike up triglycerides, and raise bad cholesterol.

To lessen your chances of a dangerous bulge, Epel suggests meditation, exercise, and plenty of sleep. "You can't prevent stressful events," she says. "But you can control how you cope with them."

What's our top psychological need?
Not money or power.
The most important factor for happiness is SELF-ESTEEM.

Q+A
how to keep from crying when you're really angry

Every time I try to express anger, I start to cry. How can I stop this?

You're not alone, that's for sure. We've often found ourselves with a lump in the throat, choking back tears when we're feeling really angry and upset. Experts say that for some women, the problem is a reluctance to feel the full weight of their fury. Almost as soon as their anger flares up, they subconsciously transform it into an emotion that they find easier to cope with—like sadness, say, or hopelessness—and start to cry.

If you think this might be your trouble, try talking with a friend soon after your next emotional episode. Reconstruct how you were feeling and how you expressed yourself. If your friend is game, you might try some role-playing in which you practice telling the object of your ire exactly how you feel—without tearing up. This ought to help you express your anger more directly the next time your blood starts to boil.

Some people's experience is a bit different; most things that make them angry tend to make them feel frustrated and hurt. It's when they try to articulate this combustible mix of emotions that they start to cry.

Here's a solution that really works: Pause for a moment to take a deep breath. This seems to shut down the tear ducts so that you can let your anger out—calmly.

yoga

the best restorative for body and spirit

If you love the way an hour of yoga makes you feel, just think what a week of it could do. Think of it as a ticket to paradise.

BY EVELYN SPENCE

Kathie Lieberman's trip to paradise came about almost by accident. Early last winter, she desperately needed an escape from her day-to-day routine. Lieberman, who's 47, was juggling the usual midlife lineup of children, parents, partner, and work.

In her case, though, the mix is a little out of the ordinary: The children in her life aren't just her own two teenagers, but also the 700 kids who attend the private school and camp that she directs in Brookville, New York. Those kids, of course, all have parents, who aren't shy about voicing their requests. Lieberman's own parents, who founded the school, are her coworkers—as are her brother and sister. A few months ago, tensions were running high among the family members about how to shift responsibilities from one generation to the next. Every day seemed to bring more demands than Lieberman could handle.

"I woke up one morning and thought, 'If I don't get out of here, I'm going to make myself sick,' " she says.

So she bought a plane ticket, announced her plans to her husband and family, and skipped town. Her destination: Rancho La Puerta, a spa nestled amid the rock-strewn hills of Tecate, Baja California. Lieberman chose the place because of the natural beauty of its location and the pampering that it offers. Little did she know that she was in for even more rejuvenation than she'd expected. By chance, Lieberman arrived when the spa was offering a weeklong yoga retreat.

Yoga, of course, has been booming in the past few years, as more and more people have discovered that stretching and strengthening the body can calm and quiet the mind. Indeed, many devotees swear it's the ultimate stress-buster. Yoga retreats—weekend or weeklong getaways that combine daily yoga classes with beautiful surroundings, healthy food, outdoor activities, and meditation—are the latest twist. And harried women are flocking to sign up.

For many, yoga retreats strike just the right vacation note. "They're a cross between laziness on the beach and go-going in Paris," says Kathryn Arnold, editor-in-chief of *Yoga Journal*. Geographically speaking, the possibilities are endless: From beach bungalows to snow-dusted peaks, a yoga vacation can take you just about anywhere.

It was great not to have to think about anything but yoga. Every day I left a little bit more stress behind.

A few centers run programs year-round, but most retreats take place at resorts or spas under the direction of well-known teachers. Some are spartan, others downright luxurious. And most can accommodate anyone from a complete beginner to a longtime yogi.

At home, Kathie Lieberman was lucky if she could squeeze an hour of exercise into a typical day, and she was rarely able to set aside quiet time for herself. But at Rancho La Puerta, free from her usual distractions, she easily settled into an alternating rhythm of activity and contemplation. Each morning at 6:30 she'd pad across the Mexican tiles of her room and join a sunrise hike. Then came a breakfast of fresh fruit or granola, enough to sustain her through the centerpiece of the morning: an hour and a half of yoga, performed in a room with glorious views of the surrounding hills and gardens.

In the afternoons, she strolled through the spa's gardens, taking in the scents of rosemary and lavender, and joined the daily guided meditations. After dinners featuring fresh fish, pasta, soups, and organic greens grown on-site, she lingered over tea with other retreat-goers, talking quietly; some nights she got a massage. "When I got back to my room, the fire was ready to be lit, and I was wonderfully tired," she says. "I sank into bed every night at 10 o'clock."

Lieberman had done yoga intermittently at home, but at the retreat, it was as if the poses took root in her body. Every day she was able to push herself further. By the end of the week, she could hold the postures longer and felt steadier than she ever had before. "It was great not to have to think about anything but yoga," she says. "Every day I left a little more stress behind."

Like many people who make yoga the focus of their vacations, Lieberman went home with a renewed commitment to keeping stress from getting the best of her. She's been taking yoga classes once or twice weekly and meditating daily.

Her new habits have helped her remain unharried in the eye of her personal hurricane. Not long after her return, for instance, one of the school's buses got into an accident. Even before she learned that no one was hurt, Lieberman was able to remain calm, pausing during the crisis to take deep breaths that kept her feeling centered and in control.

"Honestly, I feel like a changed person," she says. "I had no idea a week of yoga could be so powerful." ✳

Evelyn Spence is a former Health *staff writer.*

your path to paradise

WHETHER YOU'RE a novice or a pro, there's a yoga retreat that's right for you. They're not all as deluxe (or pricey) as those at Rancho La Puerta, which run from $1,700 to $3,000 per week (800-443-7565, www.rancholapuerta.com). The places listed here offer retreats in summer and fall (and in some cases, year-round). They fill fast, so book ahead.

FEATHERED PIPE RANCH
helena, montana
In the heart of the Rockies, this log-and-stone main lodge surrounded by yurts and tepees overlooks a private lake. Retreats feature various styles of yoga, Native American rituals, and hikes. Weekly rates range from $995 to $1,499. 406-442-8196, www.featheredpipe.com.

KRIPALU CENTER FOR YOGA AND HEALTH
lenox, massachusetts
At this center's 300 acres of meadows and hills in the Berkshires, programs emphasize the slow, gentle Kripalu style. Accommodations are basic; rates run from $85 to $256 per night, with a two-night minimum. 800-741-7353, www.kripalu.org.

WHITE LOTUS FOUNDATION RETREAT CENTER
santa barbara, california
This spot atop a steep canyon has stunning views of the ocean; yurts and cabins are within earshot of a creek. Retreats include music, dance, and discussion. Rates are $150 to $200 per night. 805-964-1944, www.whitelotus.org.

KALANI OCEANSIDE RESORT RETREAT
pahoa, hawaii
Deep within a tropical forest, this is the only coastal lodging in Hawaii's largest conservation area. Kalani offers about 30 yoga escapes per year, with hot springs, waterfalls, and black sand beaches nearby. You can camp or stay in luxury tree houses, cottages, or the lodge. Rates are $30 to $240 per night. 800-800-6886, www.kalani.com.

SPIRITUALITY
the ultimate stress-buster

Our complex lives don't just stress us out. They distract us from what's really important. Here's how women today are finding ways to build spiritual meaning into their lives.

BY KARIN EVANS

PHOTOGRAPHY BY DAN CHAVKIN

If there's a spiritual theme in Barbara Maltby's life, that theme is silence. And if there's a challenge, it's to learn to stay present, even in the hardest moments. Maltby can remember a time when she welcomed distance from difficult events. When her mother was terminally ill, for instance. The doctor didn't disclose that the diagnosis was cancer, so no one discussed what was really going on. "My mother was alone with whatever fears she had, and I was extremely grateful at the time that I didn't have to deal with those fears. But that feeling was transformed after her death into terrific guilt," Maltby says. "She was alone, and I felt as if we had abandoned her." Another pivotal moment came when Maltby's beloved dog died. "He had an old soul," she says. "He lost his eyesight, then his hearing, and finally his sense of smell. He couldn't even find his food. At that point I took him to the vet to be put to sleep. I think I was scared to see it. There I was weeping,

stretch your body, focus your mind

Yoga gives me a sense of groundedness. It is a kind of four-legged practice. You put your head and hands and different parts of your body down on the ground, not just your feet, and you connect with the earth in a different way. There's a sense of maintaining well-being, beyond the physical aspects of just trying to look good. It takes you to a state of deep quiet, focusing your awareness and concentration. When you have a sense of well-being, you are hooked into spiritual life. In the practice of yoga, the intention, classically, is to unite the individual soul with the universal soul.
—Nora Burnett, a teacher of Iyengar yoga, sometimes called "meditation in action," in San Francisco, California

weeping, weeping in the hall. But I wasn't in the room. I didn't hold him."

A former film producer who's worked on such movies as *Ordinary People* and *A River Runs Through It,* Maltby, 60, has come to see such moments as part of an ongoing spiritual journey. "You know, you have lessons in life. Mine has been to learn to be present," she says. That quest has taken her from her family's Quaker roots to meditation and Zen Buddhism. After leaving the film industry, she got a master's degree in medical ethics from Loyola University in Chicago. Today she works to improve care for dying patients and volunteers in a hospital hospice unit. "Zen Buddhism has helped me just be there," says Maltby. "If you learn to still the mind, which takes amazing discipline, in that stillness, deeper and deeper presence is possible."

Such yearning for spiritual meaning is echoed in the reflections of many women today, whether it's expressed as a desire to go deeper in life, a search for a

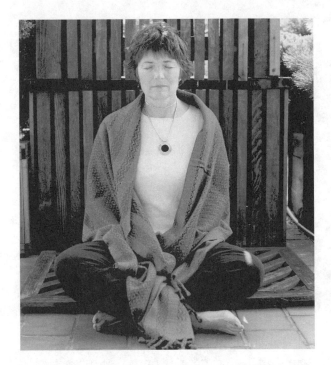

Barbara Maltby:
"You have lessons in life.
Mine has been to learn to be present."

The Art of Happiness (Riverhead Books, 1998). Even the medical establishment is taking note of the role that spirituality may play in keeping people healthy. Studies from Northwestern and Duke Universities have shown that patients with everything from gynecologic cancer to hip fracture have better outcomes if their lives include spiritual practice or beliefs. Other serious studies, examining everything from prayer and healing to religious practice and longevity, are under way.

But what does it mean to be spiritual in the new millennium? Apparently, not going to church or temple every week. Church attendance figures have been the subject of much debate (some surveyors say Americans are apt to exaggerate their habits), but the actual figure may be as low as 26 percent, down from 42 percent in 1965. For the past three decades, churches have faced a crisis of membership and funding. That doesn't mean we aren't believers: 95 percent of Americans say they believe in God; 75 percent believe in miracles.

"We have few atheists in this culture," says Wade Clark Roof, the chairman of Religious Studies at the University of California at Santa Barbara. What people mean by "believing in God," though, tends to change. "People's images of God vary enormously," Roof says. "People have moved toward more user-friendly conceptions of God: less judgmental, more comforting, supportive, nurturing, and perhaps a lot more feminine." They are replacing a distant, formal figure, Roof adds, with one that is "personal, intimate, authentic for themselves."

Where traditional churches once offered religious doctrine, gurus and leaders of every cloth now promote myriad paths to enlightenment. Yoga is enjoying unprecedented popularity. At the Omega Institute in upstate New York, spiritual seekers can sign up for classes in prayer and contemplation, qigong, rebirthing, life after death, astrology, tarot, movement as spiritual practice, and something called "being with flowers." Sufi dancing, chanting, sacred drumming, Celtic shamanism—all have their adherents.

Women seem to be leading the way down the new path. "We do 300 to 400 workshops a year, and

more authentic self, or a craving for community. Some women have a life-changing epiphany in a moment of crisis; others search for meaning quietly all their lives; still others ignore the spiritual altogether until something—illness, disappointment, a stroke of good fortune, the frantic pace of their days, or one too many hangovers—nudges them onto the spiritual road.

"Whether you think of it as a longing for a greater sense of connectedness to the whole, or to the universe, or to the divine, spirituality is on the rise," says Saki Santorelli, a director at the Center for Mindfulness in Medicine, Health Care, and Society at the University of Massachusetts Medical School. "At the same time that there's been a tremendous rise in material affluence, there is a hunger, a sense that all of that won't satisfy the deeper parts of one's being."

Pollster George Gallup, Jr., confirms that the search for spiritual moorings is a dominant trend in our society today. In 1994, when *Newsweek* pollsters asked Americans whether they felt "the need to experience spiritual growth," 58 percent said yes. Four years later, that number had surged to 82 percent. Entire bookstore sections are devoted to spiritual matters, from best-sellers rooted in the quest for simplicity, such as Sarah Ban Breathnach's *Simple Abundance* (Warner Books, 1995), to the Dalai Lama's hit,

connect with your heritage

For Sorayya Khan, 38 (right), finding a spiritual community hasn't come easily. She and her husband are Muslims raised in Pakistan. But having children in the United States has meant that Khan has had to build new bridges—to her cultural heritage, to her own values, and to her family. "My parents weren't ritualistic," Khan says. "But it was a given that God existed." Sure, when she discussed the creation of the universe with her father, a nuclear engineer, they talked about the big bang theory. Then he would ask, "But who created that first spark?"

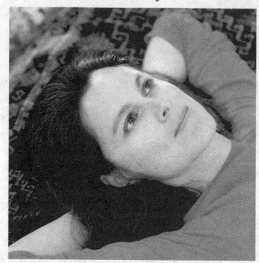

"After my kids were born, God seemed so real," says Khan. "Because of God, a miracle like them could happen." Still, the closest thing to a mosque in Ithaca, New York, was a room in the student center at Cornell University, so Khan has had to scramble for ways to fold her native culture into her family's life. She remembered how in Pakistan everyone used to deliver food to the poor during the year's two major holy days, so she and her family began to bake cookies and pies, which they take to homeless shelters.

Now when she tucks her children into bed at night, Khan repeats the rhythms of the past. Her sons, Kamal, 9, and Shahid, 5, cup their hands and say, in Arabic: *Bismillahh-i-Rahman-ir-Raheem* (In the name of God, the Merciful, the Beneficent). Then they ask, in English, for God's blessings on those who need help, and thank him for their own. Finally, they return to Arabic: *La illaha ill-allah, Muhammad-ur-rasoolullah. Ameen.*

"That is something that we completely improvised," Khan says, laughing about the challenge of mixing English and Arabic, America and Pakistan, Islam and personal belief. "The desire to have them start saying their prayers came from the desire to have them understand that they are part of something much larger—a spiritual world.

"Praying is a bit like standing atop a huge mountain and feeling humility in the face of such raw beauty," she says. "We wanted the kids to be grateful for all the blessings they have. From this knowledge the idea may grow that others have so much less. Perhaps this is a way of suggesting compassion."

---

75 percent of our students are women," says Elizabeth Lesser, who cofounded the institute 25 years ago. "There's a new sense of empowerment: We can treat spiritual longing any way we want to, and we don't necessarily have to turn to patriarchal religion."

Princeton sociologist Robert Wuthnow, who has traced the course of spirituality in America for the past five decades, is mapping the profound spiritual shift. He points to two distinct contemporary trends. In "dwelling spirituality," people still seek the safe haven of a church or established group, and their spiritual life goes on much as it did in the 1950s. But in what he calls

merge with nature

Lost in awe at the beauty around me, I must have slipped into a state of heightened awareness. Self was utterly absent. I and the chimpanzees, the earth and trees and air, seemed to merge, to become one with the spirit power of life itself.
—Jane Goodall, primatologist and author of *Reason for Hope: A Spiritual Journey* (Warner Books, 1999)

"seeking spirituality," which began to emerge in the 1960s, individuals look for meaning outside religious institutions. Seekers feel free to improvise, tailoring their practices to suit their needs and personalities, mixing mass and meditation, for instance, or alternating yoga practice with pilgrimages to Nepal. A growing community surrounds the seekers, from retreats and seminars to 12-step meetings and sacred circles.

With this new emphasis on customizing a spiritual life comes an awareness that many activities can be considered spiritual, whether walking in the woods or washing dishes. Catholic nun Madonna Buder, 70, has hardly abandoned organized religion.

But long-distance running has enhanced her commitment to spiritual life: She says she feels as if she is running with God. "There's all this expansiveness that surrounds us, so much that's greater than you are, that, really, what have you got to worry about? It helps you put everything into focus. It's such an elated feeling. When I first entered the church, it was contemplative, set apart from the world," says Buder, who lives in Spokane, Washington. "Now my path is all-inclusive."

San Francisco painter Nina Wisniewski trusts her art itself to be a guiding force. "I don't call myself a Buddhist or a this or that," she says. "There is no church that is a structure for me." In the studio, she adds, "inspirations sometimes just touch the top of my head. If I am open and listen, it will come to me. That's a rich experience for your art but also for your life. Distraction keeps people out of touch with their spirituality. You can be distracted by a zillion things that have nothing to do with your spirit or your soul."

So Wisniewski tries to let the spiritual find its way into her art workshops. "A lot of women who come have a longing to connect with an inner self," she says. "At a workshop, the rest of their lives—families, jobs—recede, and they can open up to the art. In the last class, we did tai chi and meditation before class, and it set a wonderful tone. It dispelled any competition and ego or insecurities."

do good deeds

A week after arriving in India, I gathered the courage to inquire about working for Mother Teresa. I felt shy about trying to love, if that's what I could call it—about believing I would have anything to give the struggling children in Shishu Bhavan. On my last day in Calcutta, as I am feeding a dying child, a single grain of rice falls off my spoon to the floor. I don't notice, but the boy does. His hand seizes the grain and thrusts it into his mouth. That second, my heart breaks open. I ask: Am I worthy of the trust of a starving child who notices when a single grain of rice falls? Do we, both women and men, dare open our hearts to all human beings?
—Cherilyn Parsons, a writer in Santa Monica, California

meet the unknown

After my marriage of 30 years broke up, I looked everywhere to ease the pain. All the prayers I'd learned in the Catholic church weren't enough. I turned to Buddha, I went to Al-Anon. I learned meditation. At 50, I found my true self, my true strength.
—Isabel Gomez-Bassols, psychologist and host of a Miami-based radio show called *Doctora Isabel*

what they believe, or why. They're groping, looking for pieces from various sources and traditions that give them comfort, but not necessarily from ones that challenge them or require sacrifice."

A seeking style of spirituality may suit the complexities of American society, but Robert Wuthnow, too, cautions that it may encourage dabbling rather than depth. He advocates a "practice-oriented spirituality," involving hard work and true devotion. Spiritual seeking without some kind of ultimate commitment, he says, isn't likely to satisfy the soul.

For many, that commitment boils down to a steady practice of meditation or yoga or work in a certain community. For others, old-fashioned good deeds provide satisfaction—volunteering at a soup kitchen, tutoring a teenager. "One thing I've noticed that is long overdue," says the Omega Institute's Lesser, "is a desire to be a little less self-oriented and to look more toward how this healing work and psychological transformation can be applied to help people in the world. Women are asking, 'How can we bring this spiritual awareness into schools and hospitals and daily life with our families?' So, it's not about me, me, me."

Physician Rachel Naomi Remen (author of *Kitchen Table Wisdom* [G.K. Nall & Co., 2001] and *My Grandfather's Blessing* [Riverhead Books, 2001]) says that your entire life can, in fact, be a spiritual practice. "The more you are aware of the meaning of what you are doing, the richer your life is," says Remen, whose own work as a doctor has included cofounding the Commonweal Cancer Help Program for people suffering from life-threatening illness.

"We are always on holy ground," she says, "and every relationship has a sacred dimension to it, as well as every task. Putting a bowl of soup in front of a child is a basic, spiritual act."

Some worry that a free-floating, personalized approach to spirituality may verge on the shallow and self-indulgent. "It's been called religion à la carte, the divine deli," says pollster George Gallup, Jr., who is also coauthor of *The Next American Spirituality: Finding God in the Twenty-First Century* (Chariot Victor, 2000). "Many people don't know

find a community

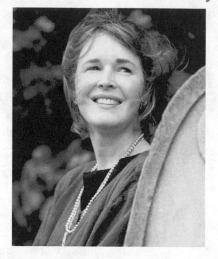

Days after her three-year-old daughter, KC, was diagnosed with cystic fibrosis, Judith Bryan (right) joined a church for the first time. As a child in Ohio, she had always felt a spiritual pull. "I would be walking down the street and suddenly have this amazing sense of oneness with the universe and all people," she says. Since her family didn't practice a religion, she talked a friend's family into taking her along to Sunday services.

Facing her daughter's health crisis with no family nearby, Bryan felt the need for a community to see her through this period of grieving and trying to cope with the disease. "I also needed a vocabulary for my latent feelings." What she found was not just a vocabulary but "a bit of grace." Cystic fibrosis was a dire diagnosis—few sufferers then reached adulthood—but KC grew up to earn varsity letters in high school and graduate from college. Bryan, 46, credits some of KC's longevity to the prayers of friends and family.

Meanwhile, Bryan's spiritual quest took a new turn when her younger daughter was diagnosed with a different, rarer genetic disorder. "I was angry," Bryan says. "But I knew it was safe to be angry, that God was big enough to handle whatever feelings I had.

"That was when I really initiated a more spiritual, as opposed to religious, journey," she adds. "I attended Presbyterian services, but I also went on retreats, read about Catholic and Buddhist and Native American spirituality. I wanted to get a clear sense of how God is present in my life.

"I try to listen to the promptings of the spirit," she says about her personal method of prayer, "sometimes taking a walk, sometimes journaling, sometimes reading a psalm until a phrase lifts up, and then I just let that phrase work on me. I love Psalm 139, which says that God has searched us out and known us. We can go to the ends of the earth and God is always with us."

A few years ago, Bryan entered divinity school. "When I started going to church, I thought it was about having a relationship with God," she says. "But more and more I believe we're meant to have relationships with others. We need to nourish our own lives, but also the people around us."

For Barbara Maltby, the two strands of spiritual life—meditation and hospice work—have not only deepened but interwoven over time. Four years ago, Maltby went to a retreat led by Pema Chrodon, an American woman who trained as a nun in the Tibetan tradition and is the author of *Pure Meditation: The Tibetan Buddhist Practice of Inner Peace* (Sounds True, 2000). "She just opened my eyes to the larger perspective of what it meant to practice," says Maltby. "To practice is to meditate, to bring certain tenets into your life and your behavior. So, as a result of those two weeks, I really integrated meditation into my life in a whole new way."

Today Maltby has what she calls her meditation shed in the backyard of her home in Connecticut. Even when she's not in it, the shed stands as a symbol, she says, for the need to take the time and be in a place where there's less distraction. "Otherwise," says Maltby, "if I walk by the kitchen, I stop to clean it up. My mind doesn't let me rest."

It's in her hospice work these days that Maltby says she feels the most profound change. "When you are with someone who is dying, you are experiencing reality about this life. I've always been a fixer, but in hospice you can't fix anything. All you can do is be there." She says, "There's the connection for me between Quakerism and Buddhism. There's a Quaker phrase that says, 'Be present where you are.' I've tried to do that for a good part of my life with greater or lesser ability and success," says Maltby. "To be present with the rareness and fullness of the human condition." ✳

Karin Evans wrote The Lost Daughters of China: Abandoned Girls, Their Journey to America, and the Search for a Missing Past *(Penguin Putnam, 2000). Additional reporting by Laura McNeal and Ingfei Chen.*

Sounds of Healing
how music relieves the stress of surgery

Sure, music can loosen up a party—but an operating table? A University at Buffalo study reports that within five minutes, music can lower patients' blood pressure to normal levels when they're under the knife. It doesn't have to be the soothing sounds of Enya, either. Any tune will do, as long the patient chooses it.

Forty patients ages 51 to 87 undergoing procedures for glaucoma or cataract removal participated in the study. All had normal blood pressure a week before the operation, but on the day of surgery experienced elevated blood pressure and stress levels—typical responses for older patients undergoing outpatient procedures. Half the people received headphones and could select from tapes of 22 types of music (from Broadway show tunes to reggae) to play before, during, and after the operation. The other half listened to the sounds of surgery.

The tune-free had elevated blood-pressure levels throughout the surgery; those who listened to music had normal blood pressure and reported lower stress levels. Study leader Karen Allen, Ph.D., suggests that the key lies in the psychological benefits of granting the patient a degree of control over his or her environment and the familiarity of a favorite melody. By allowing a patient to play deejay, doctors may be able to safely and inexpensively reduce the stress of surgery.

doubts cast on ginseng as a mood lifter

First, the credibility of Saint-John's-wort as a natural remedy for depression took a hit. Now, new evidence casts some doubt on ginseng's mood-boosting ability. A study—whose results were published recently in the *Journal of the American Dietetic Association*—found that participants who downed a pure form of ginseng saw no psychological benefits compared with those who took a placebo. The bottom line: If you're feeling low on a regular basis, talk to your doctor before you take the herbal route.

ADVICE FOR FEARFUL FLYERS

Want to make it to your destination in fine fettle? Have a light snack and a nonalcoholic drink before going on your flight, and researchers say you'll lower your chances of fainting, the most common in-flight emergency. The kind of snack you choose isn't as important as its presence; researchers believe that having something in your stomach keeps your blood oxygen, which can be affected by cabin pressure and dehydration, at safe levels. And don't forget to bring your seat and tray to their original upright positions.

learning to forgive

a prescription for better health

**Researchers say it's more than a catchphrase.
It's a path to better mental and physical health,
a way to find joy again.**

BY KARIN EVANS

Margaret McKinney sat in a chair in a Stanford University classroom, thousands of miles from her home in Belfast, with her eyes closed, breathing in, breathing out. A 69-year-old Irish mother, McKinney had lost a son to the strife in Northern Ireland more than 20 years earlier. The young Catholic man had been shot in the back of the head and left in a ditch, and every day since then, his mother had thought of little besides her boy—and the Protestants who had murdered him.

Now she was trying something most of her neighbors and family back home might have thought impossible. Having spent more than two decades weighed down by grief and rage, McKinney was learning to forgive her son's murderers. Not only that, she was doing it with two Protestants in the room—both of them mothers like herself, whose sons were killed in the conflict.

The women had all traveled from Northern Ireland to take "The Art and Science of Forgiveness" class led by Frederic Luskin, Ph.D., a Stanford psychologist

and researcher. Luskin has elevated what most people think of as a nebulous virtue to a skill that can be learned and has been teaching workshops and classes on the subject for several years. Students arrive at his classroom lugging not just backpacks but grievances: unfaithful lovers, abusive parents, harsh employers, unkind friends. Some, like the women from Northern Ireland, carry heavier burdens.

Luskin came to this work having nursed a grudge of his own for far too long, he says. "When my best friend married a woman who didn't like me, my friend withdrew," he says. "We'd been like brothers, and it was excruciating." Luskin sank into a low-level depression that lasted years. "I was letting something that had happened in 1989 give me a rainy day in 1993," he says. "And I was a psychotherapist! Why didn't I just forgive him and go on my way?"

Luskin wasn't content simply to wonder at his inability to let his friend off the hook. He set about studying everything he could find on forgiveness. He discovered that the ancient ideal had been passed down with no instruction manual. Even people who were willing to forgive often had no idea how to go about it. Eventually he came up with a plan for letting go of

Imagine a plane that has been circling for 9 or 10 years.
Think of how much energy it is taking to keep that plane up there.

Forgiveness is letting that plane land. Imagine the relief. It's about
reclaiming the power we gave to those circling planes to ruin our lives.

grudges. He put it into practice, and his own outlook—and his career—took a turn for the better. "The joy came back into my life," he says. He began to share in the classroom what he had learned. By now, a couple of thousand people have been to Luskin's classes at Stanford and elsewhere around the country.

Luskin is convinced that learning to let go of grievances can not only improve mental and physical health but literally change lives. "Think of your mind as a radar screen and you as the air-traffic controller," Luskin tells his students. "On that screen at any minute are airplanes representing all the things you need to think about and attend to at any given moment. Then imagine that on your screen is a plane that has been circling for 9 or 10 years. Think of how much energy it is taking to keep that plane up there.

"Forgiveness," Luskin says, "is letting that plane land. Can you imagine the relief? It's about reclaiming the power that we gave to those circling planes to ruin our lives."

An important step toward forgiveness is understanding where grudges come from in the first place, Luskin says. A grudge is born when something happens—you're not invited to a party, maybe, or a friend doesn't return your calls. You take it personally, blame the offender, and create what Luskin calls a "grievance story" about the incident. The more you

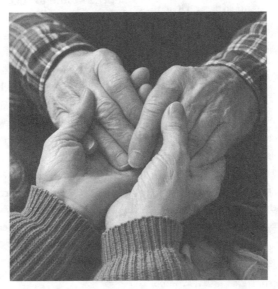

repeat the story, whether in your mind or to others, the more it becomes etched in your psyche, making it hard to look at things any other way. "When we blame something or someone else for our lack of well-being, it's very easy to slip into the role of victim, of being vulnerable and small," he says. And once the negative story becomes part of your life, it can lead to feelings of depression, mistrust, fear, and anger—emotions that can be hard on your health.

Every time the grievance comes to mind, in fact, the body can re-create the emotional and physical duress that accompanied the original hurt. You become agitated, blood pressure soars, and stress hormones are released. Nursing a grudge produces what Luskin calls "an ongoing mind-body disturbance." Forgiveness, however, can restore peacefulness and balance.

But once a grudge is embedded, it takes work to pry it loose. It doesn't simply happen, as Dana Curtis of Sausalito, California, found out. "I'd waited for it to come over me. I'd prayed for it," she says. But nothing seemed to work.

"After Luskin's workshop," Curtis says, "I thought, this is something that is within my control." And so, in an ongoing conflict with her former husband, she put the theory to work. "He's been angry at me for more than 20 years now and has never let go of it," she says. "But I had an epiphany and thought, I am

It's a misconception that if you forgive,
you have to like or accept as OK what the person did.

forgiveness 101

"Just let it go." You've probably heard this—even said it to yourself—while venting over some social slight or deeper wound. Chances are, you've discovered how difficult actually doing it is. Stanford psychologist Frederic Luskin, Ph.D., knows how tough forgiveness can be and has developed a process to make it easier for all of us. Here's an abbreviated version.

Breathe deeply in and out from your belly to relax, then visualize a time when you felt cared for and loved. Think of the situation you'd like to work on: how you wish the events had gone, the hope you had for the event or relationship that went awry. If it was a romance gone bad, for instance, you might have hoped for a deep, loving connection. Say or write down what you would have preferred to have occurred.

Take a practical look at the world around you. Has what happened to you happened to others? Is there any way you can look at it less personally? One of Luskin's students, for instance, held a grudge against her boss because he refused to transfer her to a warmer climate that would be better for her health. During Luskin's class, she learned to accept the fact that her boss put the needs of the company over her personal needs—not an unusual occurrence.

Realize that just because you didn't get what you wanted out of the situation does not mean you should give up trying to have your needs met. "The goal in this step is to appreciate that part of yourself that's lost when you get hurt," Luskin says. "If you can hold on to those loving intentions, you can reclaim your power from whoever hurt you. And you can guide your future in a much clearer way."

Make a long-term pledge to practice letting go of grudges. Luskin is careful to point out that a week—or a simple session or two on forgiveness—is not enough to work through a brutal murder or come to terms with childhood abuse. But knowing the tools to use is important. "When the old feelings come up, breathe in and out for two slow, deep breaths. Then picture something positive and wonderful in your life. That can break the cycle."

Frederic Luskin's "The Art and Science of Forgiveness" is available on tape for $16 postpaid. Write to Frederic Luskin, 730 Welch Road, Suite B, Palo Alto, CA 94304-1583. For more information, visit www.learningtoforgive.com.

just going to let go of this. I don't have any control over fixing the relationship, but I am going to choose to keep my heart open."

For all the enthusiasm about forgiveness, though, the subject has its detractors. One of the most vocal is psychologist Jeanne Safer, Ph.D., author of *Forgiving and Not Forgiving* (Avon Books, 1999). She fears that forgiveness lets offenders off the hook and that vulnerable people can be rushed or pressured into forgiving.

"It's a misconception that if you forgive, you have to like or accept as OK what the person did," Luskin says. "Another misconception is that you have to reconcile with or 'talk nice' to the person. You can forgive someone and make a clear choice to end the relationship."

I can't find it in myself anymore to hate.
—Margaret McKinney

For the women from Northern Ireland, the weeklong workshop on forgiveness was often painful. Margaret McKinney and the others learned to use deep breathing and visualization techniques when they felt overwhelmed by sad or violent memories. They tried to appreciate that it was still possible to experience love and joy in their lives, despite their losses.

And the struggle paid off. In the end, McKinney found herself laughing and smiling with the other women, something she hadn't done in decades. When the women told their stories at the last session, something had shifted. They spoke of their dead sons but said they were thinking less often about the murderers. They felt lighter, less burdened. "Before I came here, I hated all Protestants, and I never thought anything would change my mind," McKinney said afterward. "Now I see that Protestants hurt the way we do. I can't say I have fully excused the person who killed my son, but I don't look at it the same way anymore. I can't find it in myself anymore to hate." ✳

Frequent Health *contributor Karin Evans is the author of* The Lost Daughters of China: Abandoned Girls, Their Journey to America, and the Search for a Missing Past *(Penguin Purnam, 2000).*

WHAT TO DO IF THE JOB COMES ON VACATION WITH YOU

You've saved all year for this summer vacation—and then you find yourself feeling lousy the minute you get there. It could be that you're suffering from "leisure sickness," a term coined by Ad Vingerhoets, Ph.D., a psychologist at Tilburg University in the Netherlands.

According the Vingerhoets, some people, no matter how much they think they crave time off, encounter headaches, colds, nausea, and flu-like symptoms as soon as they're free from the office. After studying more than 100 men and women who reported these leisure-related symptoms, Vingerhoets found that a preoccupation with work kept the subjects from relaxing and even made them feel guilty about taking time off.

"When you are very busy, you may not even be aware you are sick," Vingerhoets says. "You may not pay attention to signals from your body. It's not until you are away from work that you feel tired, feel pain."

Leisure-sickness sufferers are typically perfectionists who are not very assertive but have a higher sense of responsibility than others, he says. The stress of preparing for travel made the subjects ill, and they thought more about their jobs during vacation than a nonsuffering control group.

The cure? Those who seemed to kick the vacation blues reported changing jobs, changing their attitudes toward work, and paying more attention to signals from their bodies. Weekend exercise and counseling also appeared to help, according to Vingerhoets. "It may help to take another view of your life, of your work situation," he says. "See things in a different perspective. Give more weight to other things that are important in life."

Feeling low? *Get silly!*

Balance—both physical and mental—is no easy feat. But injecting a little silliness into life's serious mix may be just what you need to set you straight. Don't let darkening days dampen your sense of play: Pick a childlike activity that challenges your sense of physical balance and give it a go. Borrow a pogo stick, try a handstand, or rock-hop across a stream. You may stumble—or even fall—but chances are you'll return to your routine with a new perspective.

HEALTH BUZZ

THUMBS UP

charitable giving
Brother, can you spare a lung? Thanks to an increase in the number of donors, organ transplants rose more than 5%, from 21,655 in 1999 to 22,827 in 2000.

soy
One more joy that's now linked to soy: Eating it regularly may help stave off Alzheimer's disease.

natural healing
Call it the anti-R$_x$. New research suggests antibiotics often don't help acute sinusitis in kids. So why prescribe them and raise the risk of creating antibiotic-resistant bacteria? Ask your child's doctor about alternatives.

THUMBS DOWN

unlisted allergens
Talk about your dirty tricks—25% of cookie, ice cream, and candy makers sell goodies that contain peanut and egg allergens (transferred via baking equipment that was reused without being cleaned properly) without listing them on the label.

smoking
We've come a long way— but in the wrong direction on this statistic. Smoking prevalence among women is now about equal to that of men, who traditionally have been the heavier smokers.

chunky pumps
Manolo Blahniks aren't the only culprits. Studies show that wide-heeled shoes are even more likely to strain your knees—and lead to osteoarthritis—than narrow heels. It's because women tend to wear them longer.

missing boosters
Just because she dresses like Britney doesn't mean it's time to give up the booster seat. Fewer than 10% of older kids use boosters, recommended for 4- to 8-year-olds to ensure that their seat belts fit properly.

seeking balance

How to find calm in the midst of a hectic life

BY KATRINA KENISON

On my 40th birthday, my husband and I spent the night with friends at their bare-bones lakeside cottage. It was the first week of October, the mosquitoes were gone, and so were the summer visitors. Only the loons remained, calling plaintively across the water. Before settling down to cook dinner over the fire, the four of us climbed a nearby hill to watch the autumn sunset.

As we reached the top, my friend Kerby stooped to pick up a 2-foot-long, triangular rock. Slowly, with the utmost focus and concentration, he set one of the pointed ends on top of a high, rounded stone at the edge of the path. There was a long minute as he held the rock in place and then lifted his hands away. To our amazement, the rock stayed where he had placed it, perfectly, remarkably, balanced. "This is my birthday wish for you," he announced, stepping back. "Perfect balance in all your days." In fact, there is no gift on earth that would please me more than perfect balance—nor one more elusive.

A few days later, on an early Monday morning, I woke with a headache already throbbing in my temples. With fall in full swing—work deadlines, school, music lessons, kids' sports, and countless evening meetings—I was panicking at the very thought of another over-scheduled, fast-paced week. Mentally running through my to-do list, I realized that I wasn't just tense, I was angry, too. Angry that my life had become so demanding, angry that I was once again trapped in a whirl of too many activities and too many commitments. All this angst—and I wasn't even out of bed yet!

I took a few long, deep breaths, closed my eyes again, and pictured my birthday rock. Could I possibly find balance in the midst of the never-ending demands of real life? Could I learn to juggle all my responsibilities, to prioritize and make time for everything and still keep my sense of calm?

I couldn't quit my job, make the laundry disappear, or run off to a deserted island with my husband and kids. But I knew that something had to change.

I needed to pay more attention to the life I already had.

As I lay in bed, I made a simple commitment to myself. Just for today, I would slow down and pay attention to whatever I was doing at the moment, whether it was feeding the cat, driving the kids to school, or attending my afternoon meeting. Making coffee a few minutes later, I consciously took time to savor the aroma of ground espresso beans and cinnamon. When I stepped outside for the newspaper, I paused to snap a dead blossom from the chrysanthemum and admire a flame-red maple by the driveway. I inhaled the morning air, and an unexpected wave of gratitude washed over me. Nothing in my life had changed in the last hour yet, to my surprise, I was feeling better.

For months, I realized, I had been completely caught up in doing; I had lost the knack for being. I thought again about Kerby's birthday wish for me. The truth was, perfect balance had come to seem like just another unreachable goal. It seemed like something that belonged on my to-do list, a life change I had scheduled but could never find the time to make. Now I was ready to let go of the concept of ideal balance, to discover how I could appreciate the life I already have, right now.

That was three years ago. The birthday wish still has not come true, at least not in the way I imagined it might. But my life has improved dramatically because I have recognized that, in every minute of every day, I have a choice: to be here now, fully present, or to slip away into distraction. I've come to know that when I am truly focused, I experience newfound satisfaction in the ordinary events of everyday life. That means that when I'm working, I direct all my energy to the job before me. When I'm sitting on a park bench, I try to accord those minutes of relaxation just as much importance as my work, soaking up my surroundings with all my senses. The moments I create for myself are an antidote for the rest of my hectic life. A dawn walk with a friend prepares me for a morning at my desk; 15 minutes in the garden at the end of the day is a perfect reward for six hours at the computer; a game of catch with my sons brings me out of my head and back down to earth.

Learning this hasn't been easy. I've had to become more flexible, to take each step more deliberately, and to stay open to unexpected changes in the day's emotional weather and respond accordingly. On a practical level, this means that I now say "no" more often. I do a little less than I used to, and I enjoy myself a little more. I've made my peace with slow-moving projects, a dirty kitchen floor, unexpected interruptions. I've come to accept that I'll never manage to do all the things that I'd like to. I haven't chucked my to-do list, but I'm not ruled by it, either. Instead, I give myself time to find and follow a different rhythm, time to fully inhabit my own life from one moment to the next.

I do less than I used to, and I enjoy myself more.

Learning to live this way is basic, innate, and essential, according to Jon Kabat-Zinn, author of *Wherever You Go, There You Are* (Hyperion, 1995). "When you are immersed in doing without being centered, it feels like being away from home," he writes. "And when you reconnect with being, even for a few minutes, you know it immediately. You feel you are at home no matter where you are and what problems you face."

This, I now realize, is really what it means to explore a more balanced path. Even on crazy days, I can make room for moments to choose stillness over activity,

being over doing, equilibrium over stress. I can let go of the impossible and embrace what's within reach.

When Kerby wished me perfect balance, I envisioned myself effortlessly multitasking, doing all things well. I believed that if I could prioritize and get more organized, I'd no longer feel so off-kilter. In fact, all I needed was to pay more attention to the life I already had.

Recently, I asked Kerby how he had balanced that rock. His simple reply: "First, you have to believe you can do it. And then you have to become perfectly still. If you focus on your own breathing, and pay attention, the balance comes by itself." ✳

Katrina Kenison is the author of Mitten Strings for God: Reflections for Mothers in a Hurry *(Warner Books, 2000) and editor of* The Best American Short Stories *(Houghton Mifflin, 2001). With John Updike, she edited* The Best American Short Stories of the Century *(Houghton Mifflin, 2001).*

balancing act

Every day brings a choice: to practice stress or practice peace. So writes Joan Borysenko, Ph.D, a clinical psychologist and author of *Inner Peace for Busy People* (Hay House, 2001). She offers practical advice to help even the most time-challenged find moments of balance. Some tips:

Try making two small changes every day. Take a different street, try a new restaurant, change your toothpaste, smile at someone you don't know, eat dessert first. There's a lot of landscape to explore off the beaten path.

Clear the clutter. Take a good look at where you spend your time, and start with the obvious things: dead plants, old newspapers, and the like. You can rearrange every room in your house, but you don't have to. At least have a go at reorganizing your underwear drawer.

Rediscover the simple pleasures. Do your possessions energize you, or are they a drain? If you're a habitual television watcher and want to discover more simple pleasures this week, try a TV-fast. Time will open up.

Realize not everything needs to be done today. Prioritize based on what feels right, not just what your to-do list says. If the day's rhythm favors cleaning rather than returning phone calls, that's what should get done. Tasks will still get taken care of, but the result will be more creative and elegant. And you'll surely feel more peaceful.

heartbreak
and your heart

The startling facts about chronic grief

BY KARIN EVANS

WHEN GILBERT GREEN DIED on a summer morning at the age of 89, his family, though saddened, wasn't surprised. Green, who lived in a Denver nursing home, had had a heart attack a few months earlier and had been declining visibly ever since. He had told his family that he knew he was dying and was worried about leaving his wife, Lucille, behind. Green had said that he wanted to die beside his wife, just a little bit before she did, so he wouldn't have to miss her. Not long after that conversation, Green lay in bed, holding his wife's hand, then drew a peaceful last breath. The next day, Green's son, Brent, and daughter, Julie, were at a funeral home making arrangements for their father's memorial service when an emergency call came. Their mother had suddenly taken a turn for the worse. They rushed to her side; within an hour, she, too, was dead.

Although 85 years old and suffering from Parkinson's disease, Lucille Green had been doing well before her husband died. Even in her state of grief, the nursing staff thought she was strong enough to attend her husband's memorial service. "Her vitals had been normal for years," says her daughter, Julie Bethke. "Her blood pressure was better than mine.

"We'd already called everyone about Daddy," Bethke says. "Then we had to turn around and call everyone about Mother. They all said, 'My God, that's just what they would have wanted.' " And so the children of Lucille and Gilbert Green held a double funeral, mourning two deaths but also celebrating a union that had lasted 65 years.

"Terminal dehydration and Parkinson's," read Lucille Green's death certificate. Family members offer a different explanation: "There was no way my mother was going to live without her love of a lifetime," Bethke says. "She died of a broken heart."

The Crooners Had It Right

Is such a thing possible? Poets and songwriters have long thought so. James J. Lynch, author of *The Broken Heart: The Medical Consequences of Loneliness* (Basic Books, 1977), says that hundreds of years ago grief was recognized as a cause of death, but hospitals in this high-tech millennium no longer accept such an old-fashioned notion.

Yet, recently, a topic that's long been a staple of country-western songs has become a subject of serious research. As researchers probe the mysteries of

On a scale that ranks stressfulness of life events, loss of a spouse tops the list .

when grief runs too deep

Grief is a natural and healthy response to loss. But that isn't
to say traumatic grief should be left unchecked.

How to you know when to step in and help the heartbroken?

The amount of time required for mourning can't be measured, so there's no surefire way to assess when others should step in and take action. In fact, says Arizona psychologist and grief expert Robert Wrenn, society tends to rush the grieving process. People should offer loved ones the time they need and plenty of slack. Individual symptoms vary tremendously, ranging from crying jags to numbness and disbelief. "Give up your script as to how a person is to behave," says Wrenn. Still, family members or friends who feel a grieving person may be in trouble should not be afraid to seek help. If there are signs that someone's health is declining or that he or she cannot focus on what's needed to survive, says Wrenn, it's wise to consult a professional. Therapists say the following signs may indicate a slide into trouble:

A bereaved person's health is failing,

or he or she seems unable to attend to the basics of self-care—personal hygiene, for instance, or basic nutrition. "Be on the alert for unusual behavior," says Wrenn, "particularly anything that might put the person or others at risk. "Increased alcohol intake, for example, can be a problem.

The surviving spouse,

after a few months, still takes no interest in activities that were once engaging. "Offer help," says Wrenn. "Go in with a listening ear. Ask how the person is doing and if there is anything you can do." Support groups can help immensely. The American Association of Retired Persons, or AARP (www.aarp.org), offers grief and loss programs nationwide. Other support groups may be available in your town.

Feelings of detachment from life

or futility about the future persist for more than six months. This can indicate severe, or traumatic, grief, says psychiatrist Holly Prigerson, and may warrant seeking professional help or a support group.

Friendships are falling

by the wayside. Again, says Wrenn, be available. "The best thing friends and family can do is keep the kind of relationship you had before. Don't overdo it, don't underdo it. Often people make the mistake of hovering and wringing their hands, or keeping a total distance because they don't know what to do. Treat the person as you always have." Encourage the bereaved to express any feelings they'd like to, but don't try to cheer them up. "If they don't feel like talking or visiting, let them know you would like to be there when they do." If the isolation persists after a few months—especially with someone who was previously outgoing—check with a physician or a counselor.

In all cases,

before family or friends intervene directly, Wrenn advises speaking to a professional, who may have suggestions on how to proceed. "People who are grieving may feel out of control, and they may resist someone stepping in," Wrenn says. "The more you can give people the control to get back on their feet, the better they like it."

For referrals to local grief specialists, check with a physician or hospital. The Association for Death Education and Counseling also has listings of local resources on its Web site at www.adec.org.

---

emotional distress—as well as its effects on physiology, especially the heart—poets and scientists are finding themselves in the same camp.

"Just about everybody can point to an example of someone dying of a broken heart," says Yale University psychiatrist Holly Prigerson, who has studied the ways grief does its damage to the mind and body.

"Most experienced physicians intuitively know that this happens," agrees Paul Rosch, a professor of psychiatry at New York Medical College. "Look on the walls of any synagogue. In so many instances, the names of couples are listed, with their times of death only months apart." Sometimes a grieving person volunteers the information, as did *New Yorker* editor William Maxwell, whose death in 2000 followed his wife's by just a week. "I've decided there's not much reason to stick around, now that Emmy's gone," Maxwell told a friend.

Dying of a broken heart can happen when one is young, but it probably happens more often when one is old, when the losses mount up, when one is frail to begin with.

Bill Thomas, a Harvard-trained physician who founded the Eden Alternative, an innovative system of nursing homes that emphasizes resident participation and a sense of community, says he sees the phenomenon all the time. "Dying of a broken heart can begin with the loss of a spouse, a home, or other meaningful thing in life," Thomas says. "It can happen when one is young, but it probably happens more often when one is old, when the losses mount up, when there is some physical frailty to begin with."

Fatal Distress

How is it possible for a shock that begins in the mind to strike a body down?

One answer begins with that ubiquitous culprit, stress. On a commonly used scale that ranks the stressfulness of life events, loss of a spouse or another intimate tops the list. Studying a group of widowed people in the 12 months after they'd lost a partner, Rosch says, he found they died at a rate 2 to 12 times higher than a similar group whose spouses were still alive. Among all age groups, adds Rosch, men seem more vulnerable after the loss of a partner than women. But a large Swedish study found that losing a spouse was a risk factor for mortality for both men and women. Most at risk were people under 70 and the recently widowed.

What it boils down to, says Prigerson, is that severe grief can make you sick and even kill you. Having followed a group of 150 widows and widowers for two years after they'd lost their spouses, Prigerson found that those who were hardest hit by grief also were prone to such health problems as heart trouble, high blood pressure, suicidal thoughts, and cancer. Rosch says that depression, loneliness, and social isolation—all common conditions for the bereaved—can cause damage, too, by suppressing the immune system.

For reasons only beginning to be understood, in the first days after great loss, the heart is especially vulnerable. Stress batters the heart by speeding up its rate, raising blood pressure, making blood clot faster, and negatively affecting cholesterol levels, says Robert Sapolsky, a professor of biological sciences and neurology at Stanford University. The cumulative effect is occasionally dire. "There are documented cases of sudden cardiac arrest following powerful emotional distress," Sapolsky says. Over time, both the stress and the depression that may accompany loss work their slower damage on the heart. Depression alone, reports the National Institutes of Health—in just these words—can break your heart.

A Dangerous Detachment

Fortunately, given the right kind of help, broken hearts can sometimes mend, but family—as well as physicians—have to know what warning signs to look for and when to intervene.

Although it is hard to put parameters on anything so personal and individualized as grief, researchers have realized since the time of Sigmund Freud that intense mourning that interferes with the ability to care for oneself or isolates a person from the outside world can batter both mind and body. Such a condition is called complicated or pathological grief.

But Holly Prigerson at Yale has recently identified a new category of response to loss that's deep and damaging. Traumatic grief, she calls it. "In normal grief, though there are great feelings of sadness, the person still feels emotionally connected to others and feels that life still holds meaning and purpose," Prigerson says. Traumatic grief, on the other hand, is characterized by detachment from the world and feelings of futility—a yearning for the lost person, a denial that

Traumatic grief is marked by a yearning for the lost person, a denial that he or she is gone, an inability to imagine life alone, a kind of numbness.

he or she is gone, an inability to imagine life alone, a kind of numbness.

Those most at risk? People who lack social support—those who live alone or say they feel lonely—as well as those who may have a history of depression, trauma, or other mental health difficulties. Also, in news that comes as no surprise to songwriters and romance novelists, people who are extraordinarily attached to one person and feel they've lost a soul mate seem especially vulnerable. In a national study, Prigerson interviewed couples when both partners were still living and asked them to describe their relationship. Then she looked at what happened when one partner died. "We found a significant statistical interaction between the closeness of the marriage and the decline of the surviving spouse afterward.

"If people aren't so in tune with each other, the loss is less likely to result in death," says Prigerson. "Maybe people who are really close have more to lose when one of them dies."

The Surprise of Resilience

At Lucille and Gilbert Green's funeral, Julie Bethke passed out a card that celebrated her parents' lives together. "A love affair to remember," it read. "My parents' marriage was the envy of all their friends," says Bethke. "The two were inseparable."

Could Lucille's death have been prevented? Perhaps not, because it happened so suddenly. In fact, says Arizona psychologist and grief specialist Robert Wrenn, some long-term couples are so strongly connected that the relationship seems to have a life span of its own. In many cases, however, those who suffer traumatic grief can be rescued if the severity of the trauma is identified quickly and they are offered specific treatment, such as counseling, medication, or both. Seeing a physician trained to assess depression and grief is a good way to start. Some researchers even suggest that the partner of someone facing a terminal illness be offered help early on, before loss occurs and grief begins to set in.

What separates those who are likely to die, either suddenly or by a slow downward slide, from those who bounce back? If there is a flip side to the notion of death by heartbreak, it's that other mysterious concept, the will to live. "Just as there is a letting go

when life seems to hold no meaning," says Bill Thomas, "there is the opposite effect, some force inside us that can prolong life." Even when grief hits hardest, that spark can sometimes be fanned back to life.

After George Lawton (this name has been changed) lost his wife of 30 years, he sank into despair, growing increasingly withdrawn, frail, and apparently unable to care for himself in the months following her death. When his family became concerned and suggested

Even when grief hits hardest, the will to live can sometimes be fanned back to life.

moving him to a nursing home, Lawton drove his car out on a lonely road and crashed at top speed. Somehow, though, he survived.

When he was brought to the Eden Alternative nursing home where Bill Thomas worked, Lawton was curled in a fetal position, not talking, willing himself to die. But Jude Thomas, who works with her husband, had an idea. She moved a cage of "orphaned" parakeets into Lawton's room.

A few days later she stuck her head in Lawton's door to find the widower standing by the cage, talking with the parakeets. "They're pretty perky today," he told her. Before long, Lawton discovered several dogs that needed walking and appointed himself to the task. Soon he was wandering the halls with a handful of leashes and a wide smile. Eventually, Lawton decided he wanted to live at home again. He left the nursing home on his own steam—bidding a cheery good-bye to parakeets, dogs, staff, and fellow residents.

He hadn't forgotten his loss, of course. Lawton still dearly missed his wife—and always will. But he'd moved beyond the worst of the pain. The dramatic change, Thomas says, arose from something quite simple. "He fell in love with life again." ✳

Karin Evans is a frequent Health *contributor.*

There comes a point when every woman yearns to reinvent her life. But how do you stop what you've been doing long enough to figure out what comes next?

time out:
Why a personal sabbatical is **crucial** for happiness and health

BY NANCY ROSS-FLANIGAN

PHOTOGRAPHY BY WENDY STENZEL

P romise you won't put off the things you really want to do," my father begged me a few months after I turned 21. We were sitting at the worn maple table in our family room, where Mom and I had shared after-school stories and peanut butter sandwiches, where Dad had cracked countless corny jokes. But on this April afternoon, it was only my father and I, weeping for my 58-year-old mother and her lost dreams. For years Mom had talked about someday going to college and traveling the world with Dad. Now it was too late. At the age when she was finally ready to embark on her adventures, breast cancer had killed her.

"Life is short—eat dessert first" was never just a clever T-shirt slogan to me. In my senior year of high school, I, too, had been diagnosed with cancer; while my classmates were picking out prom dresses, I was seeing doctors and undergoing treatments. When the disease spread to my lymph nodes a few months later, only ignorance saved me from despair; I didn't fully grasp the menace contained in the word metastasize. I was lucky enough to recover, but then, just before my mother died, I lost my gorgeous and wickedly witty friend Laura to the disease. One day Laura was complaining of a backache; the next thing I knew, two grieving parents were hanging her portrait in a college conference room named in her memory.

My cancer recurred in my late 20s, when I was in grad school obsessing over oral exams and lab experiments on the social lives of bees. I found another tumor in my early 40s; after chemo and radiation, it took more than a year for my body and soul to feel normal again. For a while, life had that dazzle that comes with surviving a brush with death. But eventually I got used to Technicolor, or it faded into the monochrome of everyday routine. Somehow, my plate became so heaped with commitments that it often seemed there was no time to savor the

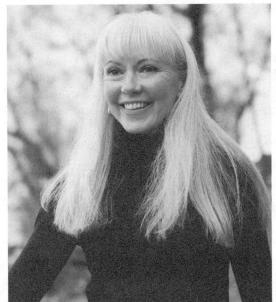

WHAT MY TIME-OUT TAUGHT ME:
i learned who i really am

Fracturing a vertebra midway through her four-month leave turned out to be a blessing in disguise for Nancy Ross-Flanigan, 52, of Belleville, Michigan. Free of the usual distractions, she gained new perspective on the many facets of her personality. She also figured out how to juggle all the things she loves and still have time to relax.

....

sweetness of a world I nearly lost, not once or twice, but three times. Life felt less precious but also more normal—and that, in a way, was a relief.

With each cancer recurrence, I felt more conflicted—determined to shoehorn meaningful experiences into whatever time I had left, yet afraid of piling on more than my immune system could handle. Friends and colleagues described me as organized, efficient, dedicated, but I wasn't always that way, and those traits seemed out of sync with my private dreams. I yearned to work with my hands instead of my head, to roam forest trails and feel the sun on my arms as I picked my way across a desert landscape. Instead I spent my days staring out an office window, enslaved by a never-ending round of deadlines. In my reveries, I would take off, traveling back roads by motorcycle or hippie van, following whims like a leaf surfing a breeze. But the prospect of actually living out my fantasies, even briefly, seemed so irresponsible, so selfish.

Then I turned 45, a birthday I had never expected to see. I had a new love, Ray; a lakeside home; and even the roaring, chromed-out motorcycle I'd dreamed of ever since Michael Parks rode his Harley across my TV screen in *Then Came Bronson*. In many ways life seemed just right. It was time to celebrate my survival, but more than that, to feel fully my happiness before it slipped away. I'd been saving money for something special:

maybe a trip to the South Pacific or replacements for the rings my mother left me, stolen before I'd had a chance to wear them. But I kept hearing the advice my father had offered at that same table where he'd handed me the rings on another tearful afternoon: Don't put off the things you really want to do.

What did I really want to do? Everything. Nothing. What I yearned for more than anything, I realized, was time. Time to think. Time to play. Time to waste. Time to fill, in ways I wouldn't regret if I did manage to grow old.

So instead of a trip or a trinket, I decided to give myself time: four months off to explore how I wanted to live the rest of my days. It wasn't a leave of absence, I told myself, but a leave of presence. As it was, I'd been absent from my life too long.

Over the years, I've had friends who took time-outs to follow a fantasy or recharge their lives. Pat, for example, moved to China for a few months and had a fling with a Frenchman she met on the plane to Beijing. A couple of years later, she took off to Paris for four months, intending to study the language but ditching her classes and exploring the city instead. Then there's my best friend from high school, who stunned me one summer by hiking nearly 700 miles of the Appalachian Trail. Cindi had always seemed more tender than tough. But as I gazed at the snapshot she'd sent me, her calves as sinewy as an Olympian's, I could see how much she'd changed.

Breaks like these, I understood, are not mere vacations. You might take along maps and guidebooks, but you never really know where you'll end up. You embrace the unexpected, and though you might come

WHAT MY TIME-OUT TAUGHT ME:
i can create my own dream job

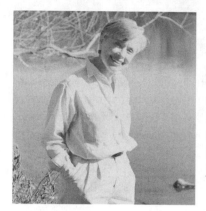

As co-owner of a busy bookstore chain based in Nashville, Tennessee, Karen Davis, 55, could barely take the weekend off. But she and her business partner yearned for extended leaves, so they decided to take turns. Davis's first break was a trip to Wales; two years later, she trekked around Europe. The sabbaticals showed her a way to combine her wanderlust with her work. Now KDavis Travels, which offers guided walking tours, is her full-time job—not that it feels like one.

home at the end of your journey, you hope to be living in a different emotional space. Still, I had no idea how challenging this trek into the unknown could be. I'd always assumed that the hardest part of taking a break would be the logistics: making room in my schedule, getting permission from my boss, setting a budget. Instead, it was the emotional roadblocks that kept tripping me up.

Until that momentous decision six years ago, my idea of a break was the five minutes I spend in line waiting for coffee to get me through the rest of the day. A four-month sabbatical seemed so extravagant that it boggled the mind. When coworkers asked how I planned to spend the time, I'd reply, "Finding out what I do when I'm not doing what I usually do." I didn't mean to be cryptic or coy; I really didn't know. I felt like a scientist again, studying myself instead of a colony of bees, curious to see how my days would develop when they were no longer organized around getting ready for work, working, and getting ready for the next day's work. I had a long wish list of places to visit, people to see, experiences to try, but except for a monthlong motorcycle trip with Ray, I had no plans. Caprice and serendipity were welcome to work their magic.

My expectations, on the other hand, were not nearly so modest or vague. I wanted to feel transformed, transcendent—not just in hindsight, when my sabbatical was over, but every moment along the way. *I want to believe that my break will lead me to be more peaceful, less anxious, less critical, more creative. In all—more the kind of person I want to be,* I wrote in my journal nine weeks before my mid-May start date. I longed for days that would feel "shimmering, delicious, orgasmic," like a perfect summer Saturday stretched out for weeks. *But I don't want to get so hung up on specialness that I can't appreciate the ordinary,* I reminded myself. Those were my hopes. My fear was that I'd just be the same cranky, impatient person I always was, only with a lot of time on my hands.

As it turned out, my worries loomed so large they almost crowded out my excitement. Grown-ups aren't supposed to goof off for four months, I told myself. And it gradually dawned on me that becoming another person would mean losing myself—or at least pieces of myself that felt comfortable and safe. Without my job, I fretted in my journal, who would I be?

April 19 *I can't figure out why I'm not more excited about the leave. Before I arranged for it, just the thought of it was so liberating. But the moment I got it approved, it became almost a burden.*

Still, the first day of my break had a texture and tone unlike any I could recall. After I woke, I ambled onto

Breaks like these are not mere vacations.
You might take along maps and guidebooks, but you
never know where you'll end up.

WHAT MY TIME-OUT TAUGHT ME:
family is what matters most

One of six Xerox employees chosen for a social service leave program in 2000, Hazel Peters-Clark, 50, spent a year with an organization for cancer patients near her Tempe, Arizona, home. She got a break from her routine, paid tribute to a sister and brother who'd died of the disease—and learned the importance of getting her priorities in order before it's too late. The result: "I've come to appreciate my time with my daughter even more. There's a calmer spirit at home."

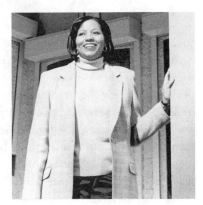

....

the deck to listen to the birds. Instead of running errands, I walked them, strolling from bank to hardware store to pharmacy. Passing a house with an open window, I heard ragtime plinking from a piano as a flabby man in boxers rocked side to side on a bench. How many days had I missed the music, I wondered. I'm determined to find a way to live like this all the time, I wrote in my journal.

But later that week, I wasn't sure I could stand my new way of life for one more day. Alone in the house on a gray morning, I wandered to my study and leafed through books on creativity. After years of working with words, I had an urge to explore other forms of artistic expression, perhaps making mosaics or collages. Problem was, I'd never tried such things before; I needed to work up the nerve. To me get started, one book suggested a "tower of pulp" exercise that was supposed to "externalize my thought processes." The idea was to create the tallest tower I could in 30 minutes, using only two sheets of newsprint and 24 inches of Scotch tape. But as I cut, folded, and twisted the paper, tangling the tape, my efficient, accomplishment-driven side wasn't buying it. This feels ridiculous, the shrill voice in my head scolded. Why don't you stop this foolishness and go clean the bathroom?

May 18 *I thought that living this way would make it easier to be mindful, but I'm finding it harder than ever. At work, I know what I need to do. Here, there are so many possibilities. Do I make soup or write a letter? Ride my motorcycle or go Rollerblading? Even when I settle on one thing, my*

mind keeps reviewing all the other possibilities.

A month passed. I filled my days pleasantly enough, yet the same conflicting emotions continued to nag. Should I explore my artistic aspirations or develop my proven talents? Spend more time with family and friends or indulge my love of solitude?

June 19 *Revelation: Chores are no less odious when one has more time for them. Another revelation: Having more time does not make one more patient. I am not in a hurry to do anything, yet . . . I still get annoyed waiting for the store clerk to write up my film processing order.*

Even without the usual forms of stress gnawing at my sleep, anxiety jolted me awake at night. Too often I lay in bed, chiding myself for not being smart enough or committed enough to my work or dedicated enough to developing my creative side. I had yearned to relive the summers of my youth, and in doing so, to become a different, better person. Yet the person I'd become felt an awful lot like the self-absorbed, insecure girl I'd been back then. I couldn't shake a growing sense of failure: In the midst of this extraordinary adventure, I was still the same scattered, obsessive mess.

And then I had a new anxiety.

July 7 *I am trying to overcome my midleave crisis—the feeling that it's going too fast. Maybe it's time for a midleave assessment to decide what it's important to do in the time left.*

I know now that almost everyone who takes a long break experiences twinges of anxiety and regret.

Toward the middle of a leave, most people feel the need for a "midterm correction" to stay on track with shifting priorities and realign their fantasies with their new reality. That's why consultants who design sabbaticals advise their clients to start with some plans and a sense of purpose but to leave plenty of room for spontaneity and chance. When you're setting off in a new direction, who knows what you'll discover along the way? When I thought about happenstance, of course, I was envisioning the merry kind that brings opportunities and delights. But when serendipity stepped in and made choices for me, it knocked me flat.

July 21 *Things have taken a most unexpected turn.*

After a weekend motorcycle trip that challenged our riding skills with thunderstorms, mud, and 100-plus-degree heat, Ray and I got home, unpacked, and gathered up our grimy clothes to put in the wash. I came up to get a few more things, and as I started down the steps, I slipped, landing on the concrete floor on my back. I lay still, afraid to move, terrified that the swelling on top of my head meant brain damage. The ambulance guys who arrived minutes later told me I'd be okay, but they strapped me onto a board and whisked me to the hospital.

Back home three days later, sporting a few bumps, a black eye, and a fractured vertebra, I could hardly be described as resting comfortably. A "turtle shell" brace—two plastic halves molded to my body and strapped together with Velcro—encased me from collarbone to pelvis. Sticky with sweat, the plastic dug into my hips whenever I moved. All I could do was prop myself up in bed or on the sofa.

The monthlong motorcycle trip was off. So were all the other activities that had filled my days. Just weeks before, I had complained of having too many options; now I had so few.

I tried to tell myself, *For now and however long it takes, my focus needs to be on healing. Everything else is secondary.* But I couldn't help feeling that serendipity had betrayed me. I had already frittered away half of my once-in-a-lifetime chance; now fate was spoiling the rest.

What I didn't realize was that fate, in fact, had intervened to give me the break I had longed for—not the way I had imagined it, but a break all the same. With my choices suddenly so limited, life had to get simpler. Time *had* to slow down.

It was my husband who started to bring me around. *Ray said this morning that he's almost glad we're staying home, because he's never had a chance to enjoy just being here. I'm trying to think that*

how to take a **time-out**

One month? Five minutes?
No matter how little time you have, there's a way to refocus and refresh.

a full-fledged sabbatical

According to a survey, 70 percent of Americans fantasize about taking off from work for several months. But few screw up the courage to approach their employer—which is too bad, because finagling a few weeks or months is often easier than people think. Here are some suggestions from *Six Months Off: How to Plan, Negotiate, and Take the Break You Need Without Burning Bridges or Going Broke,* by Hope Dlugozima, ex–*Health* senior editor James Scott, and frequent *Health* contributor David Sharp (Henry Holt, 1996):

Instead of focusing on why you can't take a break, think about what you really want to do. Read books, make lists, do research on the Internet, and brainstorm with friends until you come up with a plan that lights your fire. Next, figure out how much time you need to fulfill your fantasy. Be generous; you can always scale back. Remember: Fear of taking a risk is often the greatest impediment to getting what you desire.

Interview people who've done what you want to do. Don't just ask about the daydream—a safari in Kenya, a ceramics workshop in Japan. Pose nitty-gritty questions: "Who paid your bills while you were away? What did you do with your cat?"

If money is the main hurdle, look into grants, fellowships, scholarships, and house-swapping programs. If time is the problem, consider trading a raise or bonus for a few weeks off.

Map out as many details as necessary to make yourself feel comfortable: where to store your belongings, whether to sell your car or take it with you, and so on. Your dreams will seem more real—and more exciting. But try not to overplan the break itself; you want to allow for serendipity and spontaneity.

Before going to your boss, arm yourself with information. Find out your company's policy (official or un-) on leaves and

way—to think of this as a lovely retreat where I've come to recuperate.

August 6 *A synchronicity: One of the articles I had saved to read was on the benefits of poor health. It made the point that having to step off the*

treadmill of everyday life and let things go on without your participation can be a chance to reflect and make needed changes.

My three bouts of cancer had offered me plenty of opportunity to reflect. Yet with death so near, my impulse was not to change but to leap back on the

sabbaticals: who has taken them and under what terms, who must give the okay. Be prepared to explain how the company will benefit—or at least not suffer—from what you propose to do. (Some ideas: A rested worker is a more productive worker; varied experiences allow you to bring valuable new perspectives to the job.) Make suggestions for how your work will get done while you're away. But never, ever use the word sabbatical with your boss; it smacks of entitlement.

Get everyone on board. Loved ones and coworkers may feel envious or upset by potential disruptions in their lives. Try to involve family in the planning; stress how much happier you—and therefore they—will feel if you follow your dreams. With coworkers, point out that your absence offers an opportunity to take on more responsibility and increase their earning potential.

Don't try much during your leave. Halfway through your break, if not sooner, evaluate what you've done and give yourself permission to change direction. Make sure you have plenty of time to relax.

Take steps to fend off postsabbatical blues. Toward the end of your break, contact the office every few weeks or so. Give yourself a transition period before heading to work—the longer you've been gone, the longer the transition. Spend part of this time exploring in your journal what you learned about yourself and how you hope to change your life. Commemorate the end of your leave with some ceremony or ritual—for example, organize snapshots with your kids or hold a dinner party and slide show for friends. Ease into the grind by returning to work at midweek.

one really meaningful weekend

A long weekend vacation often just adds to overload and exhaustion. But a well-planned, seven-day "retreat"—to a spa, a mountain cabin, a plush hotel in a city you love—can be as revitalizing as a longer break (and a lot easier to arrange). The key is to clear the decks beforehand so you don't waste your time fretting about your bills or watching TV because you're too tired to do anything else. Here's some advice from Pamela Ammondson,

author of *Clarity Quest: How to Take a Sabbatical Without Taking More Than a Week Off* (Fireside Books, 1999).

Spend six weeks and months before your break making a concerted effort to get your life in order: assess your finances; declutter your home and streamline your schedule so you feel less frantic; improve your eating and exercise habits so you have more energy to make needed changes; think about your relationships and how to improve them. To accomplish these things, give yourself plenty of mental space. Get outdoors for regular doses of natural light and fresh air. Escape to a church, museum, or library for 20-minute silence and solitude breaks. Start exercising, meditating, or doing yoga.

Plan your getaway. The setting is important: It must be beautiful, restorative—and away from home (so you aren't tempted to spend time on chores). So is the season: Schedule your break at a time of year when you enjoy being outdoors.

Now, escape. Go alone. Take your journal. While you're away, spend as much time as possible in nature. Leave time to reflect on your strengths, values, dreams, and stumbling blocks.

a break in your routine

If escape is out of the question, make a full year's commitment to carve out time to do something special without disrupting your routine, suggests Mira Kirshenbaum, author of *The Gift of a Year: How to Achieve the Most Meaningful, Satisfying, and Pleasurable Year of Your Life* (Dutton, 2000). Running off to Rome might not be in the cards, but you could sign up for Italian lessons and cook a different regional menu every week.

If you can't spend the year driving cross-country, maybe you could get away for a weekend with a different friend every month .

If you can't take off all summer, at least make it more relaxing. Two ideas: Go to a four-day workweek from June through August or arrange to spend a month or six weeks working at home instead of the office. To persuade your boss to go along with it, see the advice on asking for a sabbatical.

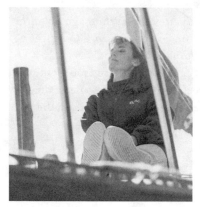

WHAT MY TIME-OUT TAUGHT ME:

i feel like a kid again

Marianne Stone, 37, of Lynbrook, New York, wanted "a summer to play" between publishing jobs. That meant figuring out how to stop chores and commitments from eating into her six-week break. Her solution: She used some vacation days before quitting work to catch up on errands. Then she spent every possible moment on the water, sailing her boat and crewing for a 72-foot tall ship.

....

treadmill as quickly as possible and get on with life as I knew it. The beauty of busyness, after all, is that it keeps your mind off your own mortality.

Now I had no choice but to change. For the first time in years, I was forced to sit still. Sometimes I stayed indoors, leafing through magazines and writing in my journal. Sometimes I sat at a table on the deck, making mosaics from shards of tile, as absorbed as a kid with crayons.

August 14 More and more, I focus on whatever I'm doing at the moment, instead of planning what I'm going to do next. I've stopped dividing up my days into impossibly short segments, trying to do a little of everything. Now, I may just read one book, not bits of several. Or I may write one letter, focusing on it, not on the half dozen I need to write next.

Before my break began, I'd wanted each day of freedom to be like a warm, sunny Saturday: so intense and delectable that it made me tingle. As my break drew to a close, those shimmering, euphoric days were now muted and melting into one another. But as their intensity faded, I realized I didn't mind at all; gone, too, was the sense of urgency and pressure. By doing less, I was somehow, magically, doing more of what I'd wanted all along—creating things for my own pleasure, caring more about satisfaction than accomplishment, letting my interests rather than my ambition drive me.

Perhaps I'd have felt this way even if I hadn't hurt my back; that's what other people who've taken long breaks tell me. Perhaps my sabbatical would have been profoundly meaningful in different ways, leading me to equally useful insights about life. All I can say is: I felt

relieved, peaceful, knowing I didn't have to wring something wonderful out of each fleeting moment. Finally, for perhaps the first time in my adult life, I knew how it felt to have all the time I needed.

I'd like to say that I haven't been the same since, that I never overload my schedule or let a day pass without claiming a chunk of it for myself. That would be a lie. Still, my life is very different these days, in ways that trace directly back to that summer. Shortly before I was due back at work, a strike put most of my coworkers, and me, eventually, on the street. When the strike went on, and on, and on, I found a new way to work, designing an eccentric five-days-in-the-office, five-days-freelancing schedule that allowed me to take new professional risks as well as creative leaps. True, I can be more oppressive than any boss, piling on assignments until I've landed, stressed out and run-down, in a doctor's office. But my schedule also lets me escape for a week if I want to or need to—and to take much of the summer off. I might never have imagined this arrangement without a respite from the nine-to-five scene.

Down in the basement workshop, meanwhile, not far from the spot where I crash-landed on my back, a couple of mosaic projects are under way. Finished ones, along with my collages, decorate all the rooms in our house. Nowadays, it seems my whole life is made up of colorful bits and pieces. But then, as my sabbatical helped me understand, so am I.

I can't point to anything concrete and say, "This is what I accomplished with my leave," but I feel so much clearer now about what is—and what is not—possible in life, I wrote as my break neared its end. *I have affirmed and clarified my priorities. I have come to accept and value all the various facets of my personality and lifestyle and to understand that I don't feel whole without all of them.*

One of the parts of me that must be honored is the dutiful worker bee who buzzes around and accomplishes like crazy. Another side is the adventurer who dreams of roaring away from responsibility on a Harley. And a third is the artist who tries to fit the

> I don't have to run away for months to be happy. I just need an occasional time-out.

pieces together in a way that pleases the eye and sustains the spirit.

The other great lesson of my break is this: I don't have to run away for months to be happy. I just need an occasional time-out—sometimes a week on my motorcycle, more often a few stolen moments here and there to breathe deeply and think.

Thank heavens I sat still long enough at least once in my life to let all the lessons sink in. ✳

Nancy Ross-Flanigan is a Health *contributing editor.*

breaking away more of life's lessons

"It's more fun to go with the flow." After nine years at a trade group in Washington, D.C., Carol Meyers, 42, took severance and spent 18 months traveling, reading, and learning to meditate, cook ethnic vegetarian dishes, and tango. A chance encounter at an art exhibit led to a trip to Ukraine, where she found long-lost relatives. One benefit of learning to trust in serendipity: She's less apt to stress out when things go wrong.

"I like being useful." A 33-year-old fitness writer (and *Health* contributor) in Santa Monica, California, Suzanne Schlosberg yearned to do something more fulfilling than telling readers how to tone their abs. Inspired by the book *Volunteer Vacations* (Chicago Review Press, 1999), she spent six months building houses in Papua New Guinea, teaching English in China, and collecting clothing for poor kids in Nebraska. Then she wrote about her hilarious adventures on www.missionimplausible.com.

"My life isn't so bad after all." A Chicago-area financial analyst with a major case of burnout, Linda Zimmerman, now 54, was granted a yearlong leave of absence to travel the world. She loved "interacting with people free of any preconceived expectations about who I ought to be." She also realized her job was more rewarding than she'd thought. So she came back early—after just nine months. Two-plus years later, she still feels refreshed.

"I don't need to be so careful." After her father's death, Susan Fitzgerald and her husband took off from work, sold their Portland, Oregon, house, and bummed around Europe for two months, following their whims. Less than a year later, at 47, she quit her job at a college to start a risky career as a freelance writer. "It's scary," she says. "But it's also thrilling."

"There's no time like the present." Terry Dorr of Milwaukee had been putting off an extended trip to her beloved France. But as she neared 49, the age of her mother's death, she realized a short visit was better than nothing. So she headed to Provence for a month with a friend to study the language and absorb the culture. Now, instead of visiting France when she retires, she hopes to live there.

"It is possible to start over." Deciding they needed "a major break," Gwendolyn Gawlick and her husband gave themselves 31 days to quit their jobs in Vancouver, B.C., and sell, store, or give away anything that didn't fit in their station wagon. Then, to relatives' horror, they set off with 18-month-old son Dallas, wandering for months before heading to Houston to visit her family. Unfettered by stuff, they gained a new appreciation for loved ones. Gawlick, 37, exults, "Life isn't written in stone."

E-therapy

Work out your issues with online counseling

Now available: online therapy with a real live shrink. Here's what happens when one woman ventures into the ether to face her issues.

BY DOROTHY FOLTZ-GRAY

"HELLO, ARE YOU THERE?" asks Dr. S. And so my therapy session begins. Yes, I respond, I'm here. Then she asks how she can help me. "I'm having trouble writing a book," I reply. I feel both excited and disembodied. It's not just because I'm about to get very personal with a complete stranger. It's because I'm not talking to my new therapist; I'm typing to her. I feel like I'm waiting for answers from a Magic 8-Ball.

I've seen a psychologist before. As a scared and suspicious 19-year-old, an identical twin thrashing through issues of separation and identity, I tried out conventional therapy. I needed to understand who I was and how I could live without depending so completely on my sister. I wound up in therapy for 12 years.

At that point, 18 years ago, I was ready to leave it

Would you try an online shrink? Sessions can be set up like a private chat room—no one but you and the therapist can see the dialogue.

behind. I didn't miss the traipsing, the fees, the commitment to a lengthy, often painful process. So when I stalled out recently on my book about being and losing a twin, I decided to try something different. I didn't think I needed intensive long-term therapy this time, but I also knew that writing about my sister's murder 19 years ago was bound to uncover emotional land mines. Online therapy beckoned.

But as Dr. S. and I met that first session, I felt skeptical. Despite her credentials, I still suspected she could be the screwball, not me. And at first I found the chat-room format annoying: I'd type an answer, and her answer to a previous comment would bubble up. Yet even within the first session, we began to find a rhythm. She asked that I put "ga"—short for go ahead—at the end of each thought to signal completion.

Although I felt like I was speaking Pig Latin, the method improved our exchange. Before long, I began to feel a listening, if ghostly, presence, and her simple phrases—"How did you feel about that?" "Tell me more."—were evoking an unexpected depth of thought. Now, instead of talking about my book, I was discussing my ambivalence about success, my father's critical eye, his own harsh father, and my mother's depression and anger. I'd come up for air and see that Dr. S. had asked a few new questions, and I would dive into those while she read my answer.

*People can use E-therapy
to work on relationships or life transitions, things
that may not warrant face-to-face therapy.*

Oddly, I couldn't see the words as I typed (a glitch the site's technical people couldn't fix). So once I started a thought, I couldn't back up. As one expert told me, online therapy can feel like writing in a diary and having the diary prod for more. I was walking a verbal plank.

I am hardly a pioneer. About a thousand therapists now offer their services on some 300 Web sites. And that doesn't count all the shrinks who augment conventional counseling with occasional E-mail sessions. The trend is fueled by people like me who have problems they'd love to iron out but who don't want long-term therapy. And for someone unnerved by the idea of face-to-face contact, it's an anonymous toe dip into counseling.

"People can use E-therapy to work on relationships or life transitions," says Storm King, past president of the International Society for Mental Health Online, an advocacy group for mental health professionals and patients, "things that may not warrant face-to-face therapy."

"Therapists are buzzing about it," says Ronnie Stangler, a clinical professor of psychiatry at the University of Washington in Seattle. "It could change the field."

Not surprisingly, online therapy isn't for everyone. Stangler says such a disembodied experience could heighten an already disturbed sense of reality, for example, or a sense of isolation. And people can easily mislead a therapist by disguising feelings. (Obviously, clients can misguide a therapist in a face-to-face

before you connect with a therapist

Say you like the sound of online therapy. Are you sure it's for you? How do you pick a shrink? And how much will it set you back? Don't fret: It's not too complicated. Here are five questions to ponder before you head to the Internet for help.

Do you belong online? Cyber-therapy is best for people who feel at home on the Web and who are able to express themselves in writing. If you're new to the Internet, E-mail, and chat rooms, online therapy may not be the place to get up to speed. And if your idea of a long letter is "Wish you were here," then take a pass.

What are your issues? Online therapy is best suited for straightforward short-term problems like career difficulties or life transitions such as moving. It can also offer people who are sad or confused a way to begin sorting through those feelings. But if you are in crisis or suicidal, contact your doctor or a local medical facility right away.

What kind of therapist? Pick a professional with a degree in a mental health field who is board-certified or has a government license. He or she should also have clinical experience obtained under supervision. If you have trouble verifying this information, you can always contact the licensing board of the state where your therapist practices to confirm his or her identity and credentials.

Should you shop around? You bet. Chat online or by E-mail with several therapists before you settle on one. Some Web sites even offer free introductory sessions. In the end, make sure you've picked somebody you can be open and comfortable with.

How mush will therapy cost? Private chat sessions can cost as much as face-to-face therapy because they tie up the doctor for just as long. Typically, half-hour sessions cost $40 to $60. Therapy by E-mail is set up differently; most professionals charge $20 to $50 per question or per E-mail exchange.

session, too, but their bodies often give their true feelings away.) An online alliance works only if both patient and therapist are bent on honesty and serious about their task.

Feeling honest and serious, I began my adventure by trolling the Web. First, I visited www.metanoia.org, a consumer guide that includes an orientation to E-therapy and a list of online counselors and their credentials. Then I checked out some sites. In the end, I picked www.here2listen.com. The site felt safe. It offers credentialed therapists whose peer references and state licenses are screened by an outside firm. And sessions can be set up like a private chat room—no one but the therapist and I could see the dialogue. (On some, therapists use E-mail rather than scheduled sessions.) I could pick a therapist by education, specialty, and a blurb each one wrote. I chose a psychologist whose focus was anxiety, low self-esteem, depression, and career issues. Me, me, me, and me.

By the third session, I was eager to chat. In therapy, I described my book as a task weighted by many burdens. No matter how well I reconstructed my sister's death, I couldn't piece back my life or hers. And what if this book never materialized, or worse, materialized and failed? How much easier to keep it hovering, perhaps like my grief, between a beginning and an end.

Dr. S. helped me untangle these problems. Slowly, the book became less ominous—a book, after all, whose pages I could work on word by word, just as I do on magazine articles. And though I had scoffed at Dr. S.'s suggestion that I write down negative thoughts as they cropped up, countering them with positive ones, I began to do just that. One day, I had a dinner party, slaving all day on Indian chicken and then obsessing that my guests hadn't liked it. Afterward, I sat up in bed, startled by my thoughts. I'd worked damn hard on that meal. It was delicious. Suddenly, it was as if Dr. S. were on my shoulder nodding. It was as easy to praise as to censor. And why not? I could like my book or not like it, fear it or not. It was my choice.

I met with Dr. S. seven times, admittedly a quick stint of therapy. Yet I felt myself relaxing, getting to

Meeting online began to feel normal, almost cozy. One day, as I chatted with Dr. S., I was lounging in my bathrobe, sipping tea.

know and trust my therapist. She had begun to ask me less generic questions that made me feel she was truly listening. As in conventional therapy, I began to feel I had an ally, someone rooting for me to retread my thinking. Meanwhile, meeting online began to feel normal, almost cozy. One day, as I chatted with Dr. S, I was lounging in my bathrobe, sipping tea. On another, I stood stretching out the kinks in my back as our session proceeded.

There were other changes, too. I was working on my book more but was being less judgmental when I needed a break. I felt more aware of how little peace I gave myself, a bully roughing my own self up at recess. If I wrote a bad line, I could hear my scolding voice rushing in to demolish my ego. So for every criticism I swallowed, I tried to respond with a positive thought.

During our last session, I told Dr. S. I'd miss her. After all, she had listened well, helping me step out of my own way. I told her I wished we could meet. And in a way we do, every time I give myself the thumbs-up. ✳

STRESS IN YOUNG WOMEN LINKED TO HEART ATTACKS

As if stress itself weren't bad enough, now there's evidence that it could put young women on a high-risk track to heart attacks later in life. Research presented earlier this year at the American Psychosomatic Society's annual meeting showed that when put in stressful situations, monkeys (which, like humans, have a 28-day menstrual cycle) produced less estrogen, a known protector against heart disease. An ongoing study of human autopsy results suggests that premenopausal women with reduced estrogen levels, which can result from stress, may react in a similar manner. So just relax—your heart will thank you.

How to ask your friends for

help

A woman under stress needn't be a damsel in distress.

BY BETH WOLFENSBERGER SINGER

Not long enough ago that I can report this without embarrassment, I found myself in an awkward place—a gutter several blocks from my house. I wasn't drunk. I wascrouched there with my two-month-old son strapped to my chest. My mission: to dangle a leash clipped to a plant-hanger hook down through a grate to snare the house keys I'd dropped while walking the dog.

The story gets dumber. I'd already returned to my house to tie up the dog and maim the plant hanger, and had observed that several neighbors were at home. I knew I should ring a doorbell, ask to phone the hubby at work, and have him drop off his keys. But no. That would disturb people. At all costs, don't disrupt anyone's day looking idiotic, I told myself as I poked through the grill, on my hands and knees, praying a car wouldn't flatten us. Just get it done. And I did.

There's something to be said for a can-do attitude, of course. This is the other thing to be said for it: patooey! Yet everywhere I look, otherwise sane women seem to suffer the same aversion to seeming needy. Personal coach Cheryl Richardson, author of *Life Makeovers* (Broadway Books, 2000) and *Take Time for Your Life* (Broadway Books, 1999), says do-it-myself-ness is so rampant among her female clients that she sometimes has them put ASK FOR HELP on their screen-savers. "We've been cultured to serve. It's

become instinctual to us. Even to think about asking for help, let alone receiving it, is foreign."

Perhaps when women spent their lives in the same village, where everybody knew one another well and had a role to play in the functioning of the community, getting help was no big deal. Going it alone was foolish, antisocial, weird. Now, though, the closest some of us come to community is the E-mail list at the office. The laborsaving, multitasking gadgets we depend on to manage our busy lives only contribute to the illusion that we can do it all—by ourselves. "We've continued to hang on to responsibility for home and family at a time when most of us work," Richardson says. "We're overwhelmed—and that just adds to our forgetfulness about asking for help. It also makes it more imperative than ever that we do it."

But how? As any woman knows, reaching out can raise issues so complicated that sometimes you'd rather just muck around in a ditch with a baby hanging from your neck. Yet this, say experts, is the point. The cure for help-o-phobia is sometimes as simple as recognizing the psychic ruts you dig for yourself and stepping around them. Here, let me give you a hand.

Jesus had 12 apostles. So go out and get 12 apostles.

You're the independent type.

Stephanie Miller, 39, is a fabulous delegator—at work. A marketing consultant in Los Angeles, she loses her chutzpah after-hours. Her mother and grandmother were very independent women. "They sure didn't ask for help," she says. Compared with them, Miller has it easy—which reinforces her sense that she has a duty to

Guess what? It's flattering to be needed.
People get tired of you always being the hero.
Asking for their help may offer them an attractive role that they don't often get to play.

fend for herself. "A feeling descends on me that I have to figure out how to do it myself. I will go to the library and research something financial, but, by God, I won't call my friend, the financial adviser. I'm the one who won't ask for directions when my husband and I are lost."

Yet being able to take care of yourself means recognizing that occasionally you do need help, experts point out. Asking a friend to give you a lift doesn't make you Rapunzel waiting to be rescued.

You're afraid of looking incompetent.

For a lot of women, this problem is especially common at the office. It starts when we get trapped in black-and-white thinking, says Sheila Heen, coauthor of *Difficult Conversations* (Penguins, 2000) and a lecturer in the art of negotiation at Harvard Law School. "We have stories we tell ourselves about ourselves," she says. " 'I'm the responsible one,' or 'I'm the person who gets things done.' If we aren't totally competent, we're totally incompetent. It becomes upsetting to ask for help then, because it's admitting you're not the person you thought you were."

Yet trying to do it all actually undermines your effectiveness and sets you up for failure. If you really want to help yourself, experts say, be realistic about what you can accomplish, set limits—and delegate early and often. Personal coach Chrissy Carew tells clients, at work or at home, to seek more support and hand off more tasks than they think they need to; this conserves time and energy for what really matters, it builds a sense of community, and serves as an example for others. "I mention Jesus," she says. "He had 12 apostles. So I have my clients go out and get 12 apostles."

You hate being obligated.

This is often related to a fear of seeming weak, says Gilda Carle, a professor of psychology and communications at New York's Mercy College and author of

Don't Bet on the Prince! (Routledge Kegan & Paul, 1989). "Women are terrified of having someone overpower us. Or we feel that we will owe someone something if we accept a favor. But in a relationship, one person is more powerful than the other at different times. If you're looking at it as people having power over you, you're doing all your relationships a disservice."

Easier said than done. One alternative is to seek help from people for whom you can do simple favors in return—for example, if you need to borrow a friend's car, offer to pick up some groceries on your way to her house. Or hire a kid to assist you and avoid that obligated feeling altogether. Carol Ann Small, of Melrose, Massachusetts, tapped a friend's 12-year-old to help her with filing and organizing. "She's very responsible, she was looking for a job, and she's the best worker," raves Small.

You don't deserve help.

As Richardson notes, women who've been trained to serve others may feel, deep down, that they don't merit the same treatment. Or they may suffer from I-made-my-own-bed-itis: They figure their busyness is their own fault—and their own problem to solve. Such women need to "take a princess pill"—to cultivate a sense of entitlement, says Lana Beckett, managing editor of an environmental newsletter in San Francisco. For Beckett, 52, this means hiring a moving company, a housekeeper, even a caterer on occasion. "Being a princess means that just because you can do something, you don't have to."

You can't stand rejection.

"Often we write a whole script in our heads," says Carle. " 'He might say no. Maybe he doesn't really like me.' We dramatize and do a number on ourselves." The first step, she says, is to train yourself to let others make their own decisions. Even very busy people may surprise you and come through. Next step: Try not to take rejection so personally. Remember, "no" usually means "no for now," not "no forever."

You don't want friends to feel pressured.

No one wants to dump their problems on harried friends and coworkers. Though this seems the opposite of hating rejection, the same advice applies. Just make it very clear that "no" is an option.

Also, start paying attention to your own tendencies to reject offers, Richardson suggests. "Do you have a friend saying to you, 'Let me take the kids for an afternoon'? Most women will turn down help out of guilt or not wanting to impose. Be generous in your willingness to let someone take care of you."

You can't trust others to do things right.

"This is a generalization, but women try to do everything themselves so it is done perfectly," says Talane Miedaner, author of *Coach Yourself to Success* (McGraw Hill, 2000). Perfectionism may work for Martha Stewart, but for the rest of us it's a prescription for anxiety, depression, and stress, psychologists say. Realize that if you spread your energies too thin and your performance suffers, you won't live up to your own high standards, either. It's easier to delegate responsibility if, instead of measuring other people against yourself at your relaxed and upbeat best, you measure them against the burned-out, crabby nutcase you become when you're overextended.

You shouldn't have to ask for help.

Many women secretly believe that if people truly cared, they'd notice when we need them. "That assumption really disables you," says Heen. "Good relationships don't mean you can read each other's minds; they mean you can share your mind. Asking for something should not diminish the worth of getting it."

finding a personal coach

Personal coaches are experts at helping people solve problems and get their lives on track. For information, contact Coach U (800-482-6224; www.coachu.com) or the International Coach Federation (888-423-3131; www.coachfederation.org).

Another reason to ask: It's flattering. "People get tired of you always being the hero," Heen says. "If you ask for help and express appreciation, it can be a very attractive role you're offering someone, a role they don't often get to play for you."

You are asking for help, but no one seems to hear.

If you're not getting results from requests, scrutinize whether you're asking clearly. Women sometimes have trouble being direct; vagueness is ineffective, and it can seem manipulative. Other common problems: feeling so defensive while making a request that you send out I-don't-really-need-you signals, and making your requests too broad.

For example, says Heen, "If you're overwhelmed at work, don't say, 'This deadline is just totally unrealistic,' because what you're saying to me is that I'm an unrealistic person, so I'm going to defend myself rather than hear that you need help."

A better approach: "I'm feeling really overwhelmed, and I'm worried that I'm not going to be able to get this done. Part of this has to do with me, and part of it has to do with our staffing right now. Let's talk about what to do."

You're out of practice.

"Ask for something small first," suggests Richardson. "Ask a waiter to serve your food differently, a friend for advice, a family member to baby-sit. It gets easier." Miedaner teaches her clients to delegate by having them list 10 chores they could hand off. The next step: farming out their least favorite.

A new puppy provided practice for Jill Silverman, of Charlestown, Massachusetts, who says her people-pleasing tendencies were her biggest impediment to asking for help. Under Carew's guidance, Silverman turned first to professional dog walkers. Next, she found kids in her building whose mother wanted them to learn responsibility and who were willing to play with the pup for a little cash. Before long, other neighbors were offering to take the dog for the night or the weekend when Silverman was away.

Now, Silverman says, "I'm really comfortable asking for help these days." Both she and her dog are happier for it. ✳

NEED A MOOD BOOSTER?
Get a whiff of this!

People have been using fragrance to cure what ails them for thousands of years. Yet until recently, scientists have viewed aromatherapy as hocus-pocus. Now, researchers are finding that some scents really can give you a psychological lift.

BOOST YOUR CONFIDENCE. In a recent study, the pungent aroma of peppermint helped college athletes perform better with less effort, or at least it made them feel like superstars. In fact, according to such measurements as heart rate and blood pressure, the athletes got just as much benefit from the scent of jasmine and a stinky chemical called dimethyl sulfite. But in sports, believing you have a mental edge can translate into the real thing—and that's all that matters, right?

CALM YOURSELF DOWN. When you're anxious, sniff something that you associate with a more relaxed time in your life, suggests Will A. Wiener, Ph.D., a psychologist and director of the Institute for Performance Enhancement in Manhattan. This strategy has helped one of Wiener's clients, a professional basketball player who gets petrified at the free-throw line. Just before he shoots a basket, the player buries his nose in a handkerchief scented with a loved one's favorite cologne. The smell allows him to block out the jeering crowd and concentrate.

KEEP YOUR FOCUS. Researchers in Miami found that adults who sniffed lavender before and after tackling simple math problems worked faster, felt more relaxed, and made fewer mistakes. The fragrant herb can also improve your nights: In a small study, a British doctor found that lavender helped elderly insomniacs fall asleep sooner and slumber longer than sedatives did.

Q+A If autumn brings depression, try this
I always get depressed when the days get shorter in the fall. What can I do?

It's not uncommon to feel a little seasonal sadness. The shorter days may leave you moody, irritable, or down. For most people, just 20 minutes a day of exposure to very bright light—10 to 20 times brighter than ordinary indoor light—is the answer. Take advantage of sunny days and have your coffee break outside, or take a walk during lunch. Regular exercise could also offer an emotional lift.

If you find that your depression is lingering for several weeks, you should consult a doctor. You may have Seasonal Affective Disorder (SAD). About 35 million Americans, women more often than men, will experience this severe depression with the onset of fall. Experts believe it is caused by the decline in the amount of light that reaches your eyes. Using a light box, which provides fluorescent, full-spectrum light, might help. Your doctor may also recommend regular light therapy or antidepressants.

chapter 8

relationships
and sex

a road map through the maze of love and family

girlfriends
the ultimate support system

Author Patricia Gottlieb Shapiro explores the rewards
and challenges of female friendship.

BY SU REID

While interviewing women for a book about life during the empty-nest years, Philadelphia freelance writer Patricia Gottlieb Shapiro was struck by how many mentioned the importance of female friendships. Curious to explore the subject further, she spent three months traveling across America to talk to women in more detail about their friendships. The result was *Heart to Heart: Deepening Women's Friendships at Midlife* (Berkley Publishing Group, 2001).

The book's subjects, women between the ages of 45 and 60, rated their friendships with other women among the most significant relationships in their lives. As one woman boldly put it, "If somebody said you couldn't have both your girlfriends and your husband, I think I'd give up my husband and keep my girlfriends. He's the kindest man going, but they fill more of an emotional need for me than he does." Another said, "Each of my friends represents a different part of me that needs nurturing."

Finding new friends is very similar to dating: It may take a while to find women you click with.

Shapiro believes friendship is an investment in the future. "Your friendships with other women are going to be longer and truer than just about any other relationship—so hold on to them," she says. "These are the people who will sustain you over the years." Shapiro took a few minutes to talk with us further about the power of female friendships.

health: Why are friendships among women so important?
Shapiro: No matter what their age, women need a sense of connection with people who are more or less their contemporaries. That's how we grow and realize who we are. A really good woman friend is very accepting, supportive, and nonjudgmental. She makes you feel as if you are understood. Your family knows you, too, but with them you play a certain role; you're looked at in a certain way. Women want to feel they can be authentic, be themselves, and friends allow them to do that.

health: What steps can women take to keep their friendships strong?
Shapiro: Rituals are really important. They help us stop and reflect on what's happening, and they are an

effective way to cement a friendship. For example, Sarah (all names Shapiro mentions have been changed) was experiencing a very difficult year: Her husband and one of her parents had died, and her daughter had left for college. On her 50th birthday, Sarah, who is a massage therapist, felt she had to do something to celebrate. So she invited her six closest friends over—all happened to be massage workers—and they each massaged a part of her body and sang songs to her. While not everyone would want that, it was just what Sarah needed.

It's important that women not only listen to and support their friends, but also share their thoughts and feelings with them. As Meg, one of the women I interviewed, said, "When someone confides in me, it's a gift. It says, 'I trust you.'"

Just saying "you're important to me" or "I value our relationship" can really strengthen a friendship.

health: What are some of the challenges that women face while trying to remain close to their friends?

Shapiro: I think that issues dealing with negative emotions—envy, anger, competition—are difficult for women. It really does benefit the friendship if the women can recognize those feelings when they have them and try to handle them openly. One woman said to me, "My friendships are more important to me than any minor annoyances," but the fact is, that minor annoyance can affect your friendship.

I'll give you an example of envy. Barbara had an undergraduate degree and was very jealous of Deena, who had a graduate degree. As a result, Barbara was very tongue-tied

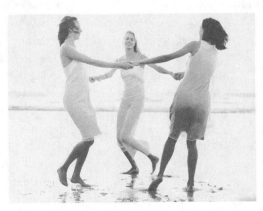

around her friend. She wasn't herself. She didn't know what to say; she was just really uncomfortable with this woman. Luckily, she finally realized that what she really wanted wasn't to take Deena's degree away but to have one of her own. So she rechanneled her energy into figuring out how to do that.

Another challenge that women, especially younger ones, often face is when a new man enters the picture. Many women get so excited when a guy comes along that they temporarily drop their friends. What they need to do is be up front with them, perhaps saying something like, "It's not that I don't care about you, but right now I need to spend a lot of time with this new person." They also need to realize in looking at the long term that relationships with friends are often truer and last longer than a relationship with a guy.

health: How can a woman with few close female friends expand her circle?

Shapiro: One thing she can do is think about who she knows and might like to know better. It might be somebody from work, a woman in her aerobics class, or a neighbor—somebody to whom she might say hello, but that's it. Some people feel comfortable saying, "I'd like to get to know you better. Let's go out and have coffee." Or "I'd like to build a friendship with you—are you interested?" But if the woman doesn't feel comfortable actually saying that, she can use her actions to show her interest. For example, she could begin to wave to her neighbor across the drive, then one day she could say, "Why don't you come in and have a cup of tea?" And then they have the opportunity to sit down and talk to each other.

Women need strong friendships with other women; those relationships often are truer and last longer than those with men. A good first step to expanding your circle is to think of someone you know casually—at work, in your aerobics class, or in the neighborhood—and ask her out for coffee.

health: It actually sounds very similar to the dating process.

Shapiro: Yes, it is. Because the two women may have coffee and find out that they're not right for each other—maybe there's no spark there. Or perhaps they have coffee and find they have 10 things in common. So it's a process of getting to know each other, but each woman has to put herself out there. That's scary for some women. They're afraid they might be rejected.

health: Talk about women's relationships with their mothers. How do they affect friendships?

Shapiro: What women learn from their mothers about friendship is often what they bring into their own relationships. A woman's relationship with her mother is the very first one she has with another woman, and it sets a sort of subconscious pattern for her. She may have certain issues relating to her mother that she isn't even aware of, and those can play out in her friendships.

health: Can you give us an example?

Shapiro: Nora grew up an only child to a mother who had no friends. For years, Nora didn't have any friends either; she just subconsciously copied her mother's pattern. As she got older, she realized something was missing in her life, so she set out to make friends and build a group around her. She looked at her two passions—photography and hiking—and then signed up for a hiking trip and joined a photography club. Eventually, she developed some good friends, and they were able to give her the support and strength she needed to face the isolation she'd felt in the past. Nora was successful because she made a very conscious effort; some people just drift along, busy with work, and never realize they don't have any friends. What we need to remember is that while our families may provide the training grounds for our friendships, in the end, it's up to us. ✳

Su Reid is a Health *assistant editor.*

TEST YOURSELF
How sex-savvy are you?

SO YOU'RE AN AVID *SEX AND THE CITY* WATCHER, and you love to browse through *Cosmo* in the grocery-store checkout line. Is everyone out there really having more sex than you are? Test your knowledge of what lies between the sheets.

1. On average, who claims to make love most often?
   A. men   B. women

2. The average number of sexual partners is:
   A. 4   B. 8   C. 12   D. 16

3. Which country's citizens claim to be enjoying the most sex—to the tune of 132 times a year?
   A. America   B. France   C. Brazil

4. Which group is the most sexually active?
   A. married people   B. singles   C. couples living together

ANSWERS

1. A. Men. Go figure. Globally, people claim to have sex an average of 96 times a year, according to the Durex Global Sex Survey. Men claim to make love more often than women, saying they have 103 sessions a year, compared with the 88 that women report.

2. B. The French topped the list with a reported average of 17 partners. Americans averaged 12 partners. Indians came in last, with 82 percent reporting just one partner.

3. A. Debunking stereotypes, Americans out-sex French and Latin lovers.

4. C. With 146 sessions a year, couples living together top the list. Married people rank next, claiming 98 sessions. Single life isn't quite so spicy—those not married or cohabitating report having sex 49 times a year.

betting on intuition

Corporate giants nationwide are investing in intuition as a management tool. But can you train people to trust their hunches?

BY KATY KOONTZ

Marcia Emery, Ph.D., has just passed a conch shell to each person at a Junior League-sponsored business seminar in Atlanta. Emery asks the sharp-suited female executives to study the shell's intricate geometric pattern as a way of helping their minds shift from the usually dominant, logical left-brain mode into the realm of the right brain, the home of creativity and imagination. She punctuates the session with deep-breathing exercises and guided visualization, all in an effort, she says, to help the participants unlock their innate intuitive powers.

Obviously, this isn't your typical how-to-deal-with-difficult-people workshop, and Emery isn't your typical business consultant. Emery, a psychologist and "intuition trainer," leads classes for some of the largest corporations in the world—Hewlett Packard and Xerox among them—who hope that encouraging their employees to develop their intuition will give their companies a competitive edge in this volatile economy.

Intuition is that gut feeling you get when you know instinctively what to do—but aren't quite sure why.

Industry giants wouldn't be investing their dwindling dollars in something so seemingly esoteric without good reason. New research is helping to legitimize intuition by expanding scientists' understanding of the phenomenon and quantifying its effects. And while their findings are still considered controversial, there is growing evidence that intuition is a teachable skill that everyone can use to make better decisions—in everything from hiring an employee to choosing a day care.

Emery, who is also the author of *PowerHunch* (Beyond Words Publishing, 2001), first discovered her own intuitive power through a series of dreams in 1970. In the first dream, she wrecked her car when her brakes failed but walked away unharmed. Exactly three weeks later, she says, the dream came true: Her brakes failed, she totaled her car, and she suffered only a few scratches.

A month after that, she had a similar dream in which her brakes went out again. Three days later, the scene unfolded just as it had in her sleep—right down to coasting to a "No Parking" sign and asking a policeman for help so she wouldn't miss a meeting.

Now Emery uses what she's since learned about intuition to train employees on such topics as how to anticipate a co-worker's needs and how to figure out the right time to make a major life change. She is one of about a dozen intuition trainers in the United States working with companies such as AT&T, Dow Chemical, and Microsoft. "Intuition has become a breakthrough management tool," Emery says. "It helps companies ride the wave of rapid change and gives leaders shortcuts for solving problems."

While experts define intuition as knowing something you have no logical way of knowing, it may help to think of it as the gut feeling you get when you instinctively know what to do in a certain situation—but you don't quite know why. Many corporations prefer words like "vision," "creativity," "innovation," and even "whole-brain training" when referring to intuition.

Semantics aside, Joyce Wycoff, co-founder of Innovation Network, a national organization enhancing creativity and innovation, says the business world has become increasingly more open to exploring this topic in the eight years since her organization was founded. "Businesses are definitely more interested in nonanalytical, nonlinear approaches to decision-making and information-gathering," she says.

Dow Chemical spokeswoman Karen Robertson says that her company has offered executives creativity courses that involve intuitive skills for about a decade. Now the company is offering the courses to all its employees. Course creator Andy Hines explains that the seminars "give employees a sense of how intuitive they may already be, teach tools for tapping into that intuition, and discuss research showing that, overall, they can trust their hunches." Although Robertson says it's impossible to know how the training has affected workers' productivity and the company's bottom line, she adds that such seminars are a valuable part of corporate growth. "We need to focus on innovation in every function," she says. "This is one way to achieve it."

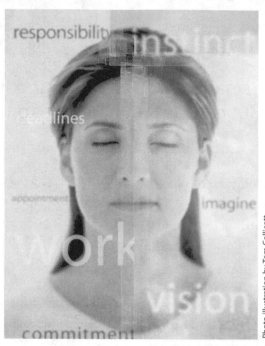

Photo illustration by Tom Collicott

Intuition began gaining legitimacy among scientists back in 1995, when Dean Radin, Ph.D., then-director of the Consciousness Research Division of the Harry Reid Center for Environmental Studies at the University of Nevada-Las Vegas, first started studying it. Radin hooked up test subjects to electrodes to monitor skin resistance—one of the methods used in lie-detector tests to measure emotional changes. Then he left them in a room alone to watch various images—some designed to provoke forceful emotions (like a car crash or mutilated bodies) and others calm emotions (like nature scenes)—flash in random order on a computer screen. "One in 10 study subjects showed a significant increase in arousal two seconds before the disturbing images appeared," Radin says, "and a drop in arousal before the calm images." These folks didn't consciously know a gruesome scene was about to pop up, but their bodies sensed it and responded subconsciously through their nervous systems.

Now, as senior scientist for northern California's Institute of Noetic Sciences, a research group that studies the brain, Radin has refined the test to measure other nervous-system responses, including skin temperature, respiration rate, and fingertip blood volume. His tests using these indicators have affirmed his earlier results.

There is no research to prove the age-old notion of "women's intuition," but there is some evidence that certain types of people are more intuitive than others. Using a test called the Ganzfeld technique, Kathy Dalton, Ph.D., a visiting scientist at the Rhine Research Center in Durham, North Carolina, found that musicians, visual artists, fiction writers, and actors seem to have stronger intuitive powers than others. In the test, two people sit in separate rooms.

One, the "receiver," is cut off from sound and visual stimulation; the other, the "sender," watches a randomly selected video clip repeatedly (anything from the tidal wave scene in *Clash of the Titans* to a Bugs Bunny cartoon). The receiver is then asked to identify the clip from four possibilities and describe any intuitive impressions. An independent judge reviews both the clips and transcripts of the receivers' comments in evaluating the results. The average person is right 34 percent of the time, a figure that has held fairly constant over the past 26 years. In Dalton's 1997 study, though, a group of creative people had a rate of 47 percent—about double the rate of random guessing.

"These people report that they rely more on hunches and gut reactions, so that makes sense," Dalton says. "They seem to process information differently than the rest of us, although we don't understand the process yet."

Now Dalton is examining the intuition skills of people who are related to one another. Early studies have suggested that parent–child pairs or sibling pairs may score an average of 60 percent. "It's possible that we all have this ability to some degree," she says. "Some of us are born with a lot, and some are born with very little, but we've probably always had it."

Larry Burk, M.D., the director of education for the Duke Center for Integrative Medicine, agrees, although he acknowledges the science of intuition has a long way to go. "There's been a startling lack of research done on intuition," Burk says. "But I believe it's starting to change. Now people feel safer talking about intuition because it's a buzzword in the business community." And while Burk thinks that the research will grow over the next few years,

seven tips for flexing your intuitive muscle

Corporate consultant and intuition trainer Marcia Emery, Ph.D., says you can strengthen your intuitive skills. Here are her tips for dialing up your natural intuitive ability.

• **Get calm.** If you can't meditate, at least do some relaxation exercises or deep breathing, take a long walk, work in the garden, or just retreat to a private room. Anything that quiets the mind will help.

• **Look at** a geometrical object or pattern (even if it is only in the wallpaper or wood grain) or listen to music that doesn't have words. These practices engage the right brain and help quiet the left brain.

• **Play with intuition.** Try to guess what someone will be wearing tomorrow, what a person you are meeting for the first time will look like, which is the quickest line at the bank, or which row has the best parking space.

• **Keep a log** of both intuitive hunches (also recording how you got them) and dreams so you can better understand the patterns of your type of intuition.

• **Beware** of emotional culprits such as wishful thinking and fear, which can sabotage your attempts. Stay as neutral as possible.

• **Lighten up.** Too much effort backfires, while laughter and fun help ideas and intuition flow more easily.

• **Avoid rigid expectations** about how intuition will come. Some people are visual, some notice different feelings in their bodies, and some may hear ideas.

Trainers claim that everyone can use intuition to make better decisions—from hiring to choosing day care.

he acknowledges that no amount of science will ever be enough to convince some people. Companies may continue to invest in intuitive trainers, and researchers may indeed make groundbreaking discoveries about the intuitive process. But for many people, the only real evidence is firsthand knowledge. "What prompts certain people to believe in something like this isn't science," Burk says. "It's personal experience." And that is one thing that isn't likely to change. ✳

Tennessee-based freelancer Katy Koontz also writes for Shape *and* Parenting.

So you've got no mate, and you're wondering who'll hold your hand in lonely times. Just when will that perfect someone finally show his face?

going solo

when looking for Mr. Right is all wrong

Four women whose lives are different from what they'd imagined discover something unexpected: Living single has helped them find out who they are—and what they want from life.

PHOTOGRAPHY BY BROWN W. CANNON III

LOOKING FOR
MR. PERFECT NO MORE

Lindsey Crittenden

Two months ago, my good friend Ann got married. She and I were supposed to grow old together, single. Two eccentric women on a park bench, we used to joke. So when she met Frank, I was a bit wary. He was recently divorced, with three kids under the age of 10. Be careful, I said, when she told me of a date spent watching the oldest child play soccer, while the ex-wife sat two rows away. Make sure you get what you need.

I'd seen marriage change some of my friends. I'd listened as Catie substituted "we" for "I," as get-togethers that once would have happened spontaneously now required weeks of advance notice. I'd heard a slight formality in Brenda's voice the night she phoned to tell me of her engagement, as if she, my best high school buddy, were going underground.

Ann in love, however, was still the Ann I loved. A forthright friend, she used to keep that best side of herself under wraps with the men she dated. But as I listened to her talk to Frank, speaking her mind with confidence, I knew the mask was off. The woman who used to fret over whether she'd said the right thing to some guy was now determined to be liked for who she is. In college, when she urged me to part my hair on the side the night of a big date, she'd expanded my sense of romantic possibilities. Now, by falling in love with a man with whom she could be utterly herself, she was doing it again.

Back in my 20s, during the first wave of weddings among my friends, I told myself (and others) that I was waiting for Mr. Right. But my fantasy groom was a blur, like a digitally altered photo of someone in the Witness Protection Program, while around him the trappings—the flowers, the receiving lines, my hair—sparkled in crisp Technicolor. I'd know him when I met him, I figured. In the meantime, I shrugged when asked why Scott and I had broken up, or why I wasn't interested in Kyle. I don't know, I'd say. Not my type. The truth was, I really didn't know. For years, my approach to dating resembled my response to overly solicitous salespeople: "Just looking, thanks."

As I moved into my 30s, I thought it might help to think in terms of specifics. He will be taller than I am and outdoorsy. He'll like diner breakfasts, stinky cheeses, and his work. He'll have a head for numbers and be gentle with little children, animals, and my moods. I dated men who appeared to fit the bill. There was Chris, who talked enthusiastically about his job—but when he went on at length about his druggy past, I couldn't ignore the feeling in the pit of my stomach. Then came Will, a swimmer with a great smile—though not great enough to make up for the fact that he was vague about an entire decade of his life.

My list of specifics, I've now realized, was only short-hand for what really matters. My college boyfriend and I had both stood 5 foot 10 in our bare feet, but that had done little to dampen our ardor. Shared food proclivities might make for a pleasant meal, but not necessarily fireworks or even compatibility. I'd pursued a few men for certain commonalities, but on the larger things—the way they talked (or didn't) about themselves, how open (or closed) they were about family and faith and future—they had let me down.

Ann, it turns out, has done more than leave me behind. By finding, at an age the odds frown upon, commitment and love without selling herself short, she's given me hope and taught me an important lesson. She found a best friend and a partner not by hunting down the embodiment of the perfect traits or by wearing bright colors (as one friend advised when I told her I'd met a man I liked), but by being comfortable with who she is and by being open to the surprise

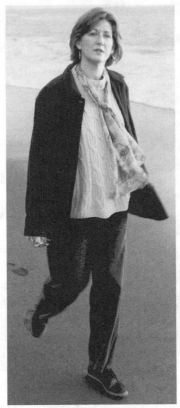

Lindsey Crittenden:
"Mr. Right is a real guy, flawed but whole."

of the unknown. Ten years ago, Ann wouldn't have looked twice at a divorced man. She'd never had a long-term relationship before Frank, but she stepped into it as if she'd been born for it. She found the perfect guy; he just happened to come with three kids.

Singlehood isn't an endurance race with a bow-wrapped mate at the finish line, any more than it is our own fault for spending too many Saturday nights with public television. It might be something that we actively choose or something we curse each and every February 14—or a little of both. But either way, it's a journey that shows us a few things, so that when the happy accident of fate or luck brings the right person into our life, we'll be more likely to recognize him.

As I approach 40 and another year of filing "Single" on my tax return and wondering if I'll ever kiss anyone again, Mr. Right is as elusive as ever. But he's no longer a gray blur amidst the silk and flowers. He's a real guy, flawed but whole—the way, on a good day, I think of myself.

Lindsey Crittenden is a freelance writer.

BABY? DEFINITELY. HUSBAND? MAYBE LATER.
Deb Levine

It is clear to me that I have none of the accoutrements considered necessary to be a successful contemporary American woman: (1) a full-time job, (2) a spouse, and (3) children. I am 38 years old, and in the eyes of my family—my mother, at least—a big disappointment.

Now, mind you, I know there are alternatives to these three imperatives. I have a busy freelance career as a sexual-health educator, an advice columnist, and a consultant. I've had several long-term relationships

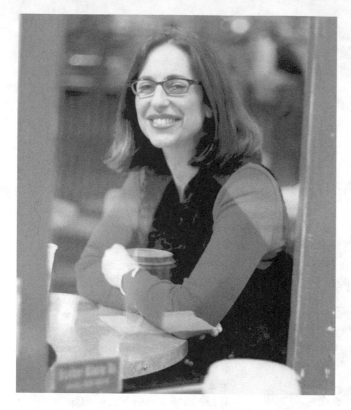

and many lovers. The family thing, though: I still haven't got a family of my own.

My salvation turns out to be my good friend Mark. He's gay. We've known each other for 20 years, but I had no idea that he wanted to have children until one day when I launched into my standard monologue about my burning desire to have a kid (or two or three). I was lamenting approaching 40 with no man—and therefore no kids—in sight, when Mark started to pout. My eyes widened. "Mark, really? You want kids?" He nodded emphatically, a nod that marked the beginning of a long journey for both of us.

And so, even though in our society the love is supposed to come first, I've made a conscious decision that it's baby first, man later. I've been testing out the idea on my friends. The responses: "But why Mark? Why not pick a good-looking guy like me?" from an old boyfriend. "Deb, this is fantastic! I owe you so much baby-sitting! Are you going to use a turkey baster or what?" from an unwed mom who has two kids of her own. And from my friend Frank: "Big

news, Deb. But don't you think you should wait one more year? I mean, to find someone to do it with?" But Frank, darling, I thought I already had.

Mark found a sample baby contract on the Web. We asked each other the suggested questions: What are your values? How do you handle your finances? What's your family's health history? Then it got tough: Do you plan to move anytime in the future? Will you have lovers? How do you think that will affect your child—and you? Even though Mark and I have been good friends for a long time, the honesty this demanded took us to a new level of intimacy.

I recently had a fantastic date with a guy my age. He told me that an ex-girlfriend had called him on her 40th birthday and asked him to father her child. Because he didn't want to get back together with her, he told her a baby was out of the question. Given my own preoccupation, it didn't strike me that she wanted to be with him again; I simply assumed she needed a sperm donor. I couldn't help but wonder if he'd understand my having a kid with someone I wasn't in love with. Not wanting to jeopardize a potential relationship on the first date, I chose to wait to tell him about Mark.

My friend Laura asked me why I'm dating at all. "You've got enough on your plate with this whole baby contracting thing," she said. "Why add the complexities of other men?" I didn't tell her the truth, which is that I want to be loved so badly that sometimes I wonder if I'm having this child for all the wrong reasons. I need to make sure I'm doing it for the right reasons, and dating helps keep the relationship thing separate from the baby thing. My biggest fear about having a kid with Mark is that it will end my chances of finding an adult partner. I'm afraid I'll be too tired, too emotionally unavailable even to look for "the one." I'm dating now because I want to know there are some guys out there (just one guy will do) who could love me—with my neuroses, my child, and the gay father of my child. You've got to admit, it's quite a package.

The contract is going back and forth

I want to be loved so badly that sometimes I wonder if I'm having this child for all the wrong reasons.

between Mark and me. Most children are conceived after a great (or mediocre) romp in the hay; our child will become part of the world under meticulously planned circumstances. I can only hope that the amount of time and energy we're putting into this before the fact sets us up for good communication once we become parents. We're equipped as fully as we can be for this one—emotionally, financially, and physically. It's a risk, but it's one we're ready to take. It's unconventional, but it's going to work for me. I'm a very practical woman.

Deb Levine lives in San Francisco.

STEPPING OFF THE MOMMY TRACK
Laura Fraser

In the back of my closet, there's a box with a set of maternity clothes inside. They're my size—or would be if I were pregnant. Each time I sift through my stuff to give away things I no longer wear, I pause and hold that box in my hand, considering. It was a little premature, I admit, to buy maternity clothes before the stick had turned blue. But five years ago, when I saw that big-bellied black minidress and tunic top, I was so sure I was soon to become one of those hip moms-to-be that I bought them anyway.

The box sat in the back of the closet while my husband and I made up baby names and debated whether we could afford to move to a neighborhood with better schools. It was still there on the day I decided to go off the Pill, which was, not coincidentally, the day my husband suggested that perhaps we should wait, that he wasn't quite sure he was ready to have a baby.

Just a few weeks later, the box got more room in the closet when my husband moved his clothes out. Not only had he realized he didn't want to have a baby, but he didn't want to be with me, period. I was 36, and

Laura Fraser: *"I think of how I'll never have a daughter my age when I'm 70, and never have grandchildren. In those moments, the loss is overwhelming."*

heartbroken. Still, I wasn't worried about not having a family. I figured it wouldn't be long before I found a new husband—a dad for the children I always took for granted I would someday have.

But it wasn't so easy to find that new guy. Being single with 40 on the near horizon was quite different from flitting about on the wide plains of 30. A lot of men seemed nervous that a woman my age might be more interested in finding a father for her unborn child than in finding a partner for herself. They seemed to have a sixth sense that a woman my age might be, well, a woman like me.

Then 36 passed, and 37, ticktock, and 38. Obviously, I've never made having children the highest priority in my life. Like many women my age, I've always paid more attention to my work, my sweetie, and my travel plans than to when I was going to have kids. I had pressed the snooze button on my biological clock, assuming I'd just wake up one day with children bouncing on the bed.

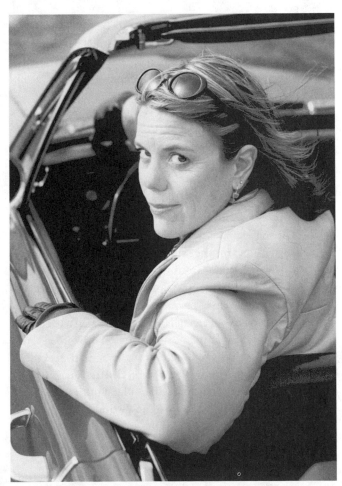

Why not reverse the order of my plans:
First have the child and then find the man? Men, after all, age better than eggs. I knew myself well enough to know that being a single mother simply wouldn't be a wise move.

But when I didn't land another mommy-track relationship right away, I had to confront the question of having a child on my own. Why not reverse the order of my plans: First have the child and then find the man? Men, after all, age better than eggs.

For months I imagined having a baby, somehow, on my own. I'd wrap her up like a papoose and take her to my office, where she would sleep quietly while I worked. I'd bundle him in his stroller, and he'd nap while I went to the gym. I'd come home, fix myself a nice dinner with a glass of wine, curl up with a long novel, and she'd be right there, snoozing along. The only problem was that in my fantasies of being a single mom, the kid slept all the time. Not a good sign.

There are people who can handle being single parents. I admire them. I just have a feeling I wouldn't be one of them. Aside from my somewhat precarious financial situation, I have an independent streak a mile wide. I've managed my career with the goal of being my own boss. Having a child might teach me patience, but I'm no saint. I'd need someone to hand the child off to once in a while. And I would have to give up many of the things I cherish—traveling, making spontaneous plans, spending time alone. I'd be willing to make those sacrifices, but not without some company. Not by myself.

Ultimately, I knew myself well enough to know that being a single mother simply wouldn't be a wise move. But I wasn't having any luck on the finding-a-dad front, either. Babies just don't seem to be in the cards for me, not in this lifetime.

I feel fine about my decision until I catch a toddler's smile while standing in line at the post office. I yearn to smell that hair, to touch those tiny toes, to feel that in a world of so many disappointed affections, someone loves me unconditionally, at least until that someone turns 13. I think of how wonderful my relationship with my parents is these days and that I'll never have a daughter my age when I'm 70, and never

have grandchildren. In those moments, the loss is overwhelming.

But letting go of the idea of having children has also brought me a sense of clarity. I want to find a partner who fits into the rhythm of my heart, not one who merely shares my interest in procreation. In the meantime, I have several nephews, a niece, and a small boy next door who adores me—and vice versa. I'm the crazy aunt who wouldn't have half as much time to bang on drums, send postcards from exotic places, and write Christmas stories if she had children of her own.

I've just turned 40, and while I know that I probably have a few years left to have a child, the chances aren't good. I've come to accept that, and I've gotten on with my life. Still, I'm not throwing away that box in the back of my closet. Not quite yet.

Laura Fraser's new book, An Italian Affair, *is published by Pantheon Books (2001).*

ON OUR OWN—TOGETHER
Louise Rafkin

Two years ago, my partner died suddenly. I was lost and, for the first time ever, afraid to be alone. It wasn't fear of external intruders but of internal demons: overwhelming grief, loneliness, and sometimes the feeling that I was incapable of caring for myself. My notions of the future evaporated; I had no idea of how I would continue on my own.

My partner and I had lived here, in this small two-bedroom cottage, for four years. Just beyond the edge of the grass and flower beds is a studio apartment we used as an office. Next to that is a one-bedroom cottage, then occupied by a couple who answered an ad I'd put in the paper. We were friendly, of course, but never even shared a meal.

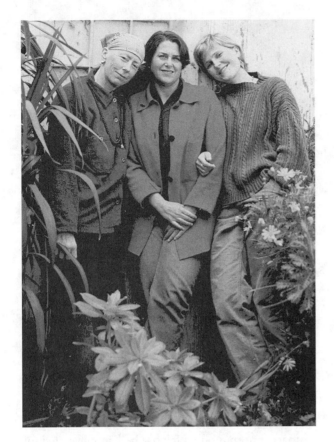

Louise Rafkin (center), with Coleen and Erika: *"We've stitched our friend-ship into something that has the distinct flavor of family."*

Coleen, who's enduring a difficult recovery from surgery. This morning, a glance across the yard reveals a perky Coleen, already on her way to the gym. Lucy greets her and, taking Col's hand in her soft retriever mouth, escorts her to the front gate.

The three of us, I believe, live with just the right amount of togetherness. We've stitched our friendships into something that has the distinct flavor of family. Expectations are few and unencumbered by the complicated emotions that come with more intimate relationships. Our back doors are usually ajar, if not wide open. We share what we can, when we can, be it an egg or an afternoon.

The give-and-take is fluid. As my sadness subsided, I was able to reach out to Coleen, shopping and driving for her during the worst parts of her treatment. She did the same for me when I had a knee operation. While I was on crutches, Erika took an ever-grateful Lucy for her daily walk. For Erika, Coleen is a new friend who shares her love of music. Coleen, I think, is comforted just by knowing that there's someone near.

My abrupt transition to solo life was eased enormously when my friend Erika moved into the back cottage. Those first months, knowing that Erika was just across the yard (and would probably be at my breakfast table) was as important to my recovery as all the hours I spent in therapy. I needed someone near, but not too close. I needed room to fall apart, but I was desperately lonely.

It's comforting to know there's someone ready to just sit on the bed and chat.

And then Coleen, a friend of 20 years who lived around the corner, was diagnosed with cancer. Knowing how hard it would be to manage alone, she left her somewhat isolated apartment and moved into the studio.

Now I share my cottage with my four-legged pal, Lucy the black Lab. My desk faces a window through which most every morning I can watch the hummingbirds practice their dainty acupuncture among the purple tendrils of the Mexican sage. Before I've brewed my first cup of coffee, I often hear Erika working on a new composition, Latin riffs rising up from the basement of her cottage. And as I open the back door to let Lucy outside, I check for the stirring of

I don't know how long our homestead will remain the way it is. There is talk of Coleen moving to a bigger place, and murmurs of Erika going to Seattle with her partner. But if I have learned anything these last years, it's that life is unpredictable. For now we are here, sharing our daily lives in ways we could not have foreseen, but that we—and I think I speak for all of us—cherish. It's impossible for me to make it through the difficult times alone, and living here—this way, with these women—has shown me that I don't have to.

Even Lucy is a convert to this way of life. From my window I watch her roam from cottage to studio, offering her company and basking in the love that comes in return. ✳

Louise Rafkin is a writer in Emeryville, California.

couples support groups
maybe the best way to stay married

A friend invited Dan and me to join a couples support group.
We feared a spousal speak-out, complete with bullhorns.
Four years later, I can't imagine life without these eight people.

BY MARIAN SANDMAIER

As marriages go, I feel pretty solid about ours. Dan and I have been together since our college days, 30 years. We still hold hands at the movies and crack up at each other's lame jokes. Most afternoons, when I hear Dan's key turn in the lock, I happily abandon my computer to join him for a walk. We talk about his students, my writing, the tangle of joy, pride, and terror that accompanies parenting our 16-year-old daughter. It's our time to reconnect. But that's only part of the picture. As surely as Dan and I give each other pleasure, we also inflict pain. Even after all these years, each of us is still equipped with fully functional hot buttons that can render us suddenly, sputteringly furious.

Like the time we were driving home from the theater. I made a casual observation about the playwright's point of view. Dan disagreed with my interpretation. I had been down this road before; I felt that my husband was so interested in asserting the incontestable superiority of his viewpoint that he hadn't even listened to me. And I told him so. Replying that he had indeed heard me correctly, he restated his position. Suddenly we were deep in battle over how we

communicated. I was fighting not only for my acumen as a theater critic, but also for some validation that what I have to say matters to my husband. "Would it kill you to just listen?" I lashed out. The more shrilly I ranted, the more professorial Dan became, analyzing our respective positions for logic and evidence. "For God's sake, shut up!" I shrieked, flipping into ice-queen mode. I felt like hell, and I wanted to make sure he did too.

We made up, and our walks continued. But after that particular fight, I felt more than usually shaken. How could this messiness still happen between us? Did we need professional intervention? Was couples counseling the sole option for two people who still genuinely loved each other but just kept tripping on the loose threads of our intertwined vulnerabilities?

My friend Brenda called a few months later. A red-headed, straight-talking psychologist in her early 50s, she had recently married her second husband, an engineer named Jim who played killer jazz saxophone and loved everything about her. She was determined, she said, to keep this marriage strong and vital. The first time around, she had tried to "do" marriage all by herself. This time, she planned on getting a little help. Would Dan and I like to join a couples support group?

Did we dare drop our mask and risk being branded the Ones With Problems? Would voicing our issues out loud cause us to doubt ourselves?

I felt instantly wary. Marital group therapy? Free-for-all gripe sessions, served up in somebody's living room with Brie and crackers? No, Brenda assured me, describing mutual support meetings for ordinary couples trying to keep their marriages in working order.

When I told Dan about Brenda's call, we contemplated whether a couples group was really a good idea. Dan and I cherished our public image as a can-do couple; did we dare drop our mask and risk being branded the Ones With Problems? My fear of exposure ran even deeper than that. Would voicing our issues out loud cause us to doubt ourselves?

An inner refrain—"Don't pass this up"—countered my fears. It dawned on me that this group might let us drop our pose of perpetual spousal cheer (an exhausting, lonely posture at times) and sink into the relief of being real. We decided to take the plunge.

Oozing apprehensiveness, we arrived at Brenda's house for the kickoff meeting. We wondered how this crew—a fund-raiser, an engineer, a photographer, a financial planner, a few teachers and writers—could help Dan and me, who had been knee-deep in each other's flotsam and jetsam for better than half our lifetimes, avoid our marital trip wires.

Four years later, I can't imagine our lives without these eight people. I remember the turning point, a meeting that centered on a seemingly innocuous topic—gift giving. This felt like such a softball that I plunged right in, abandoning my usual care when treading in our sensitive areas.

"I don't care about expensive presents, but I really love flowers," I began, turning to Dan. "Sometimes I wish you would give me flowers on special holidays." Beside me, Dan stiffened. "I do give you flowers," he pointed out. "Just not on holidays created to convince people to buy stuff." He went on to detail his distaste for our overcommercialized culture. I felt deflated. What I had hoped would be a fruitful exchange was transforming into something close to a lecture, and my familiar sense of hopelessness about being heard began to overwhelm me. Just when I thought I might burst into tears or flee the room, Dale spoke up.

"Marian," she said softly, "it took me a long time to figure out that I did a great job of telling Jeff what he was doing wrong, but he had no idea what I needed instead. Now I try to let him know what I want, and

DO-IT-YOURSELF
marriage maintenance

Help for relationship issues used to come only in the form of two-on-one sessions—a couple with a therapist. Now, couples are turning to other couples for support and encouragement.

A leaderless group isn't for everyone, cautions Sunny Shulkin, a couples therapist in Bala Cynwyd, Pennsylvania. "To create a safe structure, everyone in the group needs to be in relatively healthy relationships," she says. "Each person must be able to speak up, listen to his or her partner, and respond objectively to others without the coaching of a therapist."

If you and your partner are game, you can get a couples group going with a little advance thought and planning. Here are some seeds for a successful start.

TRY IT OUT. Consider taking a weekend workshop with your spouse to test the leaderless group format. You may even meet some couples interested in forming a group. To locate a workshop in your area, contact the Coalition for Marriage, Family and Couples Education (www.smartmarriages.com) or the Association for Couples in Marriage Enrichment (www.marriageenrichment.com or 800-634-8325).

PICK YOUR PEOPLE. Don't sign up your closest friends. Find four to six couples you're comfortable with who are committed to keeping their marriages on track. Seek couples who are basically happy together, so you don't end up performing marital CPR.

SET THE RULES. Make clear that the first meeting will be devoted to determining what everybody wants from the group—as well as what they absolutely don't want. Make sure everybody gets heard.

GET ORGANIZED. Agreeing to be "open and honest" is not enough. You'll need to set a basic format for your meetings. For ideas, check out A.C.M.E.'s workbook, *Exercises in Intimacy*.

DO IT RIGHT. Remember that a couples group is not the place for confrontation, armchair psychologizing, or advice. It *is* the place for listening as nonjudgmentally as you can, sharing your own experiences, and encouraging other couples.

why it's so important to me." Dale leaned back in her chair.

I took a deep breath and looked at my husband. "Dan," I began shakily. "When I don't feel heard, I get scared. I know it comes out angry and screeching, but inside I feel like I'm disappearing. I need to know that you care about what I have to say." I was crying openly. Surrounding us, I sensed the whole group wordlessly rooting us on as Dan took my hand. "I can do that," he told me softly.

It would be more than enough if our couples group just nudged us through such painfully stuck places, relying on neither advice nor analysis but rather on the simple, openhearted sharing of much hard-won experience.

But there is still more. During one slow meeting, Jeff boldly said, "I'd like to talk about feeling sexually attracted to other people." Oh, wonderful, I thought. Sharing our messy struggles to communicate is enough. Can we skip sex, please?

Yet after the wary silence passed, one brave woman actually spoke up. "Whenever I feel drawn to a man, it helps me to think about him as a brother. Then the sexual feelings stay down." As others joined the conversation, you could almost hear a taboo crack open. These feelings were normal—universal, even. They didn't mean our marriages were headed for the trash heap; they only meant that we needed to prepare ourselves for these inevitable stirrings. I left that meeting feeling calmer, more confident. And much safer.

It matters little whether our meetings focus on child raising, money, sex, in-laws, or the most disastrous vacation we've survived together; what matters is that this group keeps us actively attending to, and appreciating, our partnership. Pre-couples group, Dan and I raced between work, parenting, and household chores, hoping that our marriage would somehow maintain itself, like a self-cleaning oven. Now, on one precious evening a month, we call a halt to everything else and bring our full attention to the most demanding and sustaining connection of our lives. Dan and I no longer have to figure out this thing called love—mysterious, harrowing, spirit stretching—all by ourselves. Whatever made us imagine we could?✻

how to catch a liar

If you cannot tell a lie—from the truth, that is—learn from researchers at England's University of Portsmouth. They taped police interrogation of a murder suspect (who was later proven guilty) and then showed it to 65 other officers. Some were better than others at catching lies. Here's how you can apply what the researchers learned to your own interrogation technique.

Shift your attention. Ignore the person's face; watch the body or listen to the voice to sense when someone's lying. One cue to look for: Liars often move less when they lie, in an attempt to keep themselves under control.

Don't depend on eye contact. People who believed liars avoid direct eye contact were the worst lie detectors. "There's no relation between deception and gaze behavior," says study director Aldert Vrij, Ph.D.

Don't be fooled by stuttering. The notion that stuttering signals a lie is another myth. Liars don't usually stutter unless they're telling a particularly complex fib. "Most lies people tell don't require much of a mental load," Vrij says.

Let them do the talking. "A problem for liars is that they don't know what you know," Vrij says. Keep mum; the liar may keep talking until he gives himself away.

Forget that old saying. A liar's pants rarely burst into flame.

teen survey puts family first

Family—however you define it—is what really matters. A national survey of more than 1,000 high school students underscores that fact: Nearly all the teens said they have a family member in whom they can confide, and almost half named a close relative—not a pop icon or sports star—as a role model. "What our kids want from us—particularly in a year marked by national tragedy—is the reassurance that we are always there for them and will do everything within our power to keep them safe," says Kate Kelly, a parenting expert and author of *Living Safe in an Unsafe World: The Complete Guide to Family Preparedness* (NAL, 2000).

BETTER SEX =
BETTER HEALTH = BETTER SEX

MANY WOMEN KNOW an active life improves both health and self-esteem. But a busy bedroom can be a bonus too. In *Sexual Fitness: 7 Essential Elements to Optimizing Your Sensuality, Satisfaction, and Well-being* (Putnam, 2001), co-authors Hank C. K. Wuh, M.D., and Meimei Fox unite the concepts of physical health and sexual health, creating a road map to understanding and taking control of your passion and pleasure.

They explore the principle that good health equals better sex, which begets better health. They target seven key areas: diet, supplements, medications, sensual stimulation, exercise, sleep, and stress reduction. Wuh, also a surgeon and an inventor, answers our questions about women's sexual wellness.

Q: What is the greatest misconception women have about their sexuality?
A: The great myth is the belief that women have little control over their sexuality and sexual health. That is simply not true. As with physical fitness and cardiovascular fitness, we can be empowered to take charge of our sexual health and fitness by paying attention to simple yet important lifestyle factors.

Q: How closely related are physical fitness and sexual fitness?
A: There is a profound link between overall health and sexual health. Sexual dysfunction can be one of the earliest detectors of cardiovascular disease or other ailments. Similarly, a healthy lifestyle and being physically fit will have a positive impact on one's sexual health and sexual fitness.

Q: Do you think people understand the connection?
A: Actually, a lot of people do not, and many feel helpless when it comes to becoming more sexually fit. The whole concept behind this book is to help people make that connection.

Q: What are the health benefits of being sexually active?
A: A study from the United Kingdom reports that couples who engage in regular sexual activities tend to look much younger than their counterparts. People who are sexually active tend to enjoy sex more as they age. Of course, sex can be a rewarding and important part of bonding in a committed relationship.

Q: Is lack of desire a common problem among American women?
A: Lack of libido or sex drive is probably the most common sex-related complaint among women: An article from the *Journal of the American Medical Association* reported over 43 percent of women ages 18 to 59 in the United States have some form of sexual dysfunction.

Q: Many married women blame infrequent sex on careers, kids, busy schedules. What would you say to the women in these relationships?
A: I'd say to examine their lives first. It is simply impossible to isolate sexual health from the rest of our lives. If we are not happy with what's going on in our lives, it is likely that we are not happy with our sex lives either. The most important action is to find the strength within to take charge of your life, to change it, shape it, define it, alter it as necessary to feel like you are in control of your destiny.

···

high-tech wooing

Men looking to enhance their romance with candy and flowers may want to think high tech instead. Scientists at Britain's University of Hertfordshire measured women's reactions to certain gifts and found women showed the most arousal when given electronic gadgets. Such gifts keep on giving too: 6 out of 10 women said their love lives suffered when they didn't have their mobile phones or handheld computers with them.

365

walking:
good for your health and
your marriage

This could be the best way to renew your commitment to fitness—and to your relationship. The couple that strides together, stays together. So walk with your spouse.

BY DOROTHY FOLTZ-GRAY

Speed, sweat, and torture have always been my idea of exercise. Decidedly not walking. But then my family and I moved for a year to Oslo, Norway, where almost everyone walks every-where, and suddenly our bodies became our locomotives. Instead of roaring out of a garage, we swung our hips back and forth to shops, to catch the subway, to head to the library or the doctor's office. Within six weeks, my husband and I had each lost 10 pounds, and my back felt better than it had in a decade. Suddenly walking-as-exercise had my full attention.

Of course, walking has had the attention of the medical community for years. Studies show that women who walk briskly (about $3^1/_2$ miles per hour) for half an hour most days have a lower risk of stroke, heart disease, cancer, and diabetes than do couch loungers. They're also slimmer and less depressed, and they have stronger bones and less pain from arthritis. Certainly the over-50 women I met in Norway look nothing like most over-50 American women; their stomachs are flat, their skin is pink, their hair is shiny, and their energy—well, I could barely keep up.

All these gifts were compelling: weight loss, energy, the pain-free back. But they could have been lost to me had walking not bestowed another gift I hadn't expected: a resumed courtship with my husband.

In a car-free life, our two teenage sons found independence, leaving my husband and me alone for the first time in 15 years. Several times a week, we'd pick a part of the city and crisscross its streets, stopping for kaffe or to buy treats for that evening's supper. As we walked, we also talked, finding whom we'd become over the breach of frantic parenting. We discussed the city, what we'd hold onto, what we'd be happy to leave behind. We snarled about our language classes, how bad we were at turning our tongues around Norwegian. Walking, we had our worst fight in 25 years—it was about money—and then paced through our differences as steadily and evenly as if we were counting kroner into our palms. This never happened when we used to jog together. You can't run and have a serious conversation. The more we walked, the more we found answers in the footsteps. We were unwinding to each other the way the city unwound itself to us: path by path. At the end of the day, we often found we'd covered five or six miles, more than we could have mustered were we out only for exercise.

Little wonder, then, that as Dan and I resettled in Tennessee last year, we mourned the loss of our Oslo walks, the effortless way we had sneaked mileage into every day's routine.

But on lengthening summer evenings we soon found a substitute—hitting a two-mile trail when we got home from work and on the weekends. Unlike our Oslo walks, these were purely American: no purpose but fitness. We had to drive a car to the park, stride through two marked miles, then drive away. We were back to compartmentalizing our exercise as so many Americans do, and I feared that despite our renewed commitment, we'd soon find walking American-style a bore, and our motivation would fade.

Had it been up to just one of us, our evenings might have devolved into an excuse to collapse on the couch. Instead, our mutual desire for walking sessions—just the two of us, together—has spurred us on. The demarcation between the car and the trail announces a hiatus from whatever plagues us. Unlike at home, where conversations resemble a series of telegrams about dental appointments, guitar lessons, car tune-ups, or SAT test dates, on these strolls Dan and I have each other's full attention.

We start atop a hill, one of the highest and most beautiful spots in Knoxville, overlooking the Tennessee River to the hazy rise of the Smoky Mountains. We level off by the river's edge, where herons perch on fallen tree limbs. We pass huge chestnuts, oaks, and magnolias. And we relax. Dan, often laconic, even silent, turns expansive. It's here I find out about the latest chapter in his novel, the sticking point between two characters. Or here I can kvetch about my latest reportorial encounter. We sort out our son's college tuition and ruminate about the workings of teenage minds. Somehow on

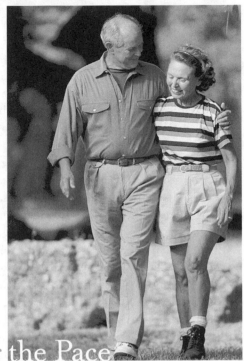

Keeping the Pace

Yes, your spouse can help provide motivation, but if you're much fitter than he is—or vice versa—he could hold you back or, worse, suffer an injury trying to keep up with you. With one of these exercise boosters, you can walk at your partner's pace and still get just as good a workout as you would on your own.

GADGETS

Powerbelt ($50; 800-797-2358): This belt has handles on the sides that are attached to coiled resistance cords. To boost intensity, grab the handles and use an exaggerated arm swing. The device can ratchet up your calorie burn by as much as 52 percent; for an average-sized woman, that's an additional 78 calories in just a half hour of walking.

IRONWEAR Vest ($80; 800-843-4444): This black Lycra-and-Velcro affair from Reebok almost looks stylish, but its real appeal is a stash of metal bars that you can slip into pockets on the front and back. Carrying extra weight will increase your heart rate and burn more calories, and you won't have to walk any faster. What's more, it'll strengthen your bones.

TRICKS

Double-time: Pick a route that takes you in a big loop from your house and plan to do two laps: One solo at your pace, and the next one with your spouse at his.

Intervals: At predetermined times—for example, every 10 minutes or perhaps when walking up hills—race-walk ahead of your partner. After three minutes, head back to your spouse and resume striding at his pace.

these walks, we have what's ordinarily lost to us: time.

What has surprised me is that no matter how tired I feel at the end of the day, I almost always feel like walking with Dan. Because we get to see each other and unwind at the same time. We get to step on that path of heron quiet and feel virtuous—and yet the evening's pleasure has already started. Once we're home the pace is less frantic. After our walk, we're in the suspended reprieve that exercise creates. We're mellow, we're fluid. Maybe we stop to pick up a loaf of bread. Maybe we decide we'll just have salad for dinner. Maybe we go home and read the paper before we fuss in the kitchen. Whatever we settle on, we share the day's rhythms, our rhythms.

Meanwhile, we're also getting fit. Last spring, Dan and I upped our measure from two miles to three, from three to four. We start out and know we'll be walking a full hour. We walk fast and feel ourselves getting faster. On weekends, we're not afraid to tackle an eight-mile hike. On weekdays, we're not afraid to step on the bathroom scale.

On these walks, we pass other people, their heads lowered. We hear snatches of their conversations and the notes of their talk match ours; a riff on the unfairness of something, the insane antics of so-and-so, the exclamation of "I told him!" and "She said what?" Couple after couple step into this space and clear the air by sweeping through. If their footsteps came to a halt, if they turned to face each other, the conversation would change, maybe halt. The legs make progress, have a goal, a timing, and like the black lines on a drawing, help us pace our psychic borders, back and forth, loud and low. It's easier to stay even and on point; the legs take the tension, the arm swing tosses out the stress. It's also easier to be romantic, to hold hands, to jostle, to reveal the sacred and yet keep walking.

This summer Dan and I will move to a house in the city where we can walk to buy our groceries or a cup of coffee. We've dubbed the neighborhood Oslo II—not for its summer sun or blustery Decembers, but because there we'll re-create a walking life. ✳

WHEN SIZE REALLY DOES MATTER

According to Trojan, 6 percent of men say condoms don't fit. So the company has come up with a new, 30 percent larger prophylactic, the Magnum XL.

Wait. A regular-sized condom can hold up to four gallons of air. That's not room enough? While supportive of anything encouraging condom use, an expert at Family Health International muses that comfort with Magnums may be more about mind than matter.

Why It's Best to Brush
before you kiss

Ah, kissing. Such a pleasant, passionate pastime that can sometimes lead to . . . tooth decay? That's right. A surprising new study published in the *Journal of the American Dental Association* tells us that the cavity-causing bacteria found in saliva may be able to travel mouth to mouth during these blissful moments. No need to abstain, though: Simply practice good oral hygiene, and persuade your partner to do the same, says Anthony Vocaturo, D.D.S., a New York City cosmetic dentist.

would you give up chocolate for sex?

Most of the 300 folks polled recently by Capresso Coffeemakers certainly would. When asked to choose among a list of monthlong sacrifices—coffee, sex, excuses, home Internet access, or chocolate—chocolate was the first to go, and sex was the last. Where did coffee rank? Just short of sex, luckily for Capresso.

your medication could be
ruining your sex life

One woman's cure cools another woman's passion. Drugs that wilt erection have been studied for decades, but the sex-busting side effects of prescription and nonprescription medications in women have only recently emerged from the shadows. It's about time: According to a 1999 survey, female sexual dysfunction—low libido, slow arousal, difficulty reaching orgasm, and painful intercourse—occurs in 43 percent of women. In the better-late-than-never category, several medications designed to combat the problem are in the pipeline, including "female Viagra," a testosterone patch, and a prostaglandin gel, all of which may counter the effects of other medications. Here's a look at drugs that can backfire in the bedroom—and what you can do to minimize their effects.

THE CULPRITS	WHY	THE ANSWER
Oral and injectable contraceptives • decrease libido • decrease vaginal lubrication • diminish orgasmic intensity	Monophasic pills (Lo/Ovral, Ortho-Cyclen, Desogen), which deliver steady doses of progestin, can short-circuit testosterone production. Depo-Provera, which delivers a higher dose of progestin, is especially likely to cause problems.	Ask about triphasic pills (Ortho-Novum 7/7/7, Ortho Tri-Cyclen, Triphasil), in which progestin levels follow a more natural cycle. Among injectables, the monthly shot, Lunelle, is less likely to whittle your libido.
Hormone-suppressing drugs such as Lupron, Zoladex, and Synarel • decrease libido • decrease vaginal lubrication	These medications (used to treat endometriosis, fibroids, and heavy menstrual bleeding) shut down the ovaries, suppressing production of estrogen and testosterone.	Researchers are investigating whether adding a low dose of testosterone via pill, cream, or gel may stimulate desire in women on these drugs. Ask your doctor if it's worth a try.
Antidepressants such as Paxil, Zoloft, and Prozac (aka Sarafem), used for depression or severe premenstrual symptoms • diminish arousal • delay or diminish orgasm	Drugs in the selective serotonin reuptake inhibitor (SSRI) family block the effects of dopamine, a brain chemical associated with pleasure, and testosterone.	For depression, a lower dose may help, or try Wellbutrin or Serzone. For severe PMS, it's worth switching between the SSRIs to see which has the least impact on your sex life.
Sedatives such as Halcion; antianxiety medications like Xanax and Ativan • prevent orgasm • decrease vaginal lubrication	These medications relax your muscles and damp down the central nervous system, both of which make it harder to climax.	The antianxiety drug BuSpar may cause fewer problems. A nightly calcium supplement can aid sleep without sexual side effects.
Blood pressure drugs: calcium channel blockers such as Procardia XL; beta-blockers such as Inderal (also used for migraines) • decrease desire • decrease vaginal lubrication • delay orgasm	These drugs lower dopamine levels in the brain and restrict blood flow to the genitals.	Cozaar may have fewer sexual side effects than other blood pressure drugs. For migraines, try Imitrex or Cafergot, which stop migraines after they start instead of preventing them. To counter the effect on blood flow, some doctors prescribe Viagra, although there's little data on its use in women.
Cold/allergy medications • decrease vaginal lubrication • delay or prevent orgasm	The chemicals that dry out a drippy nose can cause vaginal dryness too. And cold remedies may relax muscles, making orgasm difficult.	Use cold medications sparingly. Flonase fights allergies without drying you out.
Corticosteroids such as cortisone and prednisone • decrease libido	These drugs, taken for severe asthma, rheumatoid arthritis, and colitis, suppress production of sex hormones.	Low-dose testosterone may help boost desire in women whose levels are lowered.

Want better sex?
get happy!

Here's more proof that great sex starts with a healthy attitude. A survey of 3,627 women found that those who were satisfied with their bodies, regardless of their looks or shape, made love more often, reached orgasm more frequently, and were more confident about pleasing their mates.

HAVING SEX IMPROVES CHANCES OF IN VITRO SUCCESS

Until now, doctors haven't been sure how to advise patients who were undergoing in vitro fertilization (ivf) and wanted to have sex. Some experts feared that if the technique—in which ripe eggs are harvested from a woman's ovary, fertilized with sperm, and placed into her womb—resulted in pregnancy, the contractions experienced during orgasm might cause her uterus to expel the embryo. Others worried that intercourse might push bacteria to the cervix, sparking infection that could harm the embryo. But new research shows that jumping in the sack may actually improve the prospects for healthy pregnancy.

In the study, half of the couples were told to abstain from sex around the time of IVF, while the other half were encouraged to engage in intercourse, according to study author Kelton Tremellen, an obstetrician and gynecologist at Adelaide University in Australia.

After more than 1,300 embryo transfers were performed (on average, doctors implant three embryos per monthly cycle to increase the odds that at least one will develop), researchers found that women who'd had sex were about 50 percent more likely to carry a healthy embryo through the first trimester.

But before you get busy, consider this: Sex also increased a woman's chances of carrying multiple embryos. Ready for triplets?

Love:
it really is all in the brain

POP STARS AND BAD POETS AGREE: Love is one potent drug. Now, some British neurologists find themselves in accord with the balladeers after their recent study yielded evidence that the brain indeed reacts to romance as if the smitten are high.

The researchers had 17 self-professed lovesick people view pictures of their honeys as MRIS tracked their brains' activity. For comparison, subjects also viewed photos of close friends who were the same sex as their partners.

Turns out that gazing at photos of the smiling sweethearts jump-started unexpected areas of the brain. Among the stimulated regions was a trio of spots that also get turned on during drug-induced states of euphoria and a region that comes to life when you feel a rush of butterflies in your stomach. Meanwhile, the lights went off in areas active during depression and fear. And that's good news for the lovestruck. After all, even if your brain is out there playing its own tune, at least it's not singing the blues.

How good is your sex life?

According to a recent Yankelovich survey sponsored by the Adam & Eve Web site, 69 percent of adults say their sex lives are good or great. Of 922 adults questioned, 12 percent describe their love lives as poor or terrible, while 13 percent say they are fair.

THE RIGHT WAY TO TALK
TO YOUR LOVED ONES

IT'S A FACT OF LIFE: Even happy families have conflicts sometimes. Unfortunately, the way we talk to one another often aggravates those disputes rather than solving them, says linguist and best-selling author Deborah Tannen in *I Only Say This Because I Love You* (Random House, 2001). *Health* spoke to Tannen about how to ensure these conversations yield the solutions we seek.

health: Why did you write this book?
Tannen: This was my first love: the language of everyday conversation, and how it works—or fails to work—to create, reinforce, complicate, and improve family relationships. Everything family members say to each other echoes with meanings left over from the past. That can lead to misunderstandings, hurt, anger, and needless arguments.

health: How does the trouble start?
Tannen: Family members tend to get angry when they're offered unsolicited advice, not only because they don't want it, but because it makes them feel judged. Too many families operate under the tenet "I care, therefore I criticize." To the receiver, what comes through clearest is the criticism. But the one offering suggestions is usually focused on caring. The cumulative effect of minor, innocent suggestions can create major problems.

health: So how can you solve it?
Tannen: Try putting yourself in the other person's shoes. Just knowing that your actions and words will

have a resounding impact on him or her means you're not completely free to do as you please. And fight fair: Avoid sarcasm, sidetracks, and insults.

health: But it's hard to avoid frustration. How do you keep your cool?
Tannen: A crucial step is learning to separate messages from metamessages. We react not only to the meaning of the words but also to what we think those words say about the relationship based on, say, the tone of voice or the phrasing and on past associations. Don't waste time and emotional capital arguing about the message if it's the metamessage that's got your goat.

Too many families operate under the tenet
"I care, therefore I criticize."
To the receiver, what comes through clearest is the criticism. But the one offering suggestions is usually focused on caring.

health: What else can families do to break this gridlock?
Tannen: Try talking in a different way to alter the meaning of an interaction: Be wary of offering advice and try offering understanding instead. Or just change the way you interpret what is said: Regard your sibling's advice as the suggestions of a peer rather than dismissing it with resentment.

divorce

how to avoid repeating your parents' mistakes and
save your marriage

Divorce sometimes runs in families, says researcher Judith Wallerstein. But if you take the right steps, she adds, you can minimize the shock waves.

BY GINNY GRAVES

The Matriarch of Matrimony has been at it again. For 20 years, research psychologist Judith Wallerstein has been dissing divorce, citing evidence from her ongoing analysis of 131 children of split families in Marin County, California. With her third book on the subject, *The Unexpected Legacy of Divorce: A 25-Year Landmark Study* (Hyperion, 2000), her message hasn't really changed much—stay married or mess up your kids for life—except for the "unexpected" finding that the effects of divorce actually hit hardest once children reach adulthood and try to form their own romantic relationships.

I wish I could ignore this depressing news. I want to be with my husband, Gordon, until we're helping each other out of bed in the morning. But children of divorce are more likely to get divorced themselves, Wallerstein has found. My parents separated when I was in my 20s; Gordon was raised in a divorced family in the very community Wallerstein studies. Which means, statistically speaking, we're doubly screwed.

I wonder if Gordon's parents' divorce affects his role in our marriage. I wonder if my parents' breakup makes me a more devoted wife or one who is more likely to cut my losses when things get tough. I wonder if those of us from shattered families can build more durable marriages, and when we can't, if we can have less devastating divorces. When Wallerstein invites me to her home, I get the chance to ask her.

People whose parents split when they were young have no role models for what a successful relationship looks like.

Q: What can people like my husband and me do to beat the daunting odds of divorce?

A: You need to understand that people whose parents split when they were young have no role models for what a successful relationship looks like. Children from intact families—even unhappy ones—or those whose parents divorced when the kids were grown have seen their parents fight and make up, so they have a sense of the ups and downs of marriage. They don't expect to fail in relationships. But like many children of divorce, your husband probably does.

Q: Is there anything I can do to convince him that our marriage isn't going to blow up in our faces?
A: You should reassure him often that you love him and that you're happy in the marriage. It's especially important to do so during a fight because even in the best of circumstances, children of divorce are always waiting for the other shoe to drop.

Q: Makes sense. Any other advice?
A: One couple I know established a relationship with a therapist so that they could check in with her during difficult patches. At times like that, it can be extremely comforting to have someone who is psychologically knowledgeable to talk to.

When you get divorced, what you say to your kids may shape their views on marriage for the rest of their lives.

Q: When a couple is considering divorce, how should they weigh their own needs against those of their kids?
A: People who are in the midst of a divorce tend to think about what they are getting away from and not what they're getting into. But after a divorce, parenting will be more difficult. The kids will need extra attention and guidance—especially in matters of love—well into adulthood. So parents have to be prepared for those responsibilities as well as for rebuilding their own lives.

Q: Would you say that I'm better off than Gordon, since my parents waited to divorce until we children left home?
A: That all depends on whether your parents' predivorce relationship was miserable or pretty decent. Divorce causes suffering no matter how old you are. Your sense of the world as a reliable place was probably shaken just like your husband's was. But in your 20s, your life is more settled, so the impact is lessened.

Q: If you do decide to split up when your children are very young, how can you make it less traumatic for them?
A: With babies, parents who share custody need to communicate with each other. It's important to be able to say, "The baby didn't sleep last night."

Q: What if they're in preschool?
A: These are the kids who are hardest hit by divorce because it disrupts both their physical and emotional care. If you divorce when your child is preschool age, it's important to maintain continuity—to stay in the family home and, if the mother hasn't worked in the past, to postpone getting a full-time job.

Q: That doesn't seem very realistic for a lot of people. Isn't there anything else a parent can do to make it easier on kids?
A: Just do your best to make up for the fact that you're not around as much. Call often from work and spend as much time as you can with the kids. You might explain the situation by saying something like, "I have to work so I can have money to take better care of us."

The most important thing parents can do for their kids is convey that what they went through is not what marriage is all about.

Q: My husband's parents broke up when he was 12, which seems like such a brutal age. Do you have special advice for divorcing parents of teenagers?
A: You need to be respectful of teenagers' schedules when setting up custody arrangements; be flexible, but also maintain supervision. In our study, children from intact families had curfews, but children of divorce often did not. And talk to your kids about their romantic relationships, especially if there's one you think isn't positive.

Q: Don't divorced parents do that?
A: Often they don't speak up because they don't feel qualified to say anything. But divorced dads, in particular, can be helpful if they say, "I made some

serious mistakes, and I don't want you to make them too. Think long and hard about whether this is the kind of person you want to raise kids with."

Q: What's the best way to break the news to your kids?
A: They are going to remember this conversation for a very long time, and what you say may shape their views on marriage for the rest of their lives. You could say, "When Daddy and I got married, we thought we'd live together forever, and we were very happy when you were born." This is important because you don't want children to feel they were born in anger. Then say, "But now we're making each other unhappy. We've tried very hard to stay together, but we think it would be better if we separated. It's a sad time." Let them know this isn't a decision you've made lightly. Give them permission to cry and ask questions. Make sure they understand what's happening, because kids have fears and fantasies; they may worry that this means they're going to a foster home.

Q: How can you make the transition to two homes go more smoothly?
A: If your kids are school age, set up a clear schedule so they know when they'll be where. And as they get older, be flexible in relation to their changing social lives. Too often, children of divorce are treated like suitcases that are passed back and forth. So, for example, if a child is on a baseball team, ask, "What can we do during the season to make the schedule work for you?"

Q: Do you have any parting words for parents going through this tough time?
A: The most important thing parents can do for their kids is convey that what they went through is not what marriage is all about. This needs to be an ongoing conversation throughout childhood. Once they are adolescents, tell them, "Your father and I separated when you were little, so you've never seen us settle a fight, but people do." No matter what mistakes you've made, never give up your parental responsibility to help your children succeed. Instead of being embarrassed, use your experiences as an opportunity to say, "Learn from me!" ✳

Six Degrees of (Sexual) Separation

You may have more in common with the guy in front of you in the checkout line than your preference for paper over plastic. A recent survey of nearly 3,000 Swedes found that just about any two people can eventually be connected to each other via their sexual partners, even if they've had very few. Driving home the need to practice safe sex, the researchers say the results would probably be similar in other countries.

YOU CAN KEEP LUST ALIVE

Has your love life gone south? Don't despair. In 90 percent of cases, sexual dysfunction can be treated, according to Harvard Medical School professor Alan Altman and psychotherapist Laurie Ashner. In *Making Love the Way We Used to...or Better* (Contemporary Books, 2001), they discuss the full range of libido busters, from insomnia to menopause, plus how to talk about the problem without making it worse.

Low Testosterone Tip-off

If your husband seems more interested in snoozing on the sofa than in frolicking in the sack, he may be running a bit low on testosterone. You can visit www.tquiz.com to find out. Developed by doctors at the St. Louis University School of Medicine, the site's 10-question exam—covering everything from height to physical ability—will help you figure out whether your partner needs to see a doctor or if there's another reason for his low libido.

MAKING IT LAST

From deal-breakers to relationship dictionaries, Iyanla Vanzant offers advice to live by.

CULTIVATING A HEALTHY relationship requires as much knowledge and dedication as cultivating a healthy life. Iyanla Vanzant thinks it's positively possible, and she cuts through the psycho-babble and doles out frank advice to tell you how. Three of her books—*In the Meantime* (Simon & Shuster Trade, 1999), *One Day My Soul Just Opened Up* (Simon & Shuster Trade, 1997), and *Yesterday I Cried* (Simon & Shuster Trade, 2001)—are national best-sellers, and her TV talk show premiered in 2001. The author, lawyer, and formerly single parent shares her thoughts on romances that stand a chance.

Q: With women postponing marriage, dating and creating healthy relationships can be difficult as we get older. What advice do you have?
A: As opposed to looking for an equal to share the best of who we are, the best of what we know, we usually go into a relationship looking for somebody to give us something we don't have. And that's the first problem. You have to go into a relationship knowing that you are whole and complete as you are. You are the cake. The mate is the icing. You can eat cake without the icing.

Q: Do you have any guidelines for women when it comes to physical intimacy?
A: I have a 90-day rule. When you're going into a relationship with another person, you should delay physical intimacy—we're talking sex here—for 90 days. And use that 90-day period to get to know who he is. Talk about things. Share your thoughts and feelings. One thing a woman should know before she sleeps with a man is how that man feels about, talks about, treats his mother. Because that's a clear indication of how he's going to treat you. Because 99 percent of the time that's what you represent in his life. So if he's unhappy about things with her, eventually those feelings are going to be projected onto you.

Q: How do you avoid repeating mistakes from past relationships?
A: You've got to know what the mistake was. If you don't know what the mistake was, you'll repeat it until you get clear. Repetition is the mother skill. Here's one clue: Make sure you and the partner are using the same dictionary, meaning make sure you and your partner are defining the words you're using in the same way. Companionship for you may mean a walk in the park and painting the kitchen. Companionship for him may mean drinking beer and watching the basketball game. Sometimes we're reading the dictionary, and he's reading *Playboy*.

When you go into a relationship you've got to know what the deal-breakers are. Some things are deal-breakers, and very often we don't identify those. What I mean are the things that are inappropriate and unacceptable for who you are and what you know about yourself. If pizza on Thursday is a deal-breaker and he eats pizza every Thursday, then don't bother with him.

Q: How do you find a good man?
A: Be a good woman.

---

how to avoid a lonely old age

Who says the childless are destined to be lonely in their old age? A University of South Florida study of 854 retirees compared the happiness of those who had children to that of people who didn't. In terms of self-esteem, psychological well-being, and life satisfaction, the two groups came out even, leading researchers to conclude that strong social networks and engagement in activities are the key to fulfillment in the golden years.

HOW TO GET A
good divorce
OUT OF A
bad marriage

How do you know when it's time to leave?
And once you know, where do you find the courage—and the path
that will leave your emotions and your children's souls intact?

BY BARBARA HEY

In the five months since my marriage began its final descent, I have become a person strange even to myself. I am moving forward toward marital dissolution with none of the reticence with which I usually approach change—no second-guessing, no asking friends and family for validation. Instead I consult the I Ching each day, something the other me would never do. The message I receive from throwing the coins is repetitive and reassuring: "Perseverance furthers." It is a rarefied, elliptical version of what I tell my children again and again: Everything will be okay, just keep going, hang in there. Perseverance furthers.

I have no choice but to believe it. In a few weeks my family will sell our home and then divide into separate quarters. We know where we will go, and we know when, but the how is yet to be resolved—the tempers too short, the fatigue too great.

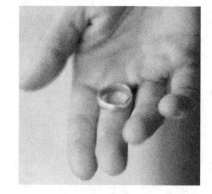

My daughter seeks refuge in her bedroom. My son cries at the least disappointment; when Burger King runs out of Rugrats toys, he is inconsolable. And I am the cause of this familial misery—because, after years of unhappiness, I have decided to vacate this airless box of a marriage for parts unknown. I am a puffy, sleep-deprived, restless, and profoundly guilty version of the person I used to be. I exercise, I shop, I work, but throughout the day I am struck down by crying fits.

I am both executioner and executed. I have done this to myself, yet I too am suffering greatly.

I am trying to be a good mother, but I am failing. I am trying to be a reasonable ex-partner, but I am failing. I am surrounded by others, but I am alone.

I am buoyed only by the Martha Stewart paint swatches—nearly 50 of them—that I carry with me, postcards

**Divorce is about learning what matters.
I love my children; the rest I can let go. I am ready to
cash it all in for the chance that I can rediscover
myself, create a life that nourishes me.**

from the other side, reminders of bright palettes that may await me once the court orders come down and the misery abates.

I believe what the coins tell me, because I must. I can't stay in my marriage. I worry: Will divorce ruin my children's lives? Will I be alone at the end of my days? Yet I'm leaving.

I know I am supposed to say something here about the sadness of parting from the man with whom I've shared my life and had two children, who has been my confidant and source of financial support, who after years of vicious, soul-destroying discord thinks he still loves me. I will say this about my husband: He is the father of my children, and they love him dearly. Me, I just want out.

I got married 13 years ago on a date that neither my husband nor I can remember exactly. That, to me, has always been a telling lapse of memory. We knew each other just four months before getting engaged, and decided to spend our lives together after the termination of an unwanted pregnancy. We were acting out of guilt and remorse, I now realize, rather than a feeling that we were destined for one another.

Even before the rings were exchanged, I had a sense I was approaching matrimony with screwed-up intentions. I had left a job I loved, ended a long-term relationship. Worse, I was, at 30, an orphan. My father had died two years before, and my mother had just succumbed after a long illness. I was looking for connection, a safe haven. But I didn't want to marry someone I would need too much; I didn't want to risk heartbreak.

I knew that every marriage requires an adjustment in expectations, a shift from the ideal to the real. In mine, that shift occurred when we had been married merely a single day. On our honeymoon, I gave my husband an overpriced bathrobe, the style of which was suited to a man wearing slippers and smoking a pipe in front of the fireplace. My husband bunched it up and stuffed it in the trunk of the car, next to the spare tire. I expressed my dismay; infuriated, he tried to rip off a Just Married totem that friends had hung on the rearview mirror. He got it off, yes, along with the mirror.

This would become the pattern in our marriage: A clash of expectations, fury on both sides, unrestrained impulse, lasting damage. We looked at each other side by side in the car, useless mirror on the seat between us. We both knew then that, for better or worse, there was no looking back.

We moved ahead, but with the same hesitancy with which we had gotten married, never successfully articulating what we needed from one another. We had children, adopted pets, established traditions, and consulted numerous therapists to try to fix what wasn't working. On the surface, we seemed like a viable match. We shared friends, a professional world, an impulsive approach to life. But there were profound differences of temperament. He has always been the kid; I've been the responsible one. His humor involved flatulence, mine neurosis.

As with so many couples, the overriding issue was intimacy. One night early on, I asked my husband an offhand question about an old girlfriend. "The past isn't your business," he said. "That's just gossip." As if I'd entertain my girlfriends with his confidences, I thought. But nothing I said through the years ever convinced him otherwise. There was to be no sharing of past experiences, of feelings, because the risk of betrayal was too great. I felt isolated, alone, uncared for. He felt cornered.

When we had children, I became a stay-at-home mother; he became the overworked dad, the guy who swooped in for bursts of hysterical fun, then picked up the remote control. I was cemented into responsibility and reviled for it—the party pooper, the keeper of bedtimes and administrator of medicine, the worrier.

Over the years, I circled away from my husband and back, through school meetings and dentist

> What I hope more than anything is that my kids will come through it without a diminished capacity for love, and without blaming me.

Pundits think the fact that so many marriages self-destruct means divorce is too easy. Divorce is never easy. It is horrible.

appointments, visits to grocery stores and therapists' offices, all the while wondering: Should I stay or should I go?

The debate ended one afternoon after I picked up a message from the elementary school: Your son fell off the swing and hurt his arm. My husband had been called, but he was some distance away. The school official suggested he remain at work; she would call me. Our child lay for hours on the couch in pain until I could be reached.

I was furious at my husband. My son had broken his elbow and needed surgery. "Imagine," my husband said as we sat in the waiting room, "Henry will never be the same." I fled to the pay phones to find solace. Despite years of intimacy, I realized, this was a man I escaped from in time of need. And at this stage of my life, I wanted someone to run to, not from. I resolved to get out before I was the one waking up in the recovery room dazed and needy—with him by my side, saying all the wrong things.

Conservative pundits think the fact that so many marriages self-destruct means divorce is too easy. Divorce is never easy. Splitting up means that every area of one's life is thoroughly examined by strangers. It is invasive and it is horrible.

easing the breakup: tools for a gentler divorce

Divorce is never easy, but fortunately new types of support—from kinder, gentler lawyers to seminars just for kids—can help you tackle this tough transition. Here are a few worth checking out.

A COLLABORATIVE DIVORCE TEAM: A good divorce begins with the right mind-set. That's the idea behind a new option called collaborative divorce, in which each party hires a team of professionals—a lawyer, a financial counselor, and a therapist—who work in a cooperative, affordable way. To learn more, log on to www.collabgroup.com (or call 415-383-5600) or www.collaborativedivorce.com (or call 888-973-8372).

A MEDIATOR: These neutral parties help a couple reach a settlement but can't give legal advice or advocate for either side. To find one in your area, log on to www.mediate.com or contact the Association for Conflict Resolution at 202-667-9700.

DIVORCE SEMINARS: Your local community center can point you toward one in your area. Or try one of these:
• Fisher's Rebuilding Seminar. The mother of all divorce seminars, it has helped more than 300,000 people worldwide deal with divorce. The 10-week program costs about $300. Log on to www.fisherseminars.com.

• Positive Divorce Resolution. In this four-hour-long course, divorcing parents learn how to communicate better with each other and their children. Call 888-747-5362 or log on to www.divorce-resolution.com.

FAMILY THERAPISTS: Consider a therapist trained in divorce issues. For a referral, call the National Board for Certified Counselors at 336-547-0607 or log on to www.nbcc.org or www.aamft.org, the site of the American Association for Marriage & Family Therapy.

PROGRAMS FOR CHILDREN: Check out these organizations or go to www.gocrc.com for articles on children and divorce.
• Kids' Turn. A six-week workshop for children ages 4 to 17. At least one parent is required to attend a separate seminar. Parents pay on a sliding scale, with a $500 maximum; the kids' seminar is free. Log on to www.kidsturn.org or call 415-437-0700.
• Rainbows. A nonprofit with over 8,000 programs for kids and parents who are grieving over a divorce or other loss. Log on to www.rainbows.org or call 800-266-3206.

Usually the first intruder is the therapist, who rakes over conflicts, looking for patterns that can be altered: Maybe the marriage can be saved. If not, other experts step in. The negotiations start: Who will make the decisions about the kids' education, religion, orthodontia? Who will pay and how much? Who gets the couch, the dog, the everyday dishes, the china? Who gets the Sarah McLachlan CD? If you can't agree, you pay someone by the hour to fight like a terrier for your rights. The outcome: more money spent, more energy wasted, more animosity for the person you'd thought you'd love forever.

For several years, since well before I decided to end my marriage, I've been a researcher of divorce. I've wanted to believe that people could come through it with dignity, honor, and psyche intact—that somehow, eventually, everyone could be all right. Now that I'm in the midst of it, I worry especially about my daughter. She absorbs things like a satellite dish. After years of listening to her parents struggle, she's decided she will never get married. I am afraid that if she does marry, she will re-create the conflict-ridden family of her birth. If therapists are to be believed, we return to the familiar dysfunction like homing pigeons, marrying a cleverly disguised version of Mom or Dad.

I know divorce will be the defining event of my kids' childhood. I was reminded of that when Judith Wallerstein's *The Unexpected Legacy of Divorce: A 25-Year Landmark Study* was published (Hyperion, 2000). Wallerstein, a research psychologist in Marin County, north of San Francisco, has been following a group of children of broken families. I kept hearing about her findings, typically and bluntly summed up as: Divorce is devastating for children. No matter what, parents should hang together. I sought her out to ask: Is the prognosis really so dire?

Once the decision has been made to split, and the logistics ironed out, the spouses can begin to get along better than they have in years. After all the issues are stripped away, what's left but rueful affection? We need to bring the kind of civility to our divorce that was absent in our marriage.

Yes, Wallerstein says—and no. The children of divorced parents generally make terrible choices in their intimate relationships when they are in their 20s. Many of the young women become promiscuous or put up walls to keep out true intimacy; the young men tend to be passive in relationships and to gravitate to women who make all the decisions. But through experience or therapy, they do learn, Wallerstein says. By their 30s, most can forge a healthy connection.

A different book, *The Good Divorce* (HarperCollins, 1994), has become my life raft. I call the author, therapist and researcher Constance Ahrons, who is currently following up on the studies that informed her book, checking in with 170 now-grown children of 1980s-era divorces. My kids will be okay, she tells me. Or at least they can be, depending on how my husband and I resolve the marriage.

"Allow your kids to remain kids," she says. That means my husband and I have to negotiate our battlefields privately, not in front of the kids. We should avoid lawyers, who generally have an adversarial approach that exacerbates animosities. We must be deliberate and considerate. In short, we need to bring the kind of civility to our divorce that was absent in our marriage.

For the sake of the children, she advises me to minimize the changes. I should stay in the same house for a while, if possible; our households should be similar enough that neither is preferred for the wrong reasons (the big-screen TV, the junk food). Explain to the kids what's happening and repeat, over and over if I need to, that their lives will be as normal as possible. Most important, tell them they're loved by both parents.

Then I ask the question whose answer I'm afraid to hear. Is there an optimal age for a child to deal with divorce? Her answer shakes me. "In my study, most couples said they waited too long to split," she says.

I imagine the future. Each room is painted a different color, and it's my voice on the messaging machine. I am not happy yet, but I have faith that happiness will come. I can wait.

"They waited it out for the kids, and damaged themselves and the kids with the waiting. If you're in a high-conflict marriage, postponing a divorce is not healthy."

So, what do I say to my children? Wallerstein

is the one with the clearest answer: As they reach mid-adolescence, she says, talk to them honestly about what you did wrong. Tell them: You are not me. You can make a good choice.

I explain that my daughter has asked, "Why did you marry Daddy anyway?" How should I respond? Wallerstein thunders back: "Tell her, 'I knew him four months before I married him. I was an idiot.' "

In the parlance of my Rebuilding Seminar—a

10-week course for people enduring or recovering from the breakup of marriage—I am a dumper rather than a dumpee. In truth, though, I feel I am carrying out the will of both of us.

These rebuilders and I share stories, write letters we will never send, cry over past hurts, dissect our relationship histories, engage in group hugs, and rehash our weeks to avoid burning out our friends. It helps to have people enmeshed in the same misery, who don't care about the shoe sale at Nordstrom. We are in terrain that demands our full attention. Finances, antidepressants, how to bolster self-esteem in a period that fosters self-loathing—this is what we speak of.

The paradox of an end-stage marriage is that once the decision has been made to split, once the negotiations are over and the logistics ironed out, the spouses can begin to get along better than they have in years. After all the issues are stripped away, what's left but rueful affection? It can mess with your mind.

I observe my husband at what he does best: being a father. He patiently puts together Lego projects too complicated for our son to handle alone, takes our daughter ice-skating, watches Cartoon Network, laughing as much as the kids do. One morning as I see

my son spooned next to his sleeping father, it occurs to me that I will never view this scene again; it may happen in a bedroom miles away, but I will not see it. This, I realize, is what it means to be a broken family.

My husband and I tread water for a while, waiting to amass the funds to physically separate. We perch in different areas of the house, come together to watch our favorite movies, the ones too stupid for us to admit that we like to future partners, too reminiscent of a failed relationship to watch by ourselves. We play one another's heartstrings. "For my last birthday dinner with you, let's make that pasta you made on our second date," my husband says. I refuse to indulge him, because to do so would be to let in some emotion that could engulf me. Instead I buy prepared foods from Costco, stuff he will later be able to procure for himself and consume without nostalgia.

I find an affordable house. My husband finds a place with a pool and a clubhouse—a single-dad pad. He won't let me see it. I sell the artifacts from my marriage to support my new life. "What name should I write on the check?" the owner of the used-jewelry store asks. I hand him my driver's license and ask him to make it out to the first two names, drop the last. "You got rid of the guy, huh?" I look again at the glass case and realize it's filled with engagement rings and 10-year diamonds.

I buy thong underwear and cover up the gray, wear a talisman around my neck for confidence, go out with girlfriends to a store filled with sexual devices, but deny that I need to purchase anything. I imagine the future. Each room is painted a different color, and it's my voice on the messaging machine. I am not happy yet, but I have faith that happiness will come. I can wait.

I realize that divorce is about learning what matters. I love my children; the rest I can let go—the financial

---

breaking up is hard to do—get help online. For help navigating the difficult road to divorce, log on to www.softsplit.com. Professionals can offer advice on everything from choosing a lawyer to telling the kids.

security, the king-sized tub, the detritus of a life of accumulation and regret. I am ready to cash it all in and endure the sadness and the terror for the chance that I can rediscover myself, create a life that nourishes me. Divorce, I admit, is about doing something selfish, for self-preservation, but trying to do it unselfishly. What I hope more than anything is that my kids will come through it without a diminished capacity for love—and without blaming me.

Two weeks ago, we filed to legally end what began all those many years ago. Where once there was a couple, there are now two separate households, both with cable TV, bubble-gum-flavored toothpaste, and matching cylinders of Pringles. My home is painted 16 colors; his is white. We have not exchanged keys.

I spend my mornings in a kind of dance class that's packed with women. We spin like Sufi dancers, punch the air and scream "no!" to imaginary opponents, reach our arms to the sky and say "yes" to the good that's out there. At the end of each class, the teacher tells us to place our hands on our hearts to feel them beating. Then we extend our arms to define a space where we can be ourselves, where we can create the life we are meant to have—where we can be happy. "Make a space and walk into your life," the teacher says. And, at last, I do. ❋

Barbara Hey is a writer in Boulder, Colorado.

A Rocky Marriage Brings *Real* Heartache

A troubled marriage could be making your heart ache in more ways than just one. New research shows that an unhappy union may increase your risk of developing cardiac disease.

To figure out whether being part of a dysfunctional couple affects a woman's health, Kristina Orth-Gomer, an internist at the Karolinska Institute in Stockholm, Sweden, interviewed 290 women who were hospitalized for heart attacks or severe chest pains. She asked them about their relationships with their partners and also about the pressures they faced in the workplace.

Five years later, she checked in with these women again. She discovered that while job stress had done no visible damage to the women's health, those in rocky relationships were almost three times as likely to have had another heart attack as women in healthy unions.

The link between a wounded heart and marital stress is still fuzzy, but more research is under way. For now, Orth-Gomer has a suggestion for women. "Take the stress of your relationship seriously," she says. "Try to get help or find a support group with other women, because stressful marriages really do impact your health."

till death do us part

Despite America's sky-high divorce rate (or perhaps because of it) nearly half of men and women ages 20 to 29 think the laws should be changed to make it more difficult to end a marriage.—*from a survey conducted for the National Marriage Project by the Gallup Organization*

commit to a new holiday spirit

Personal or national crises—even anticipating age-old family feuds—can cloud annual celebrations. Here's how to create new holiday rituals and reconnect to what really matters—family, community, and faith.

BY VERONICA CHAMBERS

Kathleen Buckley will still celebrate the holidays, but it will be quite a long time before her heart is in it. The 36-year-old mother of three is still recovering—and will be, for some time—from the September 11, 2001, terrorist attacks. Her husband worked in the World Trade Center at Cantor Fitzgerald, a financial services firm few non-Wall Street types knew about before some 700 of its employees died in the north tower's collapse. Dennis Buckley, 38, was one of them.

Kathleen is now struggling to figure out how to approach the holidays without her husband, who each year played Santa Claus for their daughters, 6-year-old Mary Kate, 4-year-old Megan, and 23-month-old Michele. "I can't take away the small things that give them joy," she says. "I want to try to make their lives as normal as possible."

Even during the best of times, the holiday season can be challenging: endless road trips with kids, pets, and gingerbread men in tow; the rush of last-minute shopping; and courtside seats to the annual sparring match between your mother and her sister, your husband and his father, or your Aunt Rose and the latest relative subjected to her dysfunctional game of family feud.

This year, thousands of families like the Buckleys will long for those petty annoyances, facing the real challenge of making it through the usually jubilant

> This is the time to ask your mom the question you've always wanted to ask. It's a time to mend fences.

season amid painful reminders of the loved ones they've lost. People in mourning have had to soldier through the season before. But this year is different.

You could certainly make the case that there is little for anyone to celebrate, with the unprecedented loss of life—and livelihood, with so many job layoffs—the displacement of thousands of military men and women, and the general uncertainty of these times.

It is possible, though, to mark the holidays in ways that reflect—and respect—the current state of affairs. Pasting on your game face and then faking your way through the typical rituals isn't one of them. Instead, experts say, this season is a chance to emphasize traditions—or establish new ones—that enhance connections with family, friends, and community. "These challenging times provide us with an opportunity to do something differently with the people we love," says psychologist Alan Lipman, Ph.D., executive director of the Center at Georgetown University for the Study of Violence.

For Kathleen Buckley and her daughters, that may mean joining other grieving families for the holidays. "It helps to see others like yourself," she says. "My older daughter asked me if she could play with some kids whose fathers have gone to heaven because of the attacks. It's too difficult to process this alone."

Even those who haven't been directly affected by the attacks can find comfort in rituals that promote community. "All cultures mark the miracle of birth and the mysteries of death through rituals," says Karen Sitterle, Ph.D., a clinical psychologist on the faculty at the University of Texas Southwestern Medical Center. "They make meaning out of where our lives have been and where they are going."

Sitterle says that "survivor guilt" can keep people from moving on because they don't think they should. "We know that so many people are affected personally, even though we're not," says Sitterle, who counseled victims' families after the 1995 Oklahoma City bombing. "We're aware that many don't have the option to move on—and feel guilty because we do."

One way to cope with survivor guilt and grief in general is to channel your emotions into action. Donna Schuurman, executive director of the Dougy Center for Grieving Children, says this is especially meaningful for kids. "The tragedy is an opportunity to educate children about what really matters," Schuurman explains. "It's about how we are loved, spending time with families, and giving back." Make "giving back" a family affair. "Take your kids to a soup kitchen, help them buy a coat for a homeless person, investigate local charities that help needy children," Schuurman suggests. "It means more to children when the giving is hands-on."

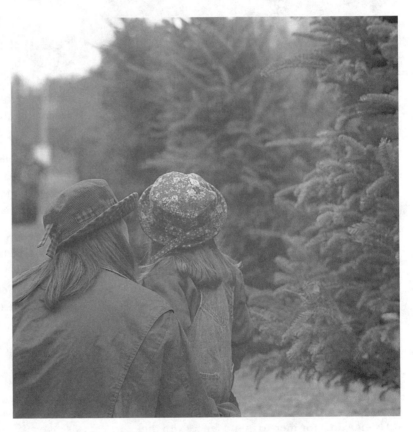

Just don't expect the heightened sense of compassion to trickle down to all family interactions, Lipman says. "If you remove the current circumstances, family conflicts and age-old differences already set the table for a certain amount of emotional tumult," he notes. "The current events will bring these feelings to the fore." Since family gatherings will be even more emotionally charged, adjust your own expectations and

One way to cope with survivor guilt and grief in general is to
channel your emotions into action.

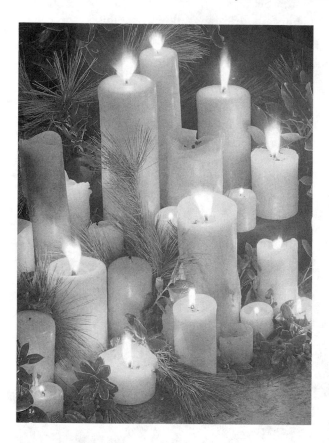

acts of healing

Coping with loss during the holiday season
does not mean abstaining from celebrations.
Here are some suggestions from Alan Wolfelt,
Ph.D., director of the Center for Loss and Life
Transition and author of the book *Healing Your
Grieving Heart: 100 Practical Ideas* (Companion
Press, 2001), for creating new family rituals that
emphasize the spirit of togetherness.

REACH OUT. Write a holiday card, send a gift, or—better
yet—stop by and visit with family or friends who have lost
a loved one. Don't forget close friends of the person who
died or anyone else outside of the primary circle of
mourners who might be trying to deal with grief alone.

SPREAD SPIRIT. What did the person love to do,
especially during the holidays? If she adored a certain
kind of cookie, bake dozens to share and include a note
explaining what this person meant to you. Or if he loved
to sing, organize a caroling party.

REMEMBER. Make the person a part of the holidays by
putting together a scrapbook of photos, stories, or other
memories. Put the album in a special place amid the
decorations. Make it part of your holiday ritual to page
through it every year.

GIVE A GIFT. Try to come up with an idea that would
have meant something special to the person who died,
and make it a family ritual. For example, donate a book
to the local library or put together a care package for
someone in need.

WALK AT NIGHT. There's something healing about
strolling in the dark on a winter's night, hand in hand with
members of your family. Breathe in, breathe out, and take
stock: In the New Year, how will you bring meaning to
your life? It's up to you.

patience level. "When conflicts arise, step in and say,
'In these times, we need to value each other,' " Lipman
says. "Only the truest cynics will continue to stir the
pot, and you have to know that cynicism is their way
of trying to hold it together."

Lipman also advises steering the conversation away
from touchy subjects and focusing on personal discovery and family ties. "This is a time to ask your mom the
question you've always wanted to ask her," he says.
"This is a time for men to mend fences with their
fathers. This is the time to ask Grandpa about his war
experiences. At family gatherings, you can crystallize
the preciousness of your time together. Emphasize the
question, 'Why not do it now?' " ✳

*Veronica Chambers is a writer-in-residence at Princeton
University. Her work has also been published in* O, Vogue,
and Newsweek. *Additional reporting by Farnaz Fassihi.*

MARILYN YALOM ON WOMEN AND "WIFEDOM"

Q+A

NOW THAT the storybook trip down the aisle is no longer a prerequisite for either sex or babies, some are asking whether women really want—or need—to be wives anymore. Marilyn Yalom, senior scholar at the Institute for Women and Gender at Stanford University and author of *A History of the Wife* (HarperCollins, 2001), isn't so sure. We talked with her about the 21st-century wife.

health: So what, really, is the purpose of marriage for women today?
Yalom: It certainly isn't to produce offspring. And we often don't need—or receive—the monetary support husbands traditionally supplied in return, either.

health: So why get married?
Yalom: For companionship. For mutual support, shared values, lifelong goals. As a partner in a marriage, you are witness to another person's life. That's the term I prefer for one's spouse—not "wife" or "husband," but "witness."

health: "Wife" does seem like a loaded term.
Yalom: It is—much more so than "husband." The role of the wife has changed much more over time than the role of the husband. As wives have moved into the workplace, their roles have expanded to include providing financial support as well as domestic services to their families. Yet most of us associate "wife" almost exclusively with domesticity. The term hasn't evolved along with the role.

health: Do you think it ever will?
Yalom: I don't. I think that the term will become anachronistic, while gender-neutral terms like "partner" and "spouse" will be used more and more in common speech. In fact, I wouldn't be surprised if 50 years from now you look in a dictionary under "wife" and see "archaic."

health: Is the role, like the term, an endangered species?
Yalom: I don't think so. People today co-habitate without marrying, they marry later—but they still get married. We haven't given up on marriage at all. When pollsters ask, they find we still want to marry and that 90 percent of us do marry in our lifetimes.

health: And the husband—is his role changing to accommodate the less-domestic wife?
Yalom: It is, but the changes are slow to develop. Women have always been very eager to take on male roles because they give us clout, whereas men resist taking on the work of women because it's traditionally low-status stuff. Little by little, however, that's changing.

VITAL STATS

54
Percentage of people who read in the bathroom

34
Percentage who talk on the phone

30
Percentage who talk to themselves

19
Percentage who make love

10,000
Number of smells an average person can detect

7
Number of primary odors that generate all those smells

10
Percentage of people who could be helped by hearing aids who actually wear them

25
Percentage of older people who wear unsuitable eyeglasses because they don't get regular eye checkups

88
Percentage of women who wear shoes that are smaller than their feet

35
Percentage of women who close the door before checking their weight

21
Percentage of men who do

Unless otherwise noted, statistics apply to the United States.

INDEX

Orthorexia nervosa, 71, 263
Osteoarthritis, 286–287
Osteoporosis, 176. *See also* Calcium.
   adding bone mass, 269
   drugs, 30
   effects of protein on, 251
   preventing, 48–51, 136, 251, 269
   slowing bone loss, 251
Overeating, 291–293, 315. *See also*
   Obesity.
Ovulation, 19

P

Pads, heating, 38
Pads (sanitary products), 27
Pain
   back, 206–211, 212–214
   during childbirth, 219, 220–221
   ear, 197
   effects of hypnosis on, 219
   foot, 205
   head, 186, 205, 224, 285–286, 298
   heel, 205
   in yoga, 130
   jaw, 197, 198, 199, 200
   joint, 201–203, 212–214
   labor, 219, 220–221
   menstrual, 38, 223
   muscle, 223
   relievers, 10, 222–224
   shin, 108
   wrist, 201–203
Pajamas, 184
"Palming," 159
Pancakes, 257 (recipe)
Panty liners, 27
Pap smears, 39, 62, 226
Pasta, 235 (recipe), 249 (recipe),
   266 (recipe)
Patches, contraceptive, 24
PCBs, 245
Peace, achieving personal, 328–329
Peanut allergies, 298–299
Pears, 254 (recipe)
Pelvic inflammatory disease, 17
Perfectionism, 347
Periods, menstrual
   asthma during, 39
   cramps, 38, 223

effects of liposuction on, 25
heavy, 24
menorrhagia, 24
mood changes before, 20–23
pads, 27
panty liners, 27
PMS, 20–23, 38
predicting, 27
premenstrual dysphoric disorder,
   20–23
premenstrual syndrome, 20–23, 38
sanitary products, 23, 27
tampons, 23
toxic shock syndrome, 23
Personality traits, 302–308, 309
Pesticides, 194, 276–277
Pesto, 267 (recipe)
Peters-Clark, Hazel, 337
Petting zoos, 64
Phthalates, 193–194
Physicians
   alternative practitioners, 191–192
   breast surgeons, 44
   cardiologists, 67
   dermatologic surgeons, 160, 161,
     162, 163–165
   frustration with, 228
Pilates, 106, 107
Pill (contraceptive), 26
Pineal gland, 40–41
Pizza, 293
Plantar fasciitis, 205
Plantar warts, 63
Plastic surgery, 25, 160–165
Plié stretches, 168–169, 172
PMS, 20–23, 38
Poise, yoga pose to improve, 131
Poison ivy, oak, and sumac, 196
Pollution, indoor, 193–195, 203
Polychlorinated hyphenyls, 245
Polyphenols, 166
Pork, 296 (recipe)
Portion control, 93, 99
Poses, yoga, 130–132, 172–173
Postpartum depression, 37
Posture, 170, 213
Potassium, 251
Potatoes, 237
   sweet, 296 (recipe)

Practitioners, alternative, 191–192
Pravachol, 29, 239
Pravastatin, 239
Prayer, 320, 322
Pregnancy
   eating fish during, 245
   ending, 27
   exercise during, 38
   increasing likelihood of, 16–18, 19
   morning sickness, 18, 286
   preventing, 24, 26
   preventing birth defects, 258, 286
Premenstrual dysphoric disorder,
   20–23
Premenstrual syndrome, 20–23, 38
Progestin, 52, 53, 369
Programs, weight loss, 13–14, 66–71,
   252, 253
Prostaglandins, 223
Protein
   C-reactive, 31
   effects on bone loss, 251
   in weight loss programs, 66
   soy, 242, 262
Protopic, 175
Prozac, 20, 22–23
Psychiatrists, 302–303, 304–305
Psychologists, 324–325, 326
Psychotherapists, 324–325, 326, 343
Psychotherapy
   cognitive-behavioral therapy, 35, 36
   online, 342–344
Psyllium, 240–241
Push-ups, 112

Q

Q10, 149
Qi, 190
Quadricep exercises, 124–125
Quercetin, 243

R

Race, 52, 352
Radiation, 44
Rafkin, Louise, 360–361
Ragout, 235 (recipe)
Rancho La Puerta, 316, 317
Ray, Cindy, 55–56
Rayon, viscose, 23

EDITORIAL CONTRIBUTORS

Elizabeth Berg

Jennifer Cadoff

Julia Califano

Holly Carter

Julie Cederborg

Veronica Chambers

Ingfei Chen

Melissa Chessher

Rick Chillot

Frank Clancy

Victoria Clayton

Treacy Colbert

Krista Conger

Lindsey Crittenden

Lynne Cusack

Lisa Davis

Catherine Dold

Laurie Drake

Paula Dranov

Daryn Eller

Mandy Erickson

Karin Evans

Laura Fraser

Susan Freinkel

Gabrielle Glaser

Megan O. Gorman

Bill Gottlieb

Fiona Gow

Ginny Graves

Jan Greene

Samantha Greene

Catherine Guthrie

Melanie Haiken

Dianne Hales

Martica K. Heaner

Barbara Hey

Jenna Hofstedt

Kelly James-Enger

Katrina Kenison

Jonathan F. King

Caroline Knapp

Katy Koontz

Len Kravitz

Elizabeth B. Krieger

Danielle Lazarin

Sally Lehrman

Karen Levin

Deb Levine

Lisa Maloof

Domenica Marchetti

Lisa Margonelli

Eliza McCarthy

Jenna McCarthy

Laura Flynn McCarthy

Maggie McKee

Tracy Minkin

Paula Motte

Peggy Nauts

Jennifer Nelson

Felicity John O'Dell

Megan Quitkin

Louise Rafkin

Victoria Abbott Ricardi

Kimberly Robinson

Leah Rosch

Anna Roufos

Susan Salinger

Marian Sandmaier

Daniela Schimmel

Sarah Schmidt

Nina Schulyer

Beth Wolfensberger Singer

Evelyn Spence

Jamie Talan

Amy Weaver

Rick Weiss

Kerri Westenberg

Nina Willdorf

Kimberly Wong

Cassandra Wrightson

Catherine Zandonella